NEW DIMENSIONS I HEALTH
From soil to psyche

J. A. Hatton
1986

Other books by David A. Phillips
From Soil to Psyche, USA, 1975
The Soil to Psyche Recipe Book, USA, 1975
Guide Book to Nutritional Factors in Edible Foods, Sydney, 1977
Guidebook to Nutritional Factors in Foods, USA, 1979
Secrets of the Inner Self, Sydney, 1980

NEW DIMENSIONS IN HEALTH
From soil to psyche

DAVID A. PHILLIPS

ANGUS & ROBERTSON PUBLISHERS

Please note: Information and suggestions in this book pertaining to diet, health, and treatment are presented only as material of general interest and not as a prescription for any specific person or any condition in a specific case. The reader is advised and encouraged to seek the aid of a qualified health practitioner for advice pertaining to his particular conditions and needs.

ANGUS & ROBERTSON PUBLISHERS
London . Sydney . Melbourne

This book is copyright. Apart from any fair dealing for the purposes of private study, research, criticism or review, as permitted under the Copyright Act, no part may be reproduced by any process without written permission. Inquiries should be addressed to the publisher.

First published in the United States and Canada by Woodbridge Press Publishing Company in 1977
First published in Australia by Angus & Robertson Publishers in 1983

© David A. Phillips 1977, 1983

National Library of Australia
Cataloguing-in-publication data.

Phillips, David A., 1934-
 New dimensions in health.

 Originally published as: From soil to psyche:
 a total plan of natural living for the new age.
 Santa Barbara, Calif.: Woodbridge Press, 1977.
 ISBN 0 207 14485 0 (paperbound)
 ISBN 0 207 14462 1 (hardbound)

 1. Health. 2. Diet. 3. Food, Natural.
 I. Title.

613.2'6

Typeset in Paladium 11/12 point by Graphicraft Typesetters
Printed in Singapore

This book is dedicated to my beloved parents, Raie and Sam, whose wisdom and dedication to their three sons is an example of perfect parentage; to my brothers, Keith and Allan, whose loving support is always on hand and to my son, Lindsay, whose constant thoughtfulness for others is a unique example of teenage understanding.

Contents

Introduction ix
To the Reader x

Stage 1 — Know Your Habits 1
　Man — The Only Suiciding Animal 1; "Threescore and Ten" 2; "How Are You?" 3; Is Sickness Inevitable? 5; Our Teachers — The Animals 6; The Era of Double Standards 7; Dare We Question Convention? 8; Old Habits Die Hard 9; The Fear of Truth 10; Habits That Hurt 10.

Stage 2 — Know Your Purpose 12
　Freedom and Awareness 12; Seek Always the Cause 14; Cause-and-Effect 15; Dangers of Fragmentation 16; The Purpose of Life 18.

Stage 3 — The Ingredients of Health 20
　A Case for De-education 20; The Secret of Long Life 21; The Essence of Life 22; The Primary Substance: Clean Air 23; Man's Lubricant: Clean Water 26; Rest and Relaxation 28; Sunshine and Shelter 31; Mental Balance and Harmony 33; Correct Food 34; Fasting 35; Exercise and Activity 36.

Stage 4 — Let's Be In Tune 40
　The Essence of Life 40; Where Is the Psyche? 41; Using the Psyche 44; Fear of the Psychic 45.

Stage 5 — The Pythagorean Ideal 47
　Silence and Meditation 50; Memory and Awareness 52; Temperance 54; Fortitude 55; Philanthropy as Compassion 56; Erudition, Creative Learning 58; Music 58; Dietetics and Fasting 60; Exercise and Activity 61; Method, Order and Efficiency 62.

Stage 6 — Man's Vegetarian Heritage 64
　Vegetarianism Defined 64; Man's Genealogical Background 65; Man's Primitive Background 65; Historical Background 66; Religious Background 67; Prominent Contemporary Vegetarians 69; Carnivore Equipment 71; World's Most Expensive Food 73; Unbelievable Savings 74; Promotional Frauds and Misunderstandings 75; The Menace of Milk 78; "Vegetarians Are Too Sensitive" 80; "Vegetarians Rob Life" 81.

Stage 7 — Not by Bread Alone 82
　Dietary Indigestion 82; Food for Confinement 83; Not by Bread Alone 84; A Garden for Every Kitchen 85; The Simple Science of Sprouting 86.

Stage 8 — Our Nutritional Needs 90
   Proteins 90; Carbohydrates 96; Fats and Oils 99; Minerals 104; Vitamins 109.

Stage 9 — Secrets of Food Combining 136
   From Table to Stomach 136; The Mouth 137; Story of the Stomach 137; Duties of the Duodenum 138; Small and Large Intestines 139; Food Classifications 141; How to Use the Food Combining Rules and Tables 144; Primary Food Combining Rules 145; Secondary Combining Rules 148; Acid and Alkaline Foods 150; Temptations of Intemperance 152.

Stage 10 — Man's Ideal Diet 155
   The Dietary Revolution 155; Abandoning Pernicious Habits 156; The Seven Basic Rules 162; A Balanced Diet 163; Breakfast 163; Lunch 165; Dinner 165; Cooking Methods 166; An Ideal General Menu 168.

Stage 11 — Uses of Health Foods and Herb Teas 171
   Genuine Health Foods 171; A Basic Guide 172; Herb Teas 202.

Stage 12 — Fasting: Abstinence Makes the Heart Grow Stronger 214
   The Physiology of Fasting 215; "Partial Fasts" 217; Preparing for the Fast 217; Fasting Facilitates Fertility 218; How to Fast 219; When to Fast 220; Fasting and Obesity 221; Breaking the Fast 222; The Spiritual Fast 223.

Stage 13 — Therapeutic Diets for Common Illnesses 225
   The Body's Disharmony 225; Some Common Symptoms 226; Psycho-sclerosis 265.

Stage 14 — The Organic Revolution 267
   Nutritional Advantages 267; Undernourished Plants 269; The Meaning of "Organic" 270; Chemicals Against Nature 271; Returning to Nature 274; Crop Selection 275; Abandoning Monoculture 276; Ground Preparation 277; Organic Fertilisers 278; Compost Formation 280; Layer Mulching 282; Fallowing 284; Crop Rotation and Compatibility 285; Harvesting 286; The Biodynamic System 286.

Into the New Age of Awareness 288

Bibliography 291
Index 293

Introduction

There is no such thing as a new idea. At best we can only bring forward a new dimension to an ageless concept — a variation on an original theme, updated to suit modern needs.

Natural health care is older than recorded history. Among its earliest attested practitioners is the famous Greek philosopher and scientist, Pythagoras, predating Hippocrates as he did by over a century. Modern research and practice has improved and refined those early concepts, but their essence remains intact — a vital legacy of our Western culture.

Modern demands on time and energy are constantly highlighting our needs for a better understanding of ourselves and of our environment. We need guidebooks to better illumine our path and focus our consciousness to the great awareness that we have within us everything we need.

In 1975, I completed the manuscript of my definitive guidebook for good health, improved happiness and the longest possible lifetime. I called it *From Soil to Psyche*, and it was enthusiastically received around the world after being released in 1977 by its Californian publishers, Woodbridge Press.

But in a further seven years of practice, research and lecturing, I have learned how much more this book could have included. And so I have updated and expanded the original *From Soil to Psyche* to embrace the newest dimensions in health. These include two entirely new chapters, plus expanded guidelines to achieving a better level of attunement, improved inner peace, revitalised energy.

David A. Phillips

To the Reader...

*Among the many views held by men
Neither reject nor accept you them.
If one speaks falsely be you calm,
For he does himself a secret harm.*

From The Golden Verses of Pythagoras (*c.* 608–520 B.C.)

We pass through this life but once. We are here because we have an important purpose to fulfil, a fulfilment which these pages will help achieve. You may be assured that it is not by chance that we meet over these words, through these pages. We are each aware that life has so much more meaning — and find that meaning we shall. What other reason has brought us together at this very point in time?

Your life has already met with some success — more, perhaps, than you realise. But as we develop an awareness of our purpose, and as we proceed to fulfil it, success becomes far more than an occasional consequence. Success, the true foundation of happiness, is the light on the path, the light which shines as we graduate from each of life's lessons.

Our life on this planet is programmed to develop in stages. These unfold as we live through its many cycles, each equipping us for the following aspect of our development.

The greatest single factor influencing our understanding of life and, in fact, our overall development, is our state of health. Not merely physical health, but our total health is the basis of our every ability and expression. This is man's most neglected asset, its abuse creating his greatest liability.

Human health has its foundation, not in the study of the physical sciences per se, but in a total study of metaphysical, as well as physical, man. All disease can be traced to disharmony; likewise, good health can only prevail in man's attunement to nature, to harmony. Man's total awakening to this principle is the cause to which this book is dedicated.

We live and thus, clearly, have chosen this life. It is therefore our responsibility to live it properly. Foremost on our list of priorities is the acquiring and maintaining of good health. This is achieved not by chance, but by our awareness of the total pattern of health as composed of its numerous physical and metaphysical facets — from soil to psyche.

David A. Phillips
North Sydney
Australia

STAGE ONE

Know Your Habits

Man causes his own sickness and suffering. In almost all cases he is more or less to blame for being sick and he as truly owes society an apology for being sick as he does for being drunk.

From a letter by Sylvester Graham,
July 13, 1840

Habit is the pattern by which most of creation lives. It provides the formula for reaction, but rarely for action. Habit is an automatic following along a known course, with rarely a thorough investigation into whether such a course is wise. Unfortunately, it often is not.

Human life, if it is to fulfil its purpose, must be characterised by action, not reaction. In that manner, it contrasts with the lives of all other creatures.

When man lives objectively, an intense satisfaction attends his efforts. When he lives by habit, he is so often a victim of uncertainties and fears. Yet man, in common with all creatures, has the vital ability of adaptation at his disposal and this he constantly employs without always understanding if it is directed towards his good. In all sincerity, could we accept that adapting to regular gastric indigestion, liquor drinking, tobacco smoking, irritability or adapting to intermittent headaches and foul body odours is either natural or desirable?

Man — The Only Suiciding Animal

Man employs the most curious use of the power of adaptability of any living creature. He can adapt to an environment or to habits which are unquestionably dangerous to him. Yet, in such circumstances, his adaptation is never complete — his body can never fully adjust to dangerous, unnatural living habits.

Could this be what Pythagoras intended to convey when he said, "Man, by his habits, sets into motion those agencies which eventually destroy him"? This warning of 2,500 years ago is no less cogent today, but how many take heed?

Most humans, by habit, live in unnatural environments which are often actually dangerous. History attests that man rarely questions his environment, electing rather to adapt than to query. "If it is good enough for my parents and their parents, it is good enough for me", is the usual attitude. But the industrial revolution has ensured that the environment is changing rapidly from that to which one's ancestors adapted. Many a young person has become aware of this and is altering the historical pattern, questioning his environment and finding it wanting.

Living in crowded cities with their polluted air and water, with their tensions and pressures, with the devitalised and stale food they offer to their inhabitants, with their disturbing noises and ugly concrete structures — this is the habit shared by an increasing percentage of mankind. Little wonder that man learns to adapt to sickness!

Man then compounds the felony by habitually administering poisonous drugs in a futile attempt to relieve his sickness, or at least the pain of it — pain which is telling him that he is slowly precipitating his premature death.

Virtually every animal has a life expectancy of around six times its maturity. Every animal, that is, except man.

Why is it that man does not live to an average 120 years and maintain active, good health for all that period? Here we find one of the greatest of all paradoxes — the most intelligent, most creative, most adaptable of all creatures has an average life expectancy of something less than three times his maturity. He is actually robbed of his most rewarding years.

At the age when man should be able to enjoy the manifold pleasures of life, he is considered too old to work, too old for life insurance and a burden on his young family. He is told to amuse himself because the state will take care of his constant sickness until he eventually ceases to be its liability and obligingly dies, his body unable to accept any more abuse.

Such "suicides" are an entrenched pattern of human life, even in the "advanced" countries where the average life expectancy is little more than the sixties, hardly more than half its intention. The rare occurrence of a man or woman living over one hundred years is invariably heralded by news publicity and an unflattering photograph. If such wrinkled, incapacitated living characterises old age, little wonder that most people prefer to die young!

But old age does not have to be miserable and decrepit. Yet, it is so as a consequence of living habits which run counter to nature, counter to the manner by which good health is maintained.

Young people tend to think of old age with pity and often hope never to reach it. Old people tend to wish they were young again (but still knew as much as they do now!) But do they really know why they are prematurely old? Sixty or seventy should really be no more than middle age. If young people would only realise that their "old age" is already being created by every unnatural living habit they entertain, their decision to objectively assess such habits would become their most urgent need.

Indeed, man can postpone old age for, while he is breathing, his body is regenerating. The pattern by which it regenerates is largely of his own making, for heredity plays a far smaller part in human health than is generally believed.

"Threescore and Ten"

As though to condone premature old age and untimely death, the human tendency, as in the case of all unsuitable habits, is to blame something or someone else. What better than an alleged predetermination from a divinely inspired source?

No matter how primitive or how cultured, man recognises a superior creative power whom he worships as his God or gods. To this source he directs his praises and excuses his habits. Races generally cultivate their religious systems in accordance with their adaptation to life — this, in turn, anchors the lifestyle to accord with the system it has evolved.

It has often been observed that as a cultural system grows in complexity, so does its moral foundation. Religions become far more complex than their founders had envisaged, and become subject to misinterpretations which actually detract from their sublime truth and potential wisdom.

The Bible is recognised as the moral foundation of instruction by most Christians. Yet, in just under two millennia since the birth of Christianity, more than twelve hundred variations of the Founder's teachings have evolved. Can we help but wonder whether most of these interpretations (for that is what they are) have arisen from personal limitations? Could this explain why so many apparent contradictions exist with regard to the Bible?

Psychologists and philosophers have always recognised the human tendency to justify one's habits by modified interpretations of natural laws. Human excuses veil the true understanding of such laws, giving rise to many complexities which detract from the basic simplicity of these same laws.

The unravelling of biblical complexities and interpretations is beyond the province of our present purpose, except where acute confusion has clouded an understanding of the Creator's simple, natural laws. But of immediate concern in aiding us to shed light on unsuitable human habits is a chapter from the Old Testament which contains one of the most commonly misquoted of all biblical instructions.

The Book of Psalms is responsible for uttering the decree which appears to conflict so acutely with natural science. If it is true that man should live at least six times as many years as his maturity, then why are we told in Psalms 90:10 that "the years of our life are threescore and ten"? And having read this, most people are inclined to accept as *fait accompli* a life expectancy of only seventy years, or little more than half that which should be natural to them.

Yet, the same Bible which appears to limit man's earthly expectation goes to great lengths in Genesis, its opening Book, to describe the lineage of the patriarchs — many of whom lived over nine hundred years.

Explanations are apparent when one reads in Psalms the preceding lines of Moses' prayer, and learns that man's years are numbered in relation to his "iniquities" and "secret sins". So if one wishes to take a single portion of a Psalm and use it in counter-scientific argument, one has to be prepared to recognise that when a quotation is out of context, it is also out of meaning. For indeed, man's years are only relegated to "three score and ten" when he sins against nature's laws and lives iniquitously, as practice proves.

Today we find that only those people who have lived a mostly natural life or those with an especially robust constitution can lay claim to a useful lifespan significantly in excess of seventy years. The vast majority of mankind is busy committing slow suicide by its unnatural daily habits.

"How Are You?"

How many people of your acquaintance appear to "enjoy" bad health? You know the type: ask them how they are feeling and be inflicted with an "organ recital" of their bodily ailments. They thrill to the opportunity, seeking your undivided attention and sympathy in return.

The common greeting of "how are you" is one you will grow less inclined to use the more hypochondriacs you meet.

It appears that man has become complacently conditioned to the acceptance of sickness in his life as an unavoidable necessity. Initially for consolation, then revelling in the pleasure of being the subject of sympathies, unnatural-living man not only identifies with a favourite set of symptoms, but also with his favourite doctor, his favourite hospital and his favourite drugs.

To the person living "conventionally" on unnatural dietary substances (which do not deserve to be called "foods") such as hamburgers, soda pop, candy confections, refined flour products, drugs and the like, life is a constant surprise. He is never quite sure if he will be sick or well the next day, or even later that very same day:

This is one type of surprise we can do without. To those of us who enjoy constant, abundant health, the assurance that every morning we awake will be the start of a day free from headache, stomach pain and the thousands of other discomforts which plague most people, is a promise which transcends all other riches. It is a most gratifying reward for sensible living — even though, sadly, one is part of a very small minority of humanity in these habits.

In the mind of the conventional person, anyone who engages in a programme of daily exercise, adopts a diet composed largely of raw, fresh fruits and vegetables, practises an occasional short fast and has a body weight below the average is considered a "health crank". Meanwhile, the intimidator has become known as a "sick crank", for there is nothing more powerful than sickness to make one cranky. Of course, for those who prefer the middle path, the compromise, they can be part-sick-part-healthy, if such were possible!

In matters of health, one is either considered healthy or sick. Anything short of pristine health has to be considered a degree of sickness. Most people maintain such a high level of toxicity in their bloodstreams that regular sickness is awaited as though no possible alternative were available.

It demands no academic qualification in psychology to become aware of the ease with which the human brain can be turned into a reactive mechanism, subject to powerful external forces. Newspaper reporters and radio and television commentators are no less aware of this than are the advertising executives who often employ subtle devices of psychology to exact specific reactions from the human brain.

Man's ability to be conditioned thus, coupled with his natural desire for adventure, makes his reaction to new products, drugs, foods and ideas generally predictable — promote it and it will sell. And most of those products are so unnecessary, so undesirable, as to result in the human body manifesting an increased level of toxicity as a result of the experience. For example, a new "TV snack" will probably be found to contain high concentrations of refined sugar with chemical flavours, colourings and preservatives; a new detergent will most probably be compounded from highly caustic chemicals which pollute waterways and ultimately the oceans.

With life so subjected to pollution, both internally and externally, it is little wonder that the human body generally runs at a level of toxicity close to the crisis point. Superimpose on this condition a sudden change in temperature or humidity, and the body acts according to its natural need to eliminate toxins at a rate beyond the capacity of its normal organs of elimination. The mucous membranes come into action to throw off unwanted toxicity by liquid elimination through the nose, mouth and/or eyes — whichever organs of that particular body can best be used. To enable this to be achieved in the most effective manner, the body temperature rises and the pulse rate quickens. The result: what is commonly referred to as a "cold" or "the flu" or some exotically named epidemic.

Man should understand how to live healthily by natural means, devoid of the superstition of ignorance that germs or viruses control his health and his destiny. Such fear is in conflict with intelligence.

How many people attend their favourite doctor regularly, even if for only a "check-up"? Do they hope to discover something excitingly new about their body, or are they so unsure of their state of health that they think some unexpected disease will suddenly overtake them? It is no surprise that many people lay claim to their "favourite doctor". "You should see MY doctor," they say. "He is such a good man."

Your reply should be: "Then why aren't you totally well?"

Is Sickness Inevitable?

The great mistake made by many people is to assume that sickness is inevitable. Some even believe that their lives will cease at some preappointed time irrespective of their mode of living. Neither belief coincides with truth.

"Accidents" excepted, the inevitability of physical death is related only to the degree of nonintelligence employed in physical life. With all animals averaging a life expectancy of six times their maturity, there is no reason for man to be the sole exception (and not live to 120). He does so only because he chooses to depart from natural living habits.

In so doing, man initiates the "inevitability" of sickness, its purpose being two-fold. First, sickness is intended to teach its sufferer the lesson that certain of his habits require correction; its second purpose is to restore good health by eliminating from the body the toxic consequences of unnatural habits.

Invariably the purposes of sickness are overlooked. People are loath to accept blame, especially when they can identify illness with some impersonal cause. This is all the easier when certain "authorities" encourage and condone such ignorance. To believe that sickness results solely from the visitation of some itinerant germ or virus and to accept treatment by some poisonous drug is to be guilty of the most naive superstition. This form of "exorcism" cannot remedy the problem because it bears no relationship to the real cause.

By palliating the symptoms, drugs tend to induce a state of euphoric ignorance of the vital cause of the sickness. As well, they induce the inevitable iatrogenic consequences of their own toxicity — "drug-induced" diseases, or "side effects", as they are more commonly known.

We should never forget that there is a purpose for everything. Sickness is no exception. The principal purpose of such physical or mental discomfort is to draw attention to a condition of disharmony which demands correction, for it interferes with the normal functioning of the being. Simultaneously, sickness is the body's attempt at self-correction, at a restoration to natural balance.

There is no other manner by which sickness can be permanently overcome than by correct understanding. The sad thing about our educational system is that it fails to teach correct, natural living. Although most schools and parents teach outer cleanliness — the soap-and-water type — very few teach the most essential form of cleanliness, inner hygiene. It seems somewhat pointless to wear clean, attractive clothing, to learn discipline and develop the art of mental investigation, when the gastrointestinal tract is laden with putrefying rubbish. Ignorance in natural living is perpetuated by its omission from the scholastic curriculum.

While most people take care of the style and presentation of their clothes, few give sufficient time to realise the internal filth they hide. Foul breath, smelly underarms, unclear eyes, dry scalp, wrinkled skin and every other tell-tale symptom of ill health might be disguised from a similarly ignorant fellow being by the temporary expedient of artificial formulations. But to the body's own intelligence and to the educated eye of those who know the simple secrets of natural living, those gimmicks are frauds and a waste of their high purchase prices.

To those who live by natural guidelines, the savings in both health and finances are huge and very real. Maybe we should be laughing all the way to the bank; but instead, we are ever trying to guide others to partake of the tremendous benefits accruing from a knowledge of the ingredients of health and their application. It is not that we have a desire to see the perfume producers, chemical companies, tobacco traders or brewery barons put out of business; but rather to deter them from poisoning themselves and humanity at large and to employ their vast resources of wealth and knowledge for the human good — so promoting health rather than disease.

Our Teachers — The Animals

Humans rely too much for their knowledge on other humans. In so doing, man has deviated from the natural, favouring the artificial. Instead of learning from effects and seeking causes, he employs disguise out of fear of changing his habits. Human life has become extraordinarily complicated in a simple, natural world.

The animals appear to know there is nothing complex about health — good health in animals is simply the result of good, natural living habits. Every wild animal knows how to live healthfully — perhaps because it cannot read advertisements or attend school! On the rare occasions of sickness, it recognises that the body must be rested and this often implies fasting until it corrects itself.

Wild animals do not normally consume processed, refined and canned foodstuffs. They do not drink chemicalised water or breathe polluted air. Their pathways are neither concrete nor asphalt and their mental environments are devoid of tension and constant rush.

By contrast, domesticated animals are far less fortunate. Likewise, their life expectancies are lower and their sicknesses far more frequent. Hence the lucrative practice of the veterinarian — a profession of comparatively recent origin without which the natural inhabitants of the jungle appear to have managed reasonably well these past millennia.

An acquaintance of the writer owned two beautiful St Bernard show dogs. For years they were grand champions until suddenly, just before a season of shows, they lost their vitality, their coats became dull and their hair started to fall out. The veterinarian could not identify the "disease" and found that all his medications were useless in the attempt to restore health to the dogs. He advised they might never be able to participate in shows again and might even have to be destroyed.

With nothing to lose and no encouragement from their vet, the owner was persuaded to fast the dogs for three days. This met with no opposition from the dogs since they had no appetite. When the dogs again started to take in nourishment, they were indeed hungry. After three days they had lost a few kilograms each, but their eyes were clearer and they certainly enjoyed the carrot juice which broke their fasts.

For the following three days, the dogs were fed fresh, organically grown vegetables, first grated, then sliced or whole. Then cheese and, alternately, sunflower seed kernels were added to the diet for protein concentrates. Four days later, raw egg yolks were added to their salad dishes.

Exactly three weeks from the day they commenced their fast, both dogs were barking happily, running around the garden with great excitement at being well again. They were still not back to their previous body weight — this took another two weeks.

Wisely, the owner rested the dogs from shows for the entire season. By the following season they were completely recovered, their coats exhibiting a lustre even brighter than previously. That season, they again won all championship ribbons and are still enjoying abundant health. They are still largely vegetarian, although they do receive occasional bones and some fresh meat, but relish their cheese and egg yolks with salad.

Many people may laugh at this as being a figment of the writer's imagination. That is their privilege, but it does not alter the facts, acceptable or not as they may be. It is true that dogs are not natural vegetarians, but neither are they naturally eaters of processed, canned, chemicalised meats. Nor are they natural showpieces, restrained in restricted and often polluted environments.

The human body possesses remarkable powers of tolerance and adaptation. It can be forced into the acceptance of poorly constituted food from its birth, extracting from it sufficient basic nutriment to develop and grow. As years pass, the penalties are exacted. Early acute childhood illnesses, such as measles and mumps, are suppressed to re-form and later compound into more chronic toxic manifestations.

Gradually, the powers of tolerance wear thin with abuse. The body manifests deficiency diseases due to inadequate nutritional balance. These are the diseases which sadly characterise modern man in spite of, or because of, his greater affluence and industrialisation. Yet, few of man's pathological problems are recognised for their true nature and rarely is nutritional intake or mental adjustment considered.

Instead, greater financial grants are directed in the open-ended warfare against germs. Illness continues to be blamed chiefly on these minute organisms of convenience, diverting man's attention from the underlying cause of disease: unnatural living habits.

Considering the intense campaign against germs, it must come as quite a shock to thinking people when they realise that human health continues to deteriorate as the lessons of sickness fail to be learned. Teachers are unqualified in this vital subject about which too much superstition, fear and ignorance still persist.

The Era of Double Standards

Since man first began to learn, experience has proven to be the best teacher. As human life grew more complex, professional teachers grew more numerous because it was found necessary for man to learn more speedily. Thus, the process of learning passed largely from one of total personal involvement to one of systematic instruction. Accompanying the transition was a growing sense of influence and power in this new profession.

In contrast to the sages and philosophers of Greece's era of influence, modern teaching has evolved with different emphasis. The ancients recognised the importance of man's gaining knowledge by experience so that he could understand his purpose in life and attempt to fulfil it. Greek teaching was intensely practical — Pythagoras allowed nothing to be committed to writing, insisting on the permanence of oral instruction, learned by practical application.

Modern teaching has developed on a more theoretical basis, often with more training of the memory faculties than a practical development of the intelligence. It is more concerned with history than mystery! Yet, paradoxically in modern education, there is more intense interest in teaching man how to make a living than how to live.

The Industrial Age inspired teaching to develop around training for remunerative work. It taught man how to conform to the machine, how to make money from his efforts; but it has not been very successful in teaching man how to use his rewards wisely and how to live happily. Rather, the enslavement of man to the machine has been found to be doubly beneficial: by inducing man to spend his rewards on machine-produced articles, more production is demanded. This discovery has persisted to such an extent that it now commands control over educational principles.

Man is encouraged, even taught, to expand his desires so that greater markets evolve for the products of his machines. Labour-saving devices reduce his physical activity and, with computers, also his mental activity; chemicals stimulate his many appetites; processed foods are promoted as superior to fresh, raw foods; copious clothing, with its ever-changing, fickle fashions encourages man to throw out rather than wear out.

The teaching of such new standards has developed a physical awareness at the expense of spiritual awareness. Man has been taught to live with processing and actively encouraged to depart from the natural. He has been taught to specialise and in so doing has cultivated the unhealthy habit of relying on other specialists to support his needs. He has been thoroughly convinced that without the medium of the lawyer, he has no chance of justice; without the medium of the physician, he has no chance of health; without the medium of the teacher, he has no chance of knowledge.

All these services demand money. Man has to develop his own standard specialisation by which to earn enough to pay for the services of others. And as the spiral increases in an ever-widening motion, man becomes more and more dependent, less and less self-sufficient.

Double standards of health versus profit enslave man to the machine and perpetuate his dependence on government. Man is taught that if he smokes tobacco, he will develop disease and may die therefrom; simultaneously governments teach farmers to grow tobacco with greater yields because governments make a very handsome profit from its sale. Man is taught that alcoholism is a killer; yet governments license its sale; for again, it ensures a very lucrative income to the state's coffers.

Man is taught that he must work to pay his expenses, but he is not taught how to reduce those expenses by removing the causes of illness from his life. Generally, man has to work for half a century to acquire sufficient net capital by which to retire and relax — by this time, he is rarely healthy enough to enjoy such freedom.

Dare We Question Convention?

It is now a well-known fact that in the single decade of the 1960s, for the first time in history the world's store of scientific knowledge actually doubled. Statistics also reveal that during the same period, the world's crime rate doubled, its hospital admission rate doubled and its expenses on public health doubled.

Obviously something went seriously wrong. That human learning could make such strides in the discovery of facts, yet could fail to improve man's life in terms of peace, harmony and health must prove that we are seeking after useless knowledge or we are not applying the knowledge we discover.

Knowledge for its own sake is useless. To accumulate multitudinous facts is of no more benefit than the accumulation of money — neither is of any value unless it is spread around in use. Yet it has become accepted as a conventional part of Western civilisation that science must continue on its uninterrupted path of research and for this purpose, huge amounts of money are devoted.

Surely we can now be convinced that to expand human knowledge, yet fail to improve the understanding or quality of human life, must be regarded as a serious breach of trust. Surely some of the millions of man-hours and billions of dollars now applied to open-ended research could be redirected to improving man's knowledge of his actual purpose on earth and in life, and how that purpose can be achieved in harmony. It is now time for man to properly know himself, his environment and how to live in happiness.

Fortunately, many people now question conventional habits and find them wanting. Habits which are known as or suspected of being injurious to health and happiness can be altered by the thinking person — in many instances, they are indeed being abandoned. By so doing, the thinking person may be branded a "nut" or "crank" or "faddist" by those of conventional habits who recognise that these habits are, by inference, being shown as unwise.

Contrary to the beliefs of some nutritionists of the traditional school, there is nothing impossible in the ability of man to live healthily on a diet which contains all essential amino acids, suitable fibres, starches and natural sugars, all vitamins and minerals, plus natural fats. All of these are obtainable from a nuts-fruit-vegetables diet — if one should wish to avoid any other food types. All too often in scientific circles do we find the personal addictions and habits of the scientists determining "expert" opinions, rather than an impartial investigation into truth.

Old Habits Die Hard

Man will do almost anything to avoid introducing radical changes to his pattern of living habits. Often these have been established at a very early age, prior to the development of the brain so that it could engage in creative thought. Thus, the formation of habits preceded any creative effort on the part of their performer, implying that they are hand-downs from parents whose own habits also were formed devoid of thoughtfulness.

Habits, then, are often the products of parents' wants, rather than the child's needs. And even as the child grows into the creative period of its youth, so deeply entrenched are these habits that very little alteration is likely. Those modifications which do transpire as youth matures into its own family responsibilities are generally minor variations on the parental theme, rarely anything more. Thus, the older the person, the more entrenched the habits and the more difficult they become to change.

This is especially evidenced as the person becomes settled into a permanent job and into family life of his own. By this time, his creative faculties generally diminish as his life proceeds with automatic regularity. He aggressively defends his habits as though they represent his total being — perhaps they do in a limited sort of way!

By the time retirement is approached and the conventional illnesses by which it is characterised manifest, man finds it the most difficult to amend his habits, even if he can be convinced of the need. It often demands sickness and intense personal discomfort to do this, a fact which was cogently demonstrated to the writer just a few years ago.

An elderly gentleman had suffered a stroke, occasioned by cerebral haemorrhage. Although previously a very active man, for weeks after his attack almost total immobility afflicted his right side. Gradually he recovered limited use of his right arm and leg, but a dullness persisted which he constantly felt and bemoaned. With a prospect of partial paralysis through the remainder of his life, with no hope of recovery offered by his physician, this uncle could think of only one possibility:

"I'll give $5000 to remove this pain and regain reasonable use of my body," he told me one day. To his surprise I offered to accept his proposition, saying that I would devote my time to him exclusively for one month, longer if needed.

"What do you intend doing to me?" he asked.

"Nothing," I replied. "Nature will do the work, given a reasonable chance. All I propose to do is to supervise you on a fast, or a series of fasts, so that your body's own healing power can go to work unimpeded. Then I'll guide you onto a balanced, natural diet."

"Does this mean I won't be able to eat anything for a time?"

"It surely does," I replied. "It will also mean that you stand a very good chance of recovering most of the use of your body while all you do is exactly nothing — just lie in bed and follow my guidance."

"What about my cups of tea and my pre-dinner cocktails?" he pleaded. "And how will I have enough strength to do anything?"

"There will be nothing to do," I assured him. "And as you don't have very much strength now, you will not be any the worse. But what I suggest in terms of a fast is only a temporary expedient to allow your body to rest totally while its healing power overcomes your enervated condition." I advised him that he would not be able to have anything to eat and could drink only pure water. As for tea and cocktails, they were finished forever, for he would lose the craving for them after he had fasted. Likewise would he lose the craving for salt and pepper, condiments, sweets and white sugar, white bread and jam, kippered herrings for breakfast, etc. Instead, I told him, he would be able to enjoy delicious fresh fruits and vegetable salads, with nuts, etc., when he came off his fast.

"Life just won't be worth living," he said. "No thanks, I'd rather stay as I am and continue enjoying my regular food." And so he refused my offer. This gentleman had worked hard all his life and, in my opinion, deserved a better opportunity to enjoy his retirement. He died from a further stroke in 1979; a happy release for, during those final years, he was often unable to talk or to taste his food.

The Fear of Truth

Human health is like a bank account — unless you contribute to it regularly, you get very little from it. Although the ingredients of good health are simple to understand and practise, most people are conditioned to complexities and refuse to accept simple natural laws which demand a change in their entrenched unnatural habits.

"He insults truth and that seems to be the reason people consume his novels — to escape not from their lives, but from truth." So quoted *Newsweek* magazine of October 27, 1969, in explaining the magic appeal of the writings of novelist Harold Robbins.

His astute observations of human habit permitted Robbins to achieve remarkable success in a short period of literary endeavour. He learned to recognise that the average citizen possessed a deep fear of truth — a fear of the unknown. Therefore, his readers apparently gained a feeling of euphoric comfort from his uncharitable pen which offered no assistance in emancipating them from the bondage of ignorance.

It is bad enough when children are afraid of the dark. But when adults are afraid of the light, this is indeed a sad situation. And it is towards the remedying of such situations that many other writers have devoted their efforts.

A century prior to Robbins, a writer who could lay claim to true literary greatness was thought too harsh in his criticism of the laziness of man. Ralph Waldo Emerson observed: "There is no expedient to which man will not resort to avoid the hard work of thinking."

In very many instances, Emerson's condemnation is all too true. The average man prefers to run a mile or chop a tonne of wood rather than sit and think constructively for five minutes about his life and its direction. Is man so afraid of his inner self, of the inner silence? Or is he merely afraid of recognising the need to amend some of his less suitable habits?

Habits That Hurt

Never before has a generation of young people been so sick. Sickness in each generation is being recorded at an earlier age than in the previous one. I believe that statistics today would undoubtedly reveal that young people show an even higher percentage of chronic illness than in 1964 when it was revealed that in the United States more than 50 per cent of youth called for military service were unfit.

As the pace of life accelerates and the quality of food deteriorates, man is left with the sad realisation that those habits into which he has evolved are doing him no good. It must therefore be time for a total reassessment of his life patterns with the object of removing those aspects which imply danger. To avoid the mental conflict many people create when they feel they are being deprived of something with which they have become familiar, we should recommend that hurtful habits be *replaced*, rather than abandoned.

Instead of giving up the drinking of alcohol, replace it with fresh fruit juices. Rather than giving up smoking, replace it with chewing dried fruits. Instead of bacon and eggs for breakfast, replace them with a fresh salad or whole grain cereal.

In terms of habit, we never really give up anything — when proven unsuitable, it is replaced. But why create habits in the first place? Habit always implies monotony, guaranteeing to remove the excitement from life. For instance, love is always exciting until it becomes a habit. A new job is always an exciting challenge until it is mastered — then it becomes automatic and loses its appeal as our creative faculties subside into disuse.

Life is potentially full of excitement and experience is the purpose that motivates us all. Habit removes the excitement, replacing it with monotony. Then we lose our consciousness of the experience and become automatons. In so doing, we lose our human individuality and identity. Then life, for the time, appears to lose its purpose.

STAGE TWO

Know Your Purpose

The man without a purpose is like a ship without a rudder — a waif, a nothing, a no man. Have a purpose in life, and, having it, throw such strength of mind and muscle into your work as God has given you.

Thomas Carlyle (1795–1881)

Everything in life, in the universe and beyond, has a purpose. Human life has its general purpose and each individual, an individual purpose.

Yet, although everyone has a purpose, very few ever come to know what it is. He who lives a life of purpose consistent with his need has invested his talents. However, he who realises his purpose but feels it to be too much to fulfil merely buries his talents; he who acts in accord with random desires and whims throws his talents away.

As man becomes aware of his purpose, he recognises that behind every event, every occurrence, is an explanation from which he can glean a little more understanding of life. Nothing occurs by chance; there is no real accident or coincidence, mystery or miracle. Everything has its explanation, its purpose, irrespective of the limitations of human perception.

What could appear more cruel or purposeless than the sudden death of a newborn infant in an automobile accident? Yet this too has its reason, remote as it may seem, when ultimately understood, devoid of personal emotion.

We realise that in the study of chemistry, reactions always follow numerous laws so that their results can be predicted when all the conditions are understood and remain constant. Thus it is with life — everything is knowable, if only life were long enough for it all to be known. But what remains unknown in this life will not remain unknown forever. Knowledge will always be revealed when the seeker is ready.

Freedom and Awareness

The outstanding faculty which is consistently found in every successful human life, and which distinguishes such a life from all others, is conscious awareness. It is the attribute of true independence; the key to personal freedom, to the extent that human life can be free. It is exemplified in such lives as Pythagoras, Socrates, Aristotle and his outstanding pupil, Alexander; in the lives of Copernicus, of Leonardo, Thomas Paine, Rudolf Steiner, etc.

The many and various laws and influences to which humans are subject exert more command on man than he is generally prepared to concede. But if he could possess total, unobstructed freedom, what would he do with it to ensure that it was not lost (for man is apt to become intensely possessive)?

Just what is total freedom? Is total freedom possible or desirable? With so many influences over physical life, is it possible to achieve every reasonable measure of freedom? Climatic influences, gravity, the law of compensation, sociological influences and especially one's immediate family, all contribute their demands so that total personal freedom in the physical sense is seen to be impossible. Yet, in the metaphysical sense, as a spiritual reality, freedom becomes as available as our awareness of it.

The inner freedom which we now discuss is an intensely personal experience. However, as we become aware of its implications, paradoxically we recognise we do not really need this freedom.

Rather, the greatest need of man is wise guidance in his choices. The nature of the source of guidance is so vast as to provide sufficient material for another entire book; so for now, let us say that the very best direction man can obtain is divine guidance.

On his journey through life, man is constantly required to choose, to decide which path he should take. One will always be the most suitable, but which one? With sufficient development of awareness of one's purpose in life, guidance will direct man's choices and he will not question its wisdom. And so a further experience and greater awareness will evolve.

Thus, as our purpose becomes clear, we have no need of choice. Rather, in accepting the responsibility for our total being, it is not necessary to have the freedom to choose, only the freedom to be able to follow guidance. And this freedom is the consequence of enlightenment based on awareness, knowledge and understanding. We learn to realise just what Pythagoras meant when he said: "Man is free only to the extent that his mind is freed from ignorance."

Now let us consider that other aspect of freedom, physical freedom. It is this material state which largely preconditions the nature of our life. Obviously, if we direct most mental attention towards material possessions, appearances and emotional demands, our prospect of freedom proportionately diminishes. Likewise, our potential reception to guidance is dulled. In being so limited, our mind is far from being freed from ignorance.

These observations are intended as general guidelines to the reader and are recognised as certainly not exhaustive. They are intended to emphasise the domination of man's thoughts in the determination of his life pattern and to illustrate the distinction which so clearly exists between the "haves" and the "have nots" — those who are fulfilling their purpose and have satisfaction in their lives; as opposed to those who neither have a clue to their purpose nor care how to discover it.

There exists perhaps no finer recent example of a purposeful public life, one in which the freedom of acceptance or rejection was more richly characterised, than that of Britain's great wartime leader, Sir Winston Churchill. His constant rejection of the decisions of his superiors, when they appeared to him unwise or untimely, brought Churchill into frequent disfavour. Yet, when the crisis of all-out war erupted, it was this man who steered his country through its many hardships, who worked untiringly as an inspiration to his people with a determination anchored in the confidence of his purpose and his ability to fulfil it.

In spite of being hailed a great leader in wartime, Churchill was rejected by his people as a peacetime leader. The loss of his first peacetime election must have been a great disappointment to one who so unstintingly gave of himself throughout Britain's darkest years. Perhaps his record of aggressive individuality, his reputation for independent decision making and his confident purposefulness were too much for a traditionally conservative electorate to risk! No doubt the British people preferred to return to their prewar habits than risk radical changes in their established life patterns.

Indeed, there is much to be said for security, but it should not be confused with habit. After years of privation, who would not wish to return to peace, comfort and security?

The tenacity and heroic fortitude of the British are legend. But such traits, if not carefully tempered, can become tantamount to stubbornness.

If a person or a nation is to fulfil its purpose, it must be prepared to learn by its experiences, for such is their reason, their *raison d'être*. To hanker for "the good old days" is to enter into spiritual decline.

As the spiritual state always determines the physical, it is conceivable that a nation which fails to evolve, to develop in accordance with its purpose and experience, must ultimately evidence apparent failure in terms of declining influence. America, no less than Britain, has suffered evidence of decline in consequence of two world wars and a few subsequent, less extensive armed crusades. Neither appears as yet to have learned that the correct path to human betterment is not to be found in aggressive conversion, but in exemplary conduct, love and wise action.

Seek Always the Cause

Man can become the master of his destiny; yet all too often, he exists as its consequence. His ability to seek the cause, recognise and act upon each purpose, determines the difference. Let us exemplify this by the most conspicuous and painful of all illustrations, the decline in human health.

That the decline in human health, ironically, has coincided with the development of scientific research is a universally attested fact. But the reason for this seeming paradox has been assiduously avoided. Whenever the cause of physical pain has been investigated, it has always been relegated to second place after the negating of the discomfort. Yet, once consciousness of the pain has been removed, its cause becomes all the more difficult to trace; in fact, to the nonthinker, the reason for tracing it no longer prevails.

By recognising the reality that behind everything lies its cause, man could avoid considerable inhumanity towards life, especially towards himself. Were science to devote its power and effort to seeking always the cause, the quality of life on earth would show marked improvement. In order for this to be possible, human investigation must discard preconceived notions and prejudices, replacing them with recognition of truth and wisdom. Emotional desires are thereupon replaced by the nobler motives of brotherhood, service and the constantly underlying aim towards perfection.

Physical illnesses such as cancer and arthritis, now so prevalent in modern society, are characteristic of ignorance. They exemplify man's failure to live nobly and naturally: his habit of being motivated by emotion, rather than awareness; by desire, rather than need; by prejudice, rather than intelligence.

Even though Winston Churchill lived to be ninety years of age, the illness and discomfort of his later years were such as to penalise rather than reward him for his earlier years of valuable service. In a period when his accumulation of decades of understanding and wisdom should have been even more priceless to mankind, Churchill was too sick, too unhappy to really care. Those who admired him in his earlier years came to pity his later incapacities. He became no different to the vast majority of mankind which fails to take care of itself when young, thereby declining into the pitiable fragility which makes most people fear old age.

Man should be alert, active and just as excited about life in his more mature years as he is in his youth. Every day should be a new experience, the successful handling of which produces happiness. If this is not the case in your life, seek the cause and correct it; accept full responsibility for your every thought and action now, for there is nothing more certain than that ultimately you must.

Cause-and-Effect

In the East it is called "The Law of Karma"; in Western science it is known as "Newton's Third Law of Motion": "To every action there is an equal and opposite reaction." The East recognises it as a basic law for all life; the West, as merely a part of physical science.

Yet, when Western science was undergoing its formation and initial development, the Law of Cause-and-Effect was as profoundly understood as it was in the East. This was in the sixth century before the current era, under the influence of the Greek philosopher Pythagoras in the West; and of Buddha, Hinduism and Confucius in the East. Cause-and-Effect became known to Pythagoras through his studies in Phoenicia, Egypt and especially under the Jewish prophet, Daniel, when both were held captive in Babylon. To the Jews it was a vital doctrine ("an eye for an eye") as it was later to the Master, Jesus, who taught that "as you sow, so shall you reap" and "do unto others as you would have them do unto you".

Since then, the mainstream of each school of thought has significantly departed from the universality of this law. The East sees Karma as a law of unavoidable penalties, a fatalistic marriage of past actions with future consequences. The West employs the principle of action-and-reaction primarily to achieve physical motion — often an exploitation of the moment.

These generalisations are not intended to overlook the more enlightened groups and individuals within each hemisphere whose code of moral conduct and thought embrace a recognition of the limitlessness of the Law of Cause-and-Effect. Total responsibility and awareness of one's thoughts, words and deeds thereby prevails, resulting in a far greater understanding of life. Improved happiness pervades the mind that comprehends the reason for things, that knows everything occurs for a purpose.

It is vital for us to recognise how this law never ceases to act as the perfect balancer. It is nature's great equaliser, setting into motion compensatory forces to remedy every imbalance. Some people call it the Law of Compensation, for indeed, it is one of the laws which cannot be broken with impunity. Every action gives rise to an equal and appropriate reaction, a rule of life that everyone must ultimately recognise. And when we do, how much happier and more successful we become. Far greater progress is always made when we swim with the current. Then we can relax and enjoy life more, sharing that enjoyment with others to whom we have shown how to swim.

Even in man's vocational pursuits does he find continuing evidence of the Law of Cause-and-Effect. Every engineer and scientist employs its principle in the development of motion or reaction in industry or research; every artist in his creative work is just as conscious of the need for balance. Yet, most fail to recognise the profound metaphysical foundation of this law, oblivious of its continual prevalence in their daily personal affairs, whether they be interrelating with others socially, in business dealings or on the sports field.

Perhaps it is the unconsciousness which underlies human habits that causes us to overlook effects which result from causes we bring into action. Is there any other reason why intelligent people sometimes act so unwisely? No matter how intelligent or well educated a person, when he smokes or administers a drug, drinks coffee or alcohol, ingests "foodless" foods or embraces any other habit which is contrary to the natural requirements of his body, he pays an ultimate penalty. Resultant reactive effects are then often registered by the nervous system as pain. Again, habit often raises its thoughtless head by seeking relief from the pain, rather than attempting to discover its cause. Such relief only tends to make one unconscious of the cause — and in so doing, it invariably causes a reaction within the body as a rebellion to the palliative drug. This is exemplified by the rocketing increase in kidney disease in Western society, the usual indirect cause of which is stress. Tension-induced headaches are fed aspirin or coffee, both of which are known irritants to the kidneys. The natural remedy would be to remove oneself from the area of tension or to learn to gain emotional control rather than be emotionally reactive.

Man often seeks to conform, rather than dare to be different and initiate a change when he recognises its need. To so conform is often to abandon one's responsibility for bringing intelligence into action. Yet, the very aspect of human life which places it beyond the monotony of the lives of other animals is man's creative ability to exercise his individuality by evolving a little more towards perfection, thereby leaving the world a better place than when he entered it. To succeed in this, he needs to understand himself and his purpose in life. This is far easier to achieve when he lives in accordance with nature than when he attempts a compromise between nature's laws and his varying whims and fancies. In fact, human purpose can *only* be fulfilled when man and nature (creature and creator) work together to achieve the same result.

It would appear that some people seek to "opt out" of this responsibility. To do so is to bury one's head in the sand for a time. Life goes on, progressing all around you, but you are not aware of it until you come out and take another look. Then you see how much catching-up you have to do. Those who thus leave the path for a time are temporarily oblivious of continuity of life, unlimited as it is to the physical. Perhaps they have to return through rebirth to discover that one can never leave the path. At best, we can only stand still for a time — until we learn the futility of such indolence.

In 1967, Australia and the Western world mourned the loss of Prime Minister Harold Holt. On that cold, wet day, he dived into the turbulent waters of Port Phillip Bay near his Melbourne home, never to be seen again. Only bravado, it would appear, could drive a man to risk such treachery as those waters and their sharks implied. Was it abandonment of responsibility for personal safety or the compelling force of the Law of Cause-and Effect in action? As a famous skin diver and shark-killer, Harold Holt may have invited the challenge once too often.

That example brought an air of finality such as can only happen once in a lifetime to any of us. Everyone is treated much more lightly by milder, less acute, early warning signals when unwise action is undertaken. Such pain and discomfort act as fuses in the body's sensory circuitry, indicating that further unwise action of that nature will be treated more harshly. All other animals and lower creatures act instinctively to avoid such recurrences; man tends to rationalise his position in any number of different ways — pain relievers, "that won't happen to me" attitude and similar. But the Law of Cause-and-Effect is never hoodwinked.

Dangers of Fragmentation

An especially unsatisfactory modern habit is that of specialisation. Such fragmentation and departmentalising of life sees only a tree, ignoring the forest. It conditions a narrowed intellect, prejudicing against balanced, unlimited awareness.

Just as the single piece of a jigsaw puzzle can never reveal the composition of the entire picture, no more can a single facet of life reveal its total purpose. The total picture of life will always exceed the sum of its individual components, for it is manifest over a vast range of expression — from soil to psyche and beyond. Fragmenting life ignores its totality and its purpose.

Nowhere is this more sadly apparent than in matters of human health. For example, how very convenient it is to blame minute germs for human illness. But who provided the toxic medium in the first place to attract the germs, for its eradication? In feeding upon our inner toxicity, is it not only natural for the germs to breed and multiply as thoughtless man continues to feed them and encourage their presence? Blaming germs is only avoiding the obvious responsibility which we must assume in our personal manner of living.

A specialist has been described as a person who learns more and more about less and less — eventually, he will know everything about nothing. Sadly, this is often so true, for in seeking to promote a specialised aim, research can lead man into many blind alleys of erudite uselessness.

This could hardly be better illustrated than by the billions of dollars spent in most Western countries on cancer research while the basic causes of cancer receive so little attention. Unnatural dietary habits with their overload of animal products, chemicals and stimulants, their deficiencies in vitamins, minerals and complex carbohydrates (whole grains particularly) have misled otherwise intelligent researchers into a detour in their witch-hunt for outside causes. Meanwhile, their pernicious habits go unconsidered. This is often illustrated when an eminent cancer researcher dies of cancer.

Similar comments can be made of the fetish about heart research and transplants. Public fund-raising for this work is almost fraudulent when the researchers fail to consider the simple causes (stress, saturated fatty acids from animal food, etc.), because the researchers themselves are rarely qualified in nutritional science and are often too addicted to their own dietary habits. The sudden death of Professor Sir John Lowenthal of a heart attack in 1980 was sad enough, but when we consider that he was head of the National Heart Foundation in Sydney, we must ask: why did he not know better?

The jealousy with which some researchers guard their discoveries is sufficient to cause one to question their motives. Research demands huge reserves of time and money to which everyone ultimately contributes, whether the organiser be government or industry, whether the funds be extracted by taxes or added onto the prices of items for sale. Yet the ultimate aim of research is invariably to make a profit for its sponsors, rarely to unselfishly improve the quality of life.

Knowledge, like love, cannot be specialised or fragmented — it must be shared to be of benefit and to develop. Fragmentation actively mitigates against the fulfilment of life's purpose by inducing disinterest beyond the confines of one's specialisation. A heart specialist was consulted recently by a friend of the writer. Despite extensive tests, her physician could find no cause for extreme tiring in the legs, severe headaches and poor lower body blood circulation. An electrocardiograph indicated a normal heart and the specialist concluded that the condition was merely one of "age". The patient had turned fifty!

With no improvement from the prescribed drugs, the patient visited a chiropractor who soon recognised the condition. With massage and spinal adjustments, the chiropractor was immediately able to correct the misalignment in the spine which was pinching certain nerves. The patient was astounded at this sudden "miracle cure" for, with the improvement of the condition in her legs, the frequency of her headaches diminished to only an occasional one when she became over-tired. Previously she thought she would be a lifelong migraine sufferer.

Let it never be forgotten that the human being can be properly guided to a full recovery of health only when it is realised that good health is the consequence of living a life which accords with the natural laws — a life which is in harmony. Only by considering the chemical, physical and metaphysical aspects of man and the totality of their interrelationships can any practitioner provide proper guidance.

As the clouds of confusion which hide reality are dispelled by awakening, let us recognise that while life pulses within our veins, there is time to return to the path. Human life in general has its purposes; individual life in particular has its special path by which its purpose can be fulfilled.

The Purpose of Life

In general terms, the purpose of human life is to learn by involvement, by experience. This can only by achieved to the degree that awareness is cultivated as life progresses in time. And of what value is time, except as a measure of experience? In the depths of reality, time has no other purpose.

Our varying stages of development indicate that each human being has a different purpose in life. It is for this primary reason that man's most reliable guidance will be that found through his own awareness. The development of this awareness will determine the fulfilment of one's purpose, an achievement based upon personal experience. And through this development, the eternal self will proceed towards perfection and a reuniting with the Great Architect of the Universe of which man is the image and likeness.

Man persistently entertains the unfortunate habit of forgetting his divine origin, allowing himself to be distracted from the pristine path into many an alley of purposelessness. He has been there before. To engage in repeated experiences of the same nature is to avoid the real purpose of life, to mark time, as it were. Such diversions are invariably motivated by sensual desires and fleeting pleasures. And it is not until his developing awareness will permit man to break these habits that he will resume further progress.

Some experiences through which we must graduate are pandemic, being shared by all members of the same nation or region. These reveal the importance of maintaining harmony with our total environment, just as personal experiences reveal the importance of maintaining inner harmony. In our association with other humans, with other forms of life and with our inanimate environment, we must recognise the need to live in peace and harmony. We must also realise that we are individually responsible for maintaining that condition.

In nature, balance is the prevailing aim of all energy. Hurricanes, storms, ocean waves and earthquakes are but natural energies directed towards maintaining balance. Man must recognise this vital leveller, for it will teach him in his own life such that every action will be guided by harmony.

By his experiences, man learns of himself. As he develops in understanding, man can assume the responsibility for his growth and commence to assist and guide others in proportion to their *needs*, not (as the unthinking do) in accordance with their *desires* or wishes for fame. The privilege of entering into the life of another human being, of assuming some measure of responsibility for guiding him at that vital time of his growth, is an experience of great mutual benefit. Wise guidance, we must realise, can only ensue if wise personal action has determined one's own living manner.

"Man know thyself, then shall you know the universe and God," Pythagoras was reputed to have instructed each of his pupils 2500 years ago. Such purpose can only bring to life that precious inner peace which passes all other possessions.

But the genius of Pythagoras extended far beyond theoretical guidance. He gave to his pupils and to the world the key to self-understanding and how to use it. All things in life are aspects of vibration, whether they are animate or seemingly inanimate. Vibrations vary from one another only by frequency and amplitude — rate of pulsation and size. These vary only by number. So number is the key to the understanding of the universe and all life within it. Thus, numbers became symbols of qualities, indicative of all aspects of life. By the understanding of numbers in our life, then, we have the key to understanding the essence of life and its purpose. This is the subject of an entire book of special interest to people seeking to know: the author's *Secrets of the Inner Self*, published by Angus & Robertson Publishers, Sydney and London, 1980.

So that is the key to self-understanding, but the science of numbers, like any important key, is of value only when we know how to use it. That knowledge is locked in the understanding of the meaning of love. This is no surprise, for every student of history and the Bible is aware of the eleventh commandment: "Love thy neighbour as thyself." This became the crux of Jesus' purpose in life and the key for all to follow, for it is impossible to "love thy neighbour" without knowing how to "love ... thyself". And the only way to love yourself is to know yourself and to realise what divine love has been poured into your own creation. There is no faster or more certain way to grow, to evolve.

It is startling to recognise the relationship between evolving and loving. The word "love" is in fact part of the word "evolve". This creates an amazing etymological clue to how intimately these two vital aspects of life are inextricably bound. They really cannot be separated. To love is to develop our own evolutionary path in the most direct way for, in so doing, our progress towards perfection receives the greatest impetus because the knowledge of our purpose, collectively and individually, is in no doubt.

So if we each undertook to express more love, life would unfold with far more purpose. Man would be kinder to man and to all creatures. Fear would be unknown, making disarmament natural and desirable. Selfishness and hunger would disappear. A new era of astounding personal growth would be upon us. It is our purpose to do everything possible to facilitate this, for that is why we have chosen this life, blending as it does into the emerging new age of awareness of purpose.

STAGE THREE

The Ingredients of Health

Health is a state of complete physical, mental and social well-being, and not merely the absence of disease and infirmity.

From Preamble to the Constitution of the World Health Organisation

There should be no surprise that the total aspects of health are recognised by the World Health Organisation; its world-wide influence in matters pertaining to health is indeed powerful. However, the surprise comes about when we realise from investigations that the WHO fails in practice to actually embrace the totality concept of health. Far too much emphasis is placed merely upon physical aspects of health, with almost general avoidance of psychic factors and failure to educate people about the natural ingredients for healthful living. Their preoccupation with germs must eventually give way to the purification of living habits if WHO is to achieve any worthwhile success with its vast influence.

For every disease combated, many others appear as testimony to man's increasing departure from natural living habits. Health and disease are not the results of chance occurrences. They are the consequences of the laws of nature in action, especially of the Law of Cause-and-Effect.

There exists an intimate relationship between man's living habits and principles on the one hand and his state of health and well-being on the other. It is no chance relationship, but one which must be understood through proper education, free from prejudices and justifications of habit.

A Case for De-education

After many years behind a school desk, an adolescent may graduate with any number of honours in academic subjects, fit to face the world of commerce, to marry and raise children; yet he usually knows precious little about life. His choice of a vocation may be restricted to the limited range of subjects encompassed by his school curriculum. His choice of a partner in matrimony is generally restricted to a small circle of acquaintances with similar interests; and he is motivated by a limited concept of love as promoted by the common culture and by his own sexual desires. The training of his children is limited to his own personal experiences — as is his knowledge of diet, exercise and the other essential ingredients of health.

Having been exposed to a formal education and limited social fraternising, young men and women mistakenly believe they are prepared for all life has to offer. If their intelligence has not been totally subjugated to an intellect crammed full of academic data, or preoccupied with achieving material success, they will soon realise that their years of scholastic effort have done very little to prepare them for an understanding of life in relation to one's purpose, or of how that purpose may be best achieved. We do not deny the importance of success in one's working career; but this should be a product of the success achieved in one's personal life (for the reverse rarely, if ever, applies).

If man has not learned to live in harmony and in permanent good health, any brilliant success he may achieve in educational establishments or industry will accord him little happiness. Yet, once life has been understood and practised according to the laws of nature, success in all other human affairs must, *ipso facto*, attend man's efforts.

Far too many otherwise well-educated persons evidence a general ignorance of the ingredients of health. They are unaware of the fact that their health is the product of their living habits; instead, they have been conditioned to the theory that ill health is solely the consequence of germ action. They have been taught the need for external cleanliness, yet the equally essential demand for inner hygiene remains ignored while chemicalised, processed substances putrefy in the gastrointestinal tract. They have been encouraged to revere the successes of science in conquering nature, in ignorance of the fact that nature remains just as unconquered as ever because man has yet to learn to live in harmony with it.

Thus, a cogent case is presented for the de-education of man to enable his conditioned intellect to unlearn some of the falsehoods which have been predicated upon unworthy motives of greed, or fame or fortune. Were education to encourage the development of man's creative faculties, his innate intelligence would be nurtured as a reliable guide by which to achieve his purpose in life. The accumulation of worldly knowledge can always be of some benefit provided a proper basis for its understanding and application has been prepared. Such is the true nature of education.

The impressing of impersonal facts, which must be remembered for later examinations, does not answer to the needs of the pupil with gastric indigestion, with a pimply face, with a migraine headache or other physical discomfort arising from the failure of education to teach him the fundamentals of healthful living.

All too often we have witnessed the school teacher or the college professor conclude an instruction in some deep scientific subject, then adjourn to the cafeteria for a meal of hamburger, cake and cola, followed by a cigarette or cigar. How ignorant even the learned can be!

A leading horse trainer was recently interviewed for his advice on the proper programme for training a thoroughbred. The reporter conducted the interview at the race track, after which the trainer suggested they go to the cafeteria "for a quick lunch". During the interview, the trainer left no doubt as to the importance of a correct and natural diet for a healthy and successful racehorse, but his own lunch consisted of the antithesis.

Drawing the trainer's attention to his selection of two hamburgers followed by a large cup of very black coffee, the reporter asked how the champion racehorse might fare on such a meal.

"Would you want to kill it?" asked the trainer!

The Secret of Long Life

The Soviet newspaper *Sotsialisticheskaya Industriy* (Socialistic Industry) published on December 24, 1971, a story about the age and life of the oldest inhabitant of the Socialist Republic of Azerbaijan. A man of 166 years, Shirali Mislimov had lived in the mountains of that region since his birth in 1805. In the poetic language for which that region is renowned, he delivered his formula for a long, healthy life:

"I was never in a hurry in my life, and I'm in no hurry to die now," Mislimov said when interviewed. "There are two sources of long life," he continued. "One is a gift of nature, and it is the pure air and clear water of the mountains, the fruit of the earth, peace, rest, the soft and warm climate of the highlands.

"The second is people. He lives long who enjoys life, and who bears no jealousy of others, whose heart harbours no malice or anger, who sings a lot and cries a little, who rises and retires with the sun, who likes to work and who knows how to rest."

This man probably learned nothing about scientific nutrition or self-discipline in school, but in life he had learned much. He may not even have had an exact record of his age, for his outlook on life did not appear to demand precision, although it does inspire agreement.

To succeed in life, one must understand and practise the requirements by which health is maintained. It is the foundation of all possessions and the only means by which the body may fully express the purpose of life. For this reason, the body's needs must be understood and supplied. And to be particular in choosing such needs is not to be regarded as a "crank" or "faddist", any more than is a person with a new car who exercises his choice in the type and grade of oil and petroleum he uses. Rightly he is very particular about his car, but that can be replaced. His body cannot.

If people would learn to be as selective in feeding their inner fuel tank as they are with their new automobiles, we could dismantle many of the world's hospitals and not worry about how we are going to accommodate increasing numbers of sick people.

A great secret which women appear to share and from which men are generally excluded is how to have a longer life expectancy. In spite of the record of their higher incidence of depression, women generally experience fewer heart attacks, strokes, ulcers and conditions of hypertension than do men. Women also tend to love more generously, cry more frequently and more readily and live in less tension than do men. Could it be that greater compassion and their ability to release pent-up emotions allow women to achieve a longer life?

Even so, women fail by many decades to achieve the life expectancy which should characterise human life, that of six times maturity — around 120 years. Instead, by unnatural living habits, human beings commit suicide by default in something around half that period. And because of those disharmonious habits, humans manifest a rapid deterioration of physical and mental condition — in sixty or seventy years, they decline at a rate far faster than they would if living twice that span in conformity with the essential ingredients of health.

The Essence of Life

It is indeed vital to man's education that he learn the rules for living a long and purposeful life. The ingredients of long life are essential to man's continual good health, and good health is necessary for his purpose to be achieved in the comparatively short number of years at his disposal. Here are the ingredients:

- **Clean air**
- **Clean water**
- **Rest and relaxation**
- **Sunshine and shelter**
- **Mental balance and harmony**
- **Correct food**
- **Fasting**
- **Exercise and activity**

This list contains nothing new. It is largely self-evident and by virtue of this, its components are constantly taken for granted. This creates unfortunate neglect in their understanding, which leads to the present generally chronic state of human health.

To believe that "near enough is good enough" attests to the general ignorance which surrounds man's recognition of the ingredients of good health. To believe that smog-laden city air, chemically charged drinking water, late-night entertainment, the wearing of heavy, tight clothes, frustrating emotional involvements, processed packaged foodstuffs and the like are near enough for man's sustenance, is to be guilty of the sort of ignorance which this book is endeavouring to dispel.

For those more fortunate people in possession of a more robust constitution, considerable abuse can be inflicted to their bodies before manifesting in illness. But when illness does finally afflict them, its consequences are invariably the more serious, as though all past abuses have been secretly accumulating in a vast toxic reservoir.

A subtle consequence of such abuse is the progressive weakening of the constitution — an undermining of the ability to tolerate unsuitable conditions. This is not always as apparent in the subject as in the offspring. Thus we observe that one human generation may have the serious handicap of a reduced lower level of initial vitality than the parents. We are, in fact, witnessing a general decline in human health which is repeatedly evidenced by the detection of such chronic diseases as cancer, arteriosclerosis and arthritis in younger and younger people.

This decline can be arrested. It is unquestionably the consequence of unnatural living conditions and will be halted, then reversed, when man recognises the essential ingredients for good health and unreservedly practises them with the same ardour with which he now avoids them.

The Primary Substance: Clean Air

There is no divergence of opinion in any school of thought that air is the most vital substance in life. However, there is frequent disagreement as to the quality of that air, with industrialists at one end of the scale and ecologists and health practitioners at the other.

While clean, fresh, pure air is universally recognised as the most desirable, few will go so far as to state that absolute purity is essential. So strong are industrial lobbyists in determining government policy that we are currently led to believe that our lungs can handle up to certain "tolerance levels" without detriment to health.

This is the sort of compromise that implies a substance is only poisonous if its concentration is of sufficient strength, ignoring its cumulative effects from sub-lethal dosages.

Pollution of our atmosphere is carelessness, laziness and thoughtlessness. It is the guilt of almost every contemporary civilisation, a by-product of the population explosion wherein excessive industrial production is engaged to cater to every whim of mankind. One now has to question whether that extra automobile (the most expensive shopping basket ever invented) is worth the sacrifice.

The laws of nature appear to have allowed for every natural contingency. The primary ingredient of life was created in such abundance that, under normal circumstances, the atmosphere of Earth would support a huge population of living organisms. But man has created an abnormality, casting these laws into imbalance. He is now realising that our atmosphere does not contain an inexhaustible supply of oxygen.

Causes of imbalance always initiate compensatory effects, as we have already reasoned. The intelligence of nature far exceeds that of man, although many will even disagree with the fact that nature is so endowed. Natural effects produced to restore the imbalance may well be working to reduce industrialisation as well as to cleanse the atmosphere. Man, by his counter-ecological actions, has set the stage whereby any manner of occurrences might yet create havoc. Time alone will prove whether the law of compensation will permit such transgressions.

Meanwhile, rather than watch and encourage those who "know not what they do" persist with their unecological activities, let us rally to the support of the rapidly growing bands of ecologists who are aware of the seriousness of our accelerating loss of vital oxygen and its replacement by poisonous gases and dangerous particles.

Introducing governmental legislation to penalise polluters is not the answer to pollution any more than it was the answer to liquor consumption or drug abuse. The answer lies in proper education. Man has to learn to live with respect for his environment and not become an "industrial Faust" by selling his balanced environment for a fast industrial profit. He must learn to produce without wastage, to recognise the laws of conservation and put them into practice — a vital aspect of industrial education which has been neglected.

Few people now question that concentration of impurities and reduction of oxygen content in the air prevail in industrial regions and areas of high population density. The question is not whether the cultural advantages of city life or the products of industry justify the physiological disadvantages of pollution, but rather how can all factors be maintained in proper balance. Effluents circulating in the city atmosphere include known carcinogens, yet most people look upon this aspect of life as they would upon Russian roulette — maybe they will not succumb to skin cancer or lung cancer or a chronic respiratory disease. However, their chances of avoiding all forms of pollution-induced illness are extremely slim.

The ideal composition of clean air, with its relatively steady proportion of gaseous elements, serves multitudinous purposes within and without the human body. Its primary physiological function is to provide oxygen to the bloodstream and to remove carbon dioxide by exchange, thereby purifying the blood somewhat and providing further potential energy for the body.

Most air contains some forms of impurity and, within certain natural limits, the human respiratory system has been designed to cope with these. The windpipe (trachea) carries air to the bronchi, which split the intake into each lung and are designed with an internal lining of hair-like projections to arrest foreign matter. If air is taken in through the mouth, its filtration depends solely upon this safeguard. If breathing is performed correctly, through the nose, long, coarse hairs in each nostril act as preliminary filters.

Even so, today's heavily polluted air is generally loaded far in excess of the body's inherent filtration ability. The rate of increase in the fouling of our atmosphere is infinitely more rapid than the human body's rate of adaptation. It requires centuries for the smallest structural modifications to transpire within the human body by natural adaptation. Therefore, the respiratory tract cannot possibly hope to cope with the sudden decrease in purity and freshness of the atmosphere. The obvious consequence is the load of impurities being taken directly into the lungs, there accumulating until it creates a condition of acute distress.

This condition is greatly magnified when the nose is bypassed and man breathes through his open mouth. It is especially dangerous when he also voluntarily inhales the effluent of a cigarette into his lungs. Human windpipes were just not constructed with sufficient cleansing equipment to filter such volumes of impurities.

Unlike the air cleaner of an automobile, human lungs possess no removable filter element which can be reconstituted or replaced when it has become clogged. Try running your car for a few years in normal city traffic without the proper servicing of the air filter — the engine will behave with increasing irregularity as it becomes progressively starved for adequate supplies of oxygen. This will be especially discernible under conditions of hard work and stress. How many people do you know who likewise become noticeably short of breath under mild conditions of stress or physical exercise?

The modern menace of industrial pollution compounds the age-old problem of atmospheric dust and smoke, which themselves often employ the body's respiratory filtration equipment to its capacity. Dust has always been a problem wherever man has denuded the soil in agricultural or pastoral development. Removal of tree protection on agricultural lands and the overstocking of pastoral areas with grazing animals has invariably resulted in wind erosion of the exposed top soil. Times of high wind have often resulted in serious dust storms which not only ruin valuable farmlands but also create grave breathing hazards.

When deprived of its natural protection, top soil can be diffused over a vast area. As dust, it can be blown many hundreds of miles and cause acute discomfort to people with a predisposition towards respiratory ailments.

The extent to which dust can be blown is expressed no more forcefully than on the snowy slopes of New Zealand's South Island mountain chain. Following periods of strong westerly winds, the snows take on a brownish hue. Winds, carrying top soil from denuded Australian farmlands, or smoke from Australian bushfires, deposit their load as dust when they rise to pass over the mountains which are more than three thousand kilometres to the east, across the Tasman Sea.

The act of breathing is another of those human habits which is rarely taught, often taken for granted. For specialised training, such as in sports competitions, singing, yoga and physical culture, varied forms of deep breathing are taught, but the most helpful is undoubtedly diaphragmatic breathing. When practised properly, this method reduces the respiratory rate while increasing the capacity of the lungs. This maintains the heart and lungs in better tone so that in times of sudden effort, both are instantly responsive without stress.

Diaphragmatic breathing also strengthens the abdominal region. It improves the functioning of all internal organs as well as the body's posture. Its manifold virtues are nowhere better exemplified than in singing, where the tone of the voice, its control and sustaining ability are discernibly improved, producing better phrasing and expression. But again, with singing, the quality of air is as important as the manner in which it is inhaled. Anyone who has ever sung in a public hall where the audience is permitted to smoke will painfully attest to this.

A further consideration of the primary substance of life is the spiritual aspect of air. Dr Rudolf Steiner, the great Austrian scientist and metaphysician who developed the biodynamic method of agriculture, proved that plants obtain a considerable amount of nourishment from the atmosphere. This, Dr Steiner stated, is both chemical and psychical. Experiments on humans are not so easily done, but those who have studied the yogic teachings of the East and the mystical teachings of the West believe in the metaphysical value of clean air — "prana", as it is better expressed. Although prana is regarded as more than air, it is descriptive of the life-giving properties associated with breathing.

As man grows in understanding and wisdom, he will apply his knowledge for the good of all. Often he will be called upon to choose between two opposing factors, but he will employ his innate intelligence and choose that which will improve the quality of life, not work to destroy it. Clean, fresh air must, at all costs, characterise our atmosphere before a condition of irreversibility develops.

Man's Lubricant: Clean Water

Second only to clean air in terms of the body's essential requirements is clean water. An average human male body, weighing 65 kilograms contains as much as 45 litres of water, accounting for 70 per cent of total body weight.

Due to considerable variations in build and body weight in humans, the actual water content of different persons has been found to vary from just over 56 per cent to nearly 80 per cent. Influencing factors include the amount of body fat, size of bones, state of health, quantity of foreign chemicals (especially hygroscopic common salt) and climatic factors to which the body is exposed. The nature of one's occupation also has an influence on the amount of water retention.

Physically, water is a lubricant vital to the body's actions; chemically, it is a compound essential to the body's many systems of functioning. When sleeping, the body uses water in its vital metabolic processes and it is evaporated through the lungs and skin. If one rested for a full twenty-four hours, about one litre of water would evaporate from the body in a temperate climate. In the tropics, up to another half litre would be given off. During that twenty-four-hour period, if the person were fasting (consuming no food or liquid), another third of a litre of water would be used in the oxidation of stored carbohydrates and fats. Thus, the minimum quantity of water required by the human adult body in a twenty-four-hour period is almost 1.5 litres.

Contrast this with the body's need for water in the same period when feeding and performing hard, manual work in a hot climate. Under such conditions, a man might evaporate up to four litres of water through his skin and lungs. He would need to pass at least another litre through his kidneys, using at least another half litre in the metabolism (oxidation) of his food. This implies that his total intake would need to be at least 5.5 litres to avoid any dehydration.

Intake of water can be from several sources. The most desirable and purest water will come from fresh fruits and vegetables which have been grown without any artificial chemicals. In the ideal diet, this source will supply the majority of the body's water needs. Supplementary water should come from drinking pure, fresh water or from fresh fruit juices drunk between meals.

As most people do not partake of the ideal diet, their intake of water from food is greatly reduced. Where much of their food supply is derived from meats, refined carbohydrates and snack "foods" (most of which are extremely low in water content), a considerable amount of supplementary fluid intake is vital. For this reason, most people are recommended to drink eight glasses of fluid daily, much of which is taken by way of soups, beverages (alcoholic and soft) and milk. None of these can compare in value with pure, fresh water.

With the average diet including such thirst stimulants as salt, spices, sugar and chemicals, man generally has to drink fairly large quantities of fluid. Little wonder, then, that drinking (often in excess and alcoholic) is accepted as a normal component of social behaviour. Can you imagine the expression on the face of your host at a party when you are asked what you would like to drink and you reply "a glass of pure water"? One can have fun doing this — and will be far healthier for the experience. To be less daring, you could ask for a glass of orange juice or mineral water — most public places and private homes do cater for this trend.

The huge general consumption of hard and soft beverages, of tea and coffee, both with meals and between, serves no purpose in satisfying thirst. Indeed, they do the opposite, inducing repeated drinking by masquerading as thirst quenchers, yet their subtle chemical components succeed in producing that delayed thirst inducement so that the drinker does not realise why he is thirsty again. Little wonder that alcoholic beverages and cola drinks, tea and coffee, are continuing to record increased consumption rates world-wide. Little wonder that premature senility, aggressiveness and kidney disease are similarly on the increase!

For the person who elects to drink city water as a "safe" supplementary fluid intake, another host of chemicals greets him. In particular, chlorine and fluoride, added to combat bacteria and tooth decay respectively. Neither chemical contributes towards health by being consumed — in fact, both are known to induce unnatural thirst, thereby increasing their intake. For safe drinking both chemicals should be removed before consumption, either by distilling or by the ion exchange method of filtration.

Fluoride deserves special mention. Added to the water either as sodium fluoride or in acid form so that it forms sodium fluoride in the water, this compound is a chemically recognised cumulative poison. The "bible" of the chemical world, *The Merck Index*, is uncompromising in warning of the hazards of this chemical:

> *HUMAN TOXICITY: Severe symptoms from ingestion of less than one gram; death from 5 to 10 gm. SUBLETHAL: Nausea and vomiting, abdominal distress, diarrhoea, stupor, weakness. LETHAL: muscular weakness, tremors, convulsions, collapse, dyspnea, respiratory and cardiac failure, death. CHRONIC: mottling of tooth enamel, osteosclerosis.*
>
> *USE: As insecticide, particularly for roaches and ants; in other pesticide formulations; constituent of vitreous enamel and glass mixes; as a steel degassing agent; in electroplating; in fluxes; in heat-treating salt compositions; in the fluoridation of drinking water; for disinfecting fermentation apparatus in breweries and distilleries; preserving wood, pastes and mucilage; manufacture of coated paper; frosting glass; in dental laboratories; in removal of HF (hydrogen fluoride) from exhaust gases to reduce air pollution.*

The dosage administered to drinking water supplies is one part per million. This is one milligram per litre, but of course this concentration cannot be regulated along the pipelines until the consumer drinks it. So the final dosage can be anything from zero to a few milligrams per litre. Now we know this fluoride to be a cumulative chemical — that is why its primary use is as an insecticide and a roach and ant poison. Thus its accumulation in the human body can reach toxicity levels with the drinking of a few hundred litres of city water. Any wonder that lethargy, heart and respiratory problems are becoming so rampant in the community?

It is startlingly serious to note among the recommended uses of sodium fluoride its value in frosting glass. The reason for this is its powerful scouring ability, for it is also used to etch glass. Now if it will do this to hard glass, what will it do to the tender lining of your gastrointestinal tract?

As important as it is to drink adequate pure water, this healthful habit is negated if water is consumed with or just after a meal. As water will dilute acid, the catabolism of protein in the stomach is slowed down by a less effective hydrochloric acid.

Without water, it is doubtful if man could live more than three or four days. However, his intake should be chosen wisely in terms of when and how much. It is wise not to drink immediately before a meal — allow at least twenty minutes' space. It is just as wise to allow time for the meal to pass from the stomach before flooding it with water — this can imply a wait of one to two hours after a fruit meal; up to four hours after a complex meal in which fats and/or proteins are consumed. The favourite American habit (which could become contagious in Australia if we are not careful) is drinking iced water with the meal. This is a nutritionally crazy act. Not only does the water dilute hydrochloric acid and render it less effective in breaking down proteins, but the freezing temperature of the water will induce cramps or spasms in the stomach, further impeding gastric digestion. So if you want the recipe for certain indigestion, iced water with a large meal is it!

Remember that the ideal way by which to obtain the majority of your water intake is from the ideal diet, comprising as it does 75 per cent fresh fruits and vegetables. These foods contain a high quantity of pure water, most of them from 80 to 98 per cent with a few as low as 60 per cent. The juiciness of these foods aids their digestion and the ease of masticating them. Compare this with the average meat and potato or fish and chip or hamburger diet, all of which are so devoid of natural juiciness and loaded with salt and seasonings that they induce avid thirsts. Hence the temptation to drink copious quantities of fluid with such a meal, exacerbating its normal indigestibility.

Some recent researches into the causes of senility have highlighted the value of water as an essential nutrient. Dr Abram Hoffer, the famous Canadian orthomolecular nutritionist, revealed this startling information during his highly successful lecture tour of Australia in October–November 1981. As Dr Hoffer is a colleague and close friend of the author, it has been possible to keep abreast of the research proving the direct connection between mental alertness and water consumption in older people. The Canadian researchers have discovered that as the body ages, it tends to dehydrate. Older people lose their desire to drink as much as when they were younger. As their bodies dry out, physical shrinking begins. The skin becomes harder and cracks, the hair drier and thinner. The body shrinking induces a reduction in height and some stooping develops.

Those are all the outside signs, but what is taking place inside? The organs grow slightly smaller — the most important organ of all, the brain, shows significant shrinking on X-ray film. Air pockets develop inside the cranium. As well, the blood becomes thicker and does not flow as freely around the body, thereby becoming less effective in nourishing the brain. The ultimate result is loss of memory, of coherence, plus the development of disorientation and confusion which become the symptoms by which senility is recognised. The treatment: drink lots of water — up to fifteen glasses (at least twelve) per day. Within six months, the condition should be significantly corrected, if not totally so.

Rest and Relaxation

Air, water and food provide the ingredients by which the body can be fuelled and lubricated to perform. Rest and relaxation, as intervals between the periods of performing, allow the stage to be cleaned, new scenery to be erected and the players (muscles and nerves) to recuperate, mustering renewed energy for the following act.

To relax is to make loose or slacken. It implies short periods of conscious inactivity. Rest goes further. It is total relaxation undertaken in a recumbent, comfortable position, permitting sleep. Relaxation is for short, conscious periods; rest for longer, unconscious hours. Inadequacy of both is the root of more than half the illnesses in the Western world.

Rest and relaxation can thus be seen as varying degrees of inactivity during which the body innervates and recharges. Short periods of relaxation are essential during waking hours to enable the mind to maintain maximum conscious control of the body. During full rest this control is temporarily abandoned, for only the involuntary muscles are working. This enables the psyche to "release itself" and engage in needed timeless activities, some of which might be consciously recalled as dreams.

Most people today live in the present — tense! So much is crammed into modern life (not all of it necessary, of course) that most people fail to allocate essential time for relaxation. This demands only occasional periods of no more than a few minutes each, during which nerves, muscles and brain are allowed to slacken. This immediately reduces tension and requires far less effort than would be employed in maintaining the tension.

The more intense the activity, the more important the time allocated to periods of relaxation. This is especially important in relation to digestion.

Food must not only provide nourishment, it must also be enjoyed. Enjoyment is initially the gratification of the taste buds, then the feeling of comfortable smoothness as the mouthful slides down the oesophagus, and finally a contentment which involves calmness in the stomach. These conditions are only possible with the aid of relaxation.

Sufficient relaxation prior to the meal will permit the gastric and salivary juices to be prepared. Relaxation during consumption of the meal allows taste sensations to be enjoyed to their fullest as the food is thoroughly masticated and slowly swallowed. Relaxation following the meal encourages the most effective gastric digestion, enabling the stomach to secrete adequate gastric juices comprising the required chemical balance.

Obviously, the more complex the meal, the longer the period of relaxation required to follow it. For a light, simple fruit meal, only a few minutes of relaxation following the final mouthful are needed to permit adequate initial digestion. This period could be extended for up to an hour following a heavy meal which might unwisely comprise a concentrated combination of fats, proteins and carbohydrates.

Failure to employ relaxation in conjunction with eating is like putting money into a bank account that not only refuses to pay interest, but also charges you for using it.

Sorrow or argument, hilarity or excitement, in fact all emotional involvements, are opposed to relaxation and antagonistic to a digestion which is generally already over-taxed by unsuitable components in the diet. These factors contribute to the multi-million dollar income of "indigestion remedy" manufacturers, whose products are of no benefit in overcoming the causes of indigestion.

Relaxation as a pause in mental activites has also proven itself constantly essential. How often have you struggled hard to remember a name, an event or a place, or to find the solution to a problem? The struggling invariably produces failure, being accompanied by tension. Yet with just a brief period of relaxation, the answer often arises, brought into consciousness by a relaxed brain which has been able to synchronise with the subconscious. The vast wealth of knowledge and wisdom inherent in the human mind can only be effectively tapped when the constrictions of tension are relaxed to permit a flow-through from the subconscious.

Relaxation should never be regarded as a future promise to be taken in the accumulated form of a vacation. Its daily employment is vital to efficient functioning of the body. It enables the blood to perform its vital task with unimpeded flowing so that cellular debris may be the more efficiently removed and replaced with nutrients to assist in growth, maintenance and repair.

The body's major house-cleaning job is performed at night during sleep. With physical activity as its lowest ebb, residues of muscular activity are minimal; this enables the bloodstream to be concentrated towards the healing of any injured part of the body. It is during such periods of total rest that the body's efforts of self-healing become the most powerful.

To a large extent, a reversal of physical activity takes place during sleep. Under conditions of rest, normalising forces come into play to lower the toxic level in the bloodstream, reduce tension in muscles and bring nerves back into harmony. In general, the effort reverts from largely physical to largely spiritual by which means the body and the psyche are brought back into phase, towards perfect harmony with each other.

Realising that any form of sickness or injury is basically a form of disharmony, we are more capable of understanding the vital need for rest. It is the essential precondition to regular and adequate regeneration by which the body is maintained in good health.

Sleep, itself, has a precondition. That is, relaxation. The most valuable aid to a good night's sleep is the body's ability to relax. For some people, this is a natural attribute which requires no conscious effort. But the ranks of such people are decreasing as tension in modern life increases. Infants and children who remain divorced from competitive activity or from stimulating chemicals are the exceptions. Sleep, to them, comes easily, for they have not lost the natural ability for instant relaxation.

Yet the penalties of modern living tend to filter down the age scale so that today we hear of more and more children who find relaxation difficult and sleep even more so. They are generally termed "hyperactive". This implies that such victims have a complex problem, when in reality it is a simple problem of parental ignorance. Unnatural stimulation of the body is more prominent in the young, being the unfortunate consequence of inept educational systems which fail to warn against the foolishness of relying on drugs and unnatural foods.

Laboratory-prepared chemicals must exert some influence on the chemical nature of the human body as it reacts to their undesirable presence. The usual reaction is directed towards removing the foreign intruder by stimulating the body into a hyperactive (over-active) condition. With more and more chemicals finding their way through industry into man's gastrointestinal tract via foods, beverages and drugs, little wonder that the body is allowed too little time to relax.

As always in life, the younger the body, the more acute its reaction. In infants it is especially noticeable and more difficult to control because they have not yet reached the age at which they respond to discipline or to understanding guidance.

As the complexity of modern life increases, humans require either longer hours of sleep or greater quality of sleep. Longer hours are rarely possible; most people getting eight hours per night regard it as a maximum period. Therefore, greater importance has to be concentrated on the need for proper relaxation prior to sleep (as well as during those vital periods through the day). The minutes of planned relaxation prior to bed will help deactivate the brain and loosen the body to enable sleep to be of greater benefit.

Anabolism, the construction of cellular tissue, is somewhat constrained during hours of normal physical activity. It is during the awakened hours that catabolism, the first half of the metabolic process (the breaking down of food from which its nutrients are extracted), is more active. Some of these nutrients are used during hours of activity; others are stored, awaiting build-up into new cellular tissue. The normal onset of tiredness is precipitated by the need for increased anabolism to repair and rejuvenate bodily tissues containing an accumulation of work-worn cells.

Cellular rebuilding is more effective and efficient when the body is at rest. To avoid rest at its required time, to stimulate into continued activity, will always result in a foundation for future disease, a condition known as enervation.

Efficient functioning of the body's organs during sleep is never questioned. People are content in the knowledge that if they sleep well they should awaken refreshed and alert in the morning. This hope is not always realised, for if the person has a high level of toxicity in the system, it is quite possible that some morning will see him awaken with an acute elimination in progress. This might be commonly referred to as a "cold", or might attract a more exotic name if one is currently in fashion, such as the Mesopotamian flu!

The body's condition on awakening will depend on many factors, all revolving around its general level of health. For the un-health-conscious person, it can be like a game of chance. For the health-conscious person living a natural life, it is always a certainty that the morning will guarantee a completed rejuvenation — the first few hours of sleep being spent in unwinding, the early morning hours in restoring.

Whatever a person's religious beliefs or understanding, when it comes to sleep, complete faith is placed in the hands of a power superior to themselves. Not even the supreme atheist will stay awake each and every night in disbelief that nothing beyond the physical could take place. He becomes tired and will, of necessity, sleep. And when he goes to sleep, he loses control of his body, placing it . . . he knows not where.

Everyone has faith that he will awaken in the morning. Habit, from infancy, prior to the brain's ability to reason, instilled this confidence. It is a soundly based confidence which should be reasoned as a natural part of life.

Then, let us not forget to look to the other natural aspects of life which are not taken for granted, which are abused because one's faith has been switched from the laws of creativity to the advertised product with the most persuasion. To divert one's faith (the precursor to understanding and wisdom) from the natural to the artificial is to invite disastrous penalties. In their chronic stages, these are called "diseases", being the body's attempts to normalise an abnormal set of conditions.

Sunshine and Shelter

Sunshine is recognised as essential for the bountiful growth of most plants, yet few humans are prepared to accord sunshine the same priority for themselves. Those who value sunshine are generally feverishly involved in acquiring a deep suntan for the sole sake of appearances.

Even less general importance is accorded proper shelter. So long as it looks expensive, withstands the weather and can receive a clear television signal, most people's ideal of a home is satisfied.

Actually, an important and traditional association exists between sunshine and shelter as vital requirements for human health and comfort.

Primitive tribes unquestioningly recognised the power of the sun. Its health-giving properties induced them to wear little or no clothes in its presence. This was also a token of submission to the spiritual power they attributed to the sun. Experience taught our ancestors that too much direct sunlight caused painful burns to their skin, dictating the need for seeking shelter.

Initially, trees provided satisfactory shelter, but they were no protection from marauding animals or inclement weather. Hence, in some places, the use of caves as shelters became highly desirable. Ultimately, huts were conceived.

When early man migrated north, the sunlight was less intense and they were also less exposed to it, owing to the necessity to clothe themselves in furs against the cold. The fairer the skin, the greater one's ability to absorb more vitamin D and the greater the risk of sunburn. Clothes, therefore, were not only demanded for warmth in winter, but also for skin protection in summer. This guaranteed that the fair skin became even fairer as the protective pigmentation diminished in successive generations.

The paleness of our Northern forebears was perpetuated by the power of those religions which designated as a moral sin the exposure of the human body. Greater emphasis on clothing became an adopted aspect of human life. Clothing thus took on a permanent role as part of man's shelter requirements.

Exposure of any part of the human body in public, except for hands and face, became a white man's taboo, contributing to a decline in his health. The comfort of the body also suffered as clothes became more and more physically restrictive. This aspect of human shelter grew to cater exclusively to appearances, involving the application of so many layers of garments over the body that it tended to take on a mummified appearance.

While restrictiveness and air-exclusion are required for corpse mummification, neither is anything but a handicap to the health of the living body. Bound by tourniquet-like, fashion-dominated clothing, with inadequate circulation of air to its skin, the human body declined further from its pristine condition of abundant health. Circulatory and skin disorders became more prevalent.

Gradually structural disorders increased as the bones were deprived of essential nutrients — in the form of composite reductions of available vitamin D and diet deficiencies of calcium and phosphorus. These effects were compounded by digestive limitations which increased as man's diet became more and more complex, less and less natural.

It never ceases to impress the observing mind how heroically the body struggles to adapt to changes of environment. With only the face and hands exposed for absorption of vitamin D, these portions of skin become so highly photosensitive that in less than an hour each day they can extract from the sunlight sufficient vitamin D to satisfy the minimum daily needs of the body.

Unfortunately, this minimum requirement became too little as man placed increased demands upon his nervous energy with tension which accompanied the world's industrialisation. The problem was further augmented as the same industrial demands created their characteristically heavy barrier of pollution which effectively filters the sun's ultraviolet rays.

Induced, perhaps, by the body's crying for more physical freedom, air and sunshine, Victorian prudishness gradually gave way under pressure of man's courageous discovery of sea and sand. Once our audacious grandparents sampled the invigoration, the unique enjoyment of bathing at the shore, their spirit of daring grew bolder.

As the body grew more open to general inspection, its possessors recognised that shape and colour were the qualities which attracted most attention. So a new health-consciousness was born as the fashion changed. Admiration for the "peaches and cream" look gave way to a fetish for suntans and their implications of greater vitality and virility.

In natural sequence, the advent of lighter clothing, both in weight and colour, presaged a general awakening to the vital, manifold benefits of sunshine in human life.

The demand for greater air circulation, light and brightness permeated throughout all human affairs. Most noticeable changes occurred in the transition of home construction with the timely employment of more extensive window areas, lighter colourings and outdoor gardens and recreational spaces. But by a curious paradox commercial buildings (inside which most people spend their daylight hours Monday to Friday) went into reverse gear in design. Fresh air was excluded as panels of fixed glass replaced opening windows and artificial air conditioning allowed everyone's carbon dioxide to be equally shared and excessive positive ions to be generated in the air.

Flushed with their successful dependence on the induced artificiality of electricity, building designers discovered more economy in removing windows altogether whenever possible. This created greater dependence on artificial light and exposed people to its tendency, in the case of fluorescent tubes, towards radiation emission. Little wonder that workers sought shorter hours as their eyes became more strained and their nerves more tensed.

It has been conclusively proved that when adequate sunshine and fresh air are denied man, he tends to become depressed and irritable. Wartime bomb shelters produced the first hint of this, but the lesson appears unrecognised if the actions of many modern architects are any criterion. They do not deserve the total blame, however, for they are reacting to the demands of greater "efficiency" in business and industry.

Mental Balance and Harmony

To the unbiased intelligence, it is obvious that all diseases are but manifestations of one basic cause: disharmony. Toxaemia is the known basis of pathological problems, but this can only be rectified when we understand the cause of toxaemia.

Some schools of human healing place too much emphasis on a treatment of the symptoms of disease, avoiding a rectification of its cause. Allegiance to such views effectively places blinkers on the intelligence, prohibiting an investigation of the broad view of human health, especially in regard to its fundamental requirements.

Some other schools of healing focus their remedial efforts on the structural (nerve) or nutritional (chemical) foundations of illness. In so doing, their rate of success is significantly higher than when treatment is directed only towards the symptoms. Even so, the increasing complexity of human life is such as to reveal that permanent rectification of ill health can rarely be achieved unless root causes are discovered and normalised.

A prevailing condition of abnormality will always create reactions of bodily discomfort for the purpose of drawing attention to the need for restoring harmony. The longer the attention is withheld, the more intense the discomfort.

Short-sighted attempts to remedy the discomfort without attention to the cause will always result in the development of further illnesses of a recurring nature or in other weakened parts of the body.

Man maintains a unique relationship to all other life by virtue of his almost limitless power of creativity and adaptability. With a significant degree of command over his affairs, man creates most of his situations in life. The degree to which these situations harmonise with his purpose and being will determine the nature of his success as well as the condition of his health. Man is thus in greater command of his life than is conventionally accepted — the use or abuse of his power being no more forcefully apparent than in his condition of health.

One of the greatest lessons in human life is for man to develop the ability to adjust to the vast range of environmental influences. This demands keen awareness so that constant mental balance guides his activities. Only in this manner can man achieve and maintain that state of harmony which guarantees success and happiness, the rewards of wise living.

The secret of man's success will be measured by the degree of harmony between his ideals and his actions, between awareness and expression. This is the art and science of natural living, vital aspects of the requirements for good health.

Correct Food

The famous English librettist and humorist, W.S. Gilbert, once said something to the effect that it was not that which was upon the table that mattered as much as that which was upon the chair.

The intimate relationship between diet and health is an aspect of life which is becoming more and more accepted in circles which once attributed health almost exclusively to the whims of capricious germs. The next stage in this unfolding awareness is the realisation that diet is all too frequently the result of habit, rather than conscious choice guided by an understanding of the body's needs. Such needs rarely succeed in the battle of choices against man's whims of addiction.

In spite of the huge variety of fresh foods available to man, his choice is invariably distracted from the natural to processed offerings promoted by extensive and expensive advertising. These offer a limited variety to a diet which has basically evolved from the eating habits of the parents.

Conventional dietary habits are more restrictive than their adherents realise. This is the consequence of food being ignorantly relegated to a place of minor importance to human health. So long as its function is considered to be satisfied if sufficient enjoyment, satiety and energy are the results, the inclusion of only correct foods for man in his daily dietary will continue to be ignored. Indeed, enjoyment is an essential aspect of diet, but the ability of that diet to provide a balanced selection of essential nutrients must rate for equal consideration in its composition.

Consideration of diet is generally limited to its immediate effects. If it provides energy, most people are satisfied, yet they fail to realise the importance of the quality of that energy and what residues it might produce.

Few people would consider buying a new automobile for many thousands of dollars, then skinflinting for a few cents to run it on a fuel inferior to that for which it was designed. They know that by so doing, their precious possession will still run, but with less power, efficiency and comfort. Inferior fuel will also result in the accumulation of excessive residues, inducing excessive wear on all moving parts. So, too, with the human body.

The car can be replaced. Not so the body. Many surgeons are constantly called upon to replace certain organs (invariably without working to rectify the cause of collapse of the original), yet the body never functions as well as with a set of healthy original organs.

The appearance and performance of the human body is always directly responsive to the suitability and quality of its diet, both in the long and short terms. The texture and appearance of the skin is no less dependent on dietary nutrients than are vitality, virility, endurance and elimination. What we eat becomes our very appearance and mode of expression, with a vital influence on our state of happiness. The responsibility for our actions must commence with our thoughts and the determination of what, when and how we eat. The body's power of adaptability is by no means limitless and will accept just so much abuse before registering strong disapproval.

Man's choice of correct food is simple. The soil produces it; man has only to employ his faculty of discrimination to choose suitable products.

Not everything produced from the soil is suitable for man's diet. Certain plants possess poisons or irritants which can be most harmful to the delicate gastrointestinal tract. But it is not difficult to learn which these are, recognising that reliance upon suitable fruits, vegetables, nuts, seeds and grains provides a very extensive choice, far more than most people enjoy on the conventional diet revolving around animal meats and bread.

The methods by which food is grown are determinants in its nutritional quality; so too is the stage at which the food is harvested and its method of storage. Once selected, the food must then be prepared in the most nutritious manner, combined with other ingredients in the diet for easiest digestion and eaten in the most harmonious environment. These factors all contribute to correct food comprising the ideal diet.

The avoidance of unnatural substances in the diet cannot be too highly stressed. Refined sugars, flours and starches as well as chemical additives, strong herbs and spices commence their trail of damage by stimulating false appetites and inducing overeating (especially pernicious when unsuitable foods are gormandised). Irritation, with eventual ulceration of the gastrointestinal tract, is a regular result of the modern diet, testifying forcefully to its unsuitability.

A balanced diet of natural foods will provide all the nutrients required by the body. It will be abundant in delicious flavours and perfumes, creating pleasure for the taste buds as the natural sugars and mineral salts give advice of their presence. The correct diet for man requires no false inducements to satisfy the appetite — unnatural appetite stimulations are the spices of gluttony.

Fasting

In the ancient teachings of esoteric numerology, the number seven represents learning by experience and is the symbol of sacrifice. It is no coincidence that the seventh essential ingredient of health is that which involves the body and mind in the process of "giving up", of total rest called "fasting".

Just as the plan for creative, healthy living is of nature, so too is there a plan for correcting, for normalising any tendency which has departed from the natural.

The remedy for such undesirable effects is a reversal of habit known as "fasting". It is the process of total physiological and mental rest, one which is known and practised by all forms of life in time of need. Man alone refuses to acknowledge such a simple, natural, corrective plan, preferring to persist with the pattern which created the illness or abnormality and resort to oral palliatives in vain efforts at relief.

Complete fasting implies a totally subjective state of doing nothing. It is a combination of total rest and abstinence from any food or stimulation, water being the only intake. Fasting is not a system of restrictive diets, such as the "grape fast" or "juice fast", when only grapes or juices are consumed for a certain period of time. It is no more possible to undertake a partial fast than it is to dig a partial hole.

Fasting can be employed for an almost endless list of reasons, be they physical or metaphysical. It will restore one's appetite for food and pleasure; sharpen the senses; revitalise the memory, vigour and virility; normalise the emotions; clear the skin, eyes and thoughts; and, more surprisingly, develop one's powers of awareness by clearing away the dross which accumulates in most heads. Fasting is nature's great gift of recuperation to man, demanding of him no effort except to find a place to rest in comfort and peace. The more complete the rest, the more beneficial the fast and the shorter need be its duration.

Limitations of fasting are incurred when disease has reached a stage of irreversibility so that the body no longer possesses any reserves of energy. This advanced state of degeneration is rarely incurred, but when it is an investigation into the patient's history will always reveal a long trail of abuses, compounded by drugging and surgery. Yet, even under such conditions of near hopelessness, some measure of benefit can be achieved as the fast minimises pain such that the end becomes more endurable. Undertaking a fast will cause no added complications, but will certainly delay the arrival of the undertaker.

Being the simplest solution to most pathological and psychological problems, fasting is usually the last to be considered. Such is the nature of the complexity to which modern humans have been conditioned in their living habits. For mental and emotional disturbances, illness or recovery from injury, fasting is the ideal remedy and the only one offered by nature. For changing diet or losing weight, fasting also provides the ideal solution. For the development of increased psychic faculties and the improvement of memory, fasting offers guaranteed benefits. And while all these purposes are being achieved through fasting, so too is bodily toxicity being reduced with the bonus of significant health improvement.

Fasting proves the wisdom of the modified proverb: "Abstinence makes the heart grow stronger."

Exercise and Activity

In Washington, London and Canberra, it is said that politicians are learning to exercise with yoga. This is the only way they can sit on the fence and keep both ears to the ground!

For the purpose of teaching correct living, it is necessary to differentiate between exercise and activity. While both are important in that they involve the body in vital physical movement, they vary in degree, benefit and time. Both employ the body in voluntary movement. Activity uses the body to a limited degree and generally to achieve another purpose. Exercise employs the body over the widest possible range of movement for the particular purpose of maintaining or acquiring muscle tone and control with maximum joint flexibility.

When man lived in a simpler, natural manner, his body was engaged in a wide variety of such activities as to make the need for supplementary exercise almost unnecessary. His farming methods were not simplified by machinery; he had to fell trees prior to building shelters; to climb, bend and stretch far more than is required today.

As the employment of machinery grew more widespread, so did the waistline of man. Although he employed his brain more, man's muscles were needed less. He thus became indolent and fat. This gave rise to the vital need for supplementary exercises being incorporated in man's programme of living to enable his body to be maintained in a state of optimum fitness.

Activity requires less physical effort and often little conscious effort, once the routine has been established. Exercise demands considerable physical effort and is the more beneficial to the degree that mental concentration is simultaneously employed.

Many of my patients tell me they "get plenty of exercise". They walk, play golf, have lots of housework to do, work on the waterfront, swim in their pool occasionally and some even play table tennis. None of these classifies as exercise. The participants rarely get breathless, employ one side of their body more than the other, use their joints over a limited degree of movement and their muscles over a limited range of contraction and expansion. What they have been doing are activities, not exercises, engaging in the activities either for casual fun, as part of a work programme to achieve a desired conclusion or competitive games designed for winning.

By contrast, exercise is vigorous with concentrated intention. Rather than being pursued for the outcome, the desired result is the actual involvement in the exercise for the flexibility, strength and endurance it develops while it takes place and between it and the next exercise period. The fun is one's attitude towards exercise and this directly produces greater benefits.

Activities are important, but so is exercise. The two work ideally together.

Competitive sports can often be regarded more as activities than exercise; but the training for them is usually very much exercise oriented. Calisthenics, gymnastics, distance or fast swimming, competitive cycling and athletics, etc, are good examples of exercises, but by themselves are not sufficient for the body to maintain total physical toning and flexibility. Each muscle group and joint needs to be included in a complete exercise programme, so those which are inadequately exercised by the particular mode employed need to be supplemented by other appropriate exercises.

Many people regard cycling, for example, as a good exercise. It can be that, but it does almost nothing for the upper body. So a suitable exercise programme for a cyclist would include a weight-lifting or isometric routine for the chest, arms and shoulders, plus abdominal exercises on the slant board, or similar. A competitive golfer or tennis player should concentrate supplementary exercises towards the opposite side of their body to that used in the sport.

A suitable and comprehensive exercise programme for each person should be tailored to their individual needs and lifestyle. It should embrace, in general, three primary styles — calisthenics, flexibility exercises and muscle-toning exercises. There should never be any strain, but there should be adequate stretching and muscular expansion and contraction.

Many variations to this theme are possible, but a wisely chosen programme should be undertaken at a regular time each day or, as a minimum, every second day. Different lifestyles dictate different preferences, but the most suitable time of day to exercise is usually the morning, before breakfast.

Exercise is always best performed when the stomach is empty, but after adequate warming-up has been undertaken. This will certainly help the day commence with improved vitality, dispelling that feeling of morning blues which is so common among under-exercised people. For those people to whom the morning is unsuitable, early evening, before dinner, is perhaps their most suitable time, especially if they have been engaged in intense mental work while sitting most of the day.

Every effort should be made to exercise in the morning. If it means getting up half an hour earlier to make adequate time, then get to bed half an hour earlier (most people go to bed far too late, preferring to sit in front of that addictive square-eyed monster and be entertained with inane insults to the intelligence). After getting out of bed and completing one's teeth, scalp and skin brushing, exercise time is at hand. Yet never overlook the importance of brushing the scalp and the skin — they are just as vital as brushing the teeth. Most women already recognise the importance of hair brushing, but scalp brushing is the deeper activity of maintaining the skin's flexibility over an area which gets insufficient sun or massage.

Ideal for scalp massage is the round, plastic massager which can usually be purchased at the chemist or supermarket for around fifty cents. Bend the body over the bath tub or into the shower recess so the head is lower than the heart. This helps the blood to flow into the scalp region, where the brushing will induce some worthwhile stimulation. Brush for a few minutes thoroughly over the scalp, then use the fingers to move the scalp by applying pressure in all parts consecutively. Follow this by vigorously massaging the scalp with the fingers. Then stand upright and brush the hair into place. This early morning routine will be your best insurance against dandruff and baldness, keeping the scalp flexible enough for the hair to luxuriate through the follicles — the fact that people talk a lot keeps the follicles of the jaw flexible, ensuring that the face never goes bald!

Follow the scalp massage and hair brushing with a vigorous brushing of the skin. Use a pure bristle, dry skin brush on a detachable handle. They are available at most health food stores. Remove all clothes and brush the skin all over the body — using the brush on the handle for your back, removing the handle to use the brush in your hand for all other parts. Apply just sufficient pressure to ensure the skin receives good toning, but not so that it hurts. This will help keep the skin soft, smooth and flexible — just as important for men as for women.

After that five to ten minutes of vital skin and scalp toning, you are ready to undertake your warm-up exercises. Running, cycling, swimming, calisthenics or whatever mode suits you and your location will contribute to getting the blood flowing freely through the body. Spend a few minutes warming-up and when you get breathless, go straight into deep breathing. This will further improve blood circulation and will, most importantly, oxygenate the blood to vitally aid its purification and energy distribution processes. It will also clear from the lungs the accumulated carbon dioxide which always resides in the lower lungs during shallow breathing (especially during sleep). This regular extension of the lungs and rib cage will significantly improve posture, breathing and endurance. Always remember that when deep breathing, inhale through the nose with mouth closed; exhale through the open mouth.

The body is then ready for some stretching and mobility exercises. Hatha yoga is extremely adaptable to these exercise needs; it is that practice of the ancient Hindu philosophy which concentrates on the development of body flexibility and its mental control. Hatha yoga offers many suitable postures (asanas) to achieve suppleness, balance and an attractive figure, but care has to be taken to employ such movements with wisdom as they are designed for the light-framed, slower-moving Eastern anatomy. It is this writer's opinion, one proved by years of teaching and practice, that yoga should be modified to Western needs by reducing the period during which a posture is held, to approximately ten seconds. It is also wise to alternate a yoga posture with a dynamic stretching exercise to give a balanced programme.

The final aspect of the balanced exercise programme should involve muscle-toning exercises. These can embrace moderate weight-training, isometric movements or dynamic body movements. Weight-training should employ adequate weights for resistance to muscle contraction so that eight to ten repetitions can be achieved with each exercise using either a bar or a set of dumbbells. Isometrics are static exercises which pit one set of muscles against a corresponding set, one used in contraction, the other in expansion until an equilibrium is reached when both sets are at equal tension. This position is held with a deep breath for up to eight seconds, then released slowly.

A deep breath should be taken prior to any exercise being performed, as a means of providing plenty of oxygen and to support the diaphragm. For this reason, it is wise to exercise in an atmosphere of clean, fresh air.

Dynamic body exercises include the well-known push-ups, deep knee bends, abdominal raises (for which a slant board is most suitable, otherwise over the end of a bed with feet held firmly) and the like. A high, horizontal bar is also amply suited to body exercising, being ideal for chinning movements as well as stretching.

Exercises for muscle tone are intended to improve blood circulation so that energy can be swiftly taken to the muscle region and residues of muscle action rapidly removed. As well as improving bodily strength, this will greatly assist in maintaining a good temperature equilibrium in the body during times of atmospheric extremes. Remember, it is the efficiency of blood circulation, *not* abundant fat, which ensures warmth in winter and coolness in summer. The body does not require excessive fat insulation, it needs blood circulation for efficient functioning and temperature control.

A complete exercise programme would include specific exercises for the toning of each major muscle group. Especially important are the abdominal muscles, for they are at the centre of the body's movements. This is vital for women, for if they were to maintain good muscle tone in the abdominal region, their chances of requiring major internal surgery in later years would be greatly minimised. If time does not permit a programme which covers all muscle groups, plan your exercises so that over a two- or three-day period full coverage is achieved, exercising upper body one day, lower body next.

Everyone needs to exercise. Women need never worry about acquiring bulging muscles, for such is the nature of the female body that only attractive curves will result. Exercise will provide instant energy when required, strength in reserve for almost any need and an excellent blood circulation and nutrient appropriation.

Exercise requires time. Therefore, it is wise to go to bed just that much earlier each night, allowing the earlier rising next morning for a regular programme — it is the ideal way to say "good morning". A good exercise programme is an indispensable part of healthful living and is much more than jumping to conclusions and running up accounts!

STAGE FOUR

Let's Be In Tune

To love, to laugh, to run and be free
Are the joys of life and attune you and me.

In tune with what? In tune with ourselves, with our environment, with our associates, in tune with all life — this is what we need to achieve. Of primary importance is that the body and psyche are attuned, for without this, everything in life is dull.

Many people pass through life with a closed mind and an open mouth. The purpose of wise education is to reverse this condition, for it is never too late to start, or restart, learning.

Scientific advances in our age have been remarkable for their improvement of the physical well-being of mankind and equally remarkable for their ignorance of man's psychical needs. Consequently a state of serious imbalance has been created in which physical progress has greatly outstripped the spiritual.

With material concerns occupying so much of man's consciousness, it must come to him as a great shock to learn that more powerful forces exist beyond the physical which exert far greater influence over his life. By their nature, these forces are called "metaphysical", for they are, literally, beyond the physical. Not readily detectable by the physical sense organs, their influence on man's physical being is nevertheless vast and significant.

The Essence of Life

Let us suppose, for a crazy moment, that man consisted only of a physical body. He would not be able to reason; he would be devoid of emotions, of ideals, of ethics. He would be unable to create, his actions being nothing more than responses to external stimuli — they would be reactions only. Man would thus exist only to procreate, to eat and to engage in whatever immediate activities he could find, for reasons he would not understand.

But this does not describe man, nor does it describe any of the higher animals. To experience pleasures, pride, ideals and emotions is to acknowledge that man is far more than a physical being, for these are metaphysical functions. To go even further and recognise that man has a brilliant intelligence by which he can create from abstract ideas, by which he can deduce conclusions from remote experiences, is to confirm that great power is associated with the metaphysical components of being.

Again, when we note the apparent extrasensory powers of some, more adept, humans, we are made aware of the great potential which remains largely untapped. Unfortunately, such potential attracts comparatively little interest in scientific circles; indeed, many academicians are inclined to ignore its very existence, even to ridicule it.

To limit one's understanding of life to the physical is to ignore the very essence of being.

As age and wisdom develop, man's earlier years of virile urges for procreation and diversion should moderate and translate into vibrant powers of creativity. This natural transition distinguishes man from all other animals. Every creature has the desire to live — man alone possesses the creative potential to improve the quality of his life, to understand its purpose and to guide others on their paths.

This is the expression of man's *psyche*, a term derived from the old Greek verb meaning "to breathe". Psyche, therefore, implies the life force in man, the very essence of his being, the "I am".

Man can choose to ignore his psychic abilities or to cultivate them. To ignore them is to create a state of imbalance or disharmony, caused by too much emphasis on the physical forces in life. To cultivate one's psychic forces in conjunction with the physical is to achieve balance and harmony, to gain attunement. By such means, man can acquire a mastery of life which is rare in this materialistic society, but which will characterise the coming New Age.

Even now some aspects of this new age are beginning to be realised. Important among these is the recognition that life must revert to the natural, become again a simple, balanced fulfilment, free of the complications which over recent years have enslaved man to industrial avarice.

As man grows in psychic awareness, understanding will replace fear and love will oust envy. A developing knowledge of the finer forces of life will take man's understanding into higher realms; he will replace his fear of death with an understanding of what lies beyond. Man will see his purpose more clearly and be able to better develop his ability to more successfully fulfil that purpose. His thoughts will always be constructive and compassionate, and sickness will diminish in rapid retreat as natural living patterns determine his habits.

Call this prophetic, call it wishful thinking, call it "hogwash", call it what you will. That is the prerogative of human individuality. But realise that by your attitude shall you be known, if only to yourself! Attitudes do not alter facts; attitudes are only the way we interpret facts.

Where Is the Psyche?

There are narrow and well-defined limits to the detection ability of each of our physical organs. Ears, eyes, nose, brain, fingers, tongue, etc can each recognise specific rates of vibration, but only over a narrow band-width, termed the frequency spectrum.

"Vibration" is the movement of energy through a medium or space. Vibrations basically vary from each other by force (amplitude) and frequency, which is measured by a rate of cycles per second.

Human ears can generally detect sounds which vibrate at rates between 16 and 16,000 cycles per second. The human brain emits vibrations of around eight to ten cycles per second, a range not detectable by the ear. At the other end of the scale, it is known that dogs can hear sounds in excess of the human upper limit and it is probable that some other animals share this faculty.

Rates of vibration detectable by the eyes and nose are very much higher in frequency than the audible. The following scale of frequencies shows some uses to which science has already put some of these vibrations. It also shows the light and perfume rates, as well as those vibrations emitted by chemicals. But notice those band widths which contain waves of unknown nature, the higher ones going on *ad infinitum*.

Space does not permit every octave to be shown. Omitted are those within the ranges already defined by their upper and lower frequencies.

With his limitless ingenuity, man has utilised most of the frequencies to transmit messages or as power for physical purposes. But what of the many frequencies of the spectrum already in use by man for communication of a metaphysical nature?

To understand the psyche, we must expand our physical awareness. Important in this regard is the understanding of the emotions, of the nervous system and of the brain. A basic knowledge of electricity is of great value here, for nerve impulses function in much the same manner. Neither space nor the intent of this book will permit this subject to be expanded here as I would like. However, a subsequent book is planned in which this vital aspect of life (and life after death) will be the theme.

For now, let me suggest to the reader that many excellent popular books are available to provide a guide to the human essence of life, the psyche. Books such as *The Afterdeath Journal of an American Philosopher* by Jane Roberts (Prentice-Hall, New Jersey, 1978), *Journeys Out of the Body* by Robert Monroe (Anchor Press/Doubleday, New York, 1977), *Many Mansions* by Gina Cerminara (New American Library, New York, 1967), *Life After Life* and its sequel, *Reflections on Life After Life*, both by Dr Raymond Moody (Stackpole Books, Harrisburg, USA, 1975 and 1977 respectively) and many similar books offer a wealth of information giving clues to the expression of the psyche in its many facets. My recent best-selling publication *Secrets of the Inner Self* (Angus & Robertson Publishers, Sydney, 1980) offers some of the most unusual aspects of the psyche and how it relates to others and to life's circumstances to provide vital lessons in human evolution.

The presence of these and similar books on best-selling lists attests that emerging New Age awareness is far more influential now than declining Middle Age narrowness. But the transition is a very recent one, barely twenty years old. Such books would never have been popular in the 1950s. In fact, in the early 1960s when I commenced teaching psychic development through improved nutrition, classes were very small, rarely over ten in number. Now, the interest is so encouraging that classes have become seminars of up to forty students, many booking over two months in advance.

Rocketing interest in human self-awareness is restoring to man a level of understanding virtually unknown for 2500 years. Not since the days of the Pythagorean University at Crotona, when Western culture had its birth, has there been so much growth away from the spiritual tourniquet which has, for centuries past, engendered fear, ignorance and misunderstanding. Thus have confining prejudices so stifled the progress of man through his religious and scientific development that only those "acceptable" phases of belief and discovery were, until very recently, allowed voice. But religion and science are both yielding to the pressure of modern man's craving for *total* knowledge. No longer are blind faith and materialistic science acceptable. They are too limited, found far too wanting. They have certainly proved incapable of guiding man to the happiness to which he should surely be entitled after all these centuries of "progress".

Since the Middle Ages, history has revealed many scientists who have dared to be different. Those who sought to reveal truth through scientific revelations, who sought to guide mankind to a better life through an improved understanding of himself and his universe, have been cruelly victimised for their efforts. Galileo Galilei, Leonardo da Vinci, Copernicus and Christopher Columbus were all considered crackpots by the "authorities" of their day because they dared to embrace lateral thinking, dared to question established science. But such constraining parochialism did not end with the development of the Industrial Revolution.

Many scientific and religious bodies, outwardly most respected even today, fail to recognise their prejudices when condemning conclusions of intelligent people whose investigations have revealed a totally different solution to that expected by other researchers. When orthodox bodies feel their prestige threatened, they respond like a cornered animal by reacting viciously, intimidatingly or in any way to justify their prevailing prejudices. Such actions are neither scientific nor honourable and therefore have no place in genuine science or religion.

Modern victims of such prejudices are Dr Linus Pauling, Dr Herbert Shelton and Dr Abram Hoffer, to name but a few. Dr Pauling, although a dual Nobel Prize winner, has been regularly criticised for his discovery relating vitamin C to the common cold. Dr Shelton, although, like Pauling, not a medical practitioner, has helped thousands of patients recover from terminal cancer and arthritis by supervised fasting and improved nutrition; yet his health school in Texas has been closed. Dr Hoffer has been the world's most successful megavitamin practitioner with thousands of cases of previously incurable schizophrenia, multiple sclerosis, etc., rectified under his treatment of massive doses of suitable vitamins (he *is* a medical practitioner as well as a nutritionist).

Energy Frequencies as Registered in Cycles per Second

Cycles per second (c.p.s.)

The fundamental frequency	1	
1st Octave	2	Animal and human bodily vibrations
2nd "	4	
3rd "	8	
4th "	16	Audible sound
5th "	32	[Middle C is approximately
8th "	256	252 c.p.s.–261 c.p.s. (it is usually
14th "	16,384	256 c.p.s.)]
19th "	524,288	Radio transmission — 550,000–
20th "	1,048,576	1,650,000 c.p.s. on "medium wave
21st "	2,097,052	broadcast frequencies"
25th "	33,554,432	Electronic transmission — television,
28th "	268,435,456	radar, etc.
35th "	34,359,738,368	
40th "	1,099,511,627,776	UNKNOWN
45th "	35,184,372,088,832	
46th "	70,368,744,177,664	Heat — infra-red spectrum
48th "	281,474,976,710,656	
49th "	562,949,953,421,312	Light — colour spectrum
50th "	1,125,899,906,842,624	Chemical rays — ultraviolet spectrum
51st "	2,251,799,813,685,248	Perfumes — smell spectrum
57th "	144,115,188,075,855,872	
58th "	288,230,376,151,711,744	X-rays
60th "	1,152,921,504,606,846,976	
61st "	2,305,843,009,213,693,952	
62nd "	4,611,686,618,427,389,904	UNKNOWN
63rd "	9,223,373,236,854,779,808	

But, dare it be said that colds, cancer, arthritis, multiple sclerosis, etc: are not supposed to be curable — maybe if such cures became regular, too much surgical and drug-based income would be lost!

If these and other pioneer health practitioners find difficulty in having their successful diagnoses and practices recognised by the orthodox associations now appearing to control health practice, how much more difficult is it for people at large to accept them? Theoretically, such acceptance is thwarted by the destructive propaganda of the associations. Yet the many thousands, probably millions, of people aided back to health by simple, natural techniques as described above, plus their friends and associates, have no problem in attesting to the efficacy of these new systems.

With shock treatment rarely effective, often injurious and no longer needed to be inflicted upon poor sufferers of schizophrenia, their recovery of health will allow the *causes* of the disease to be self-investigated and remedied. Their responses to suitably prescribed and administered large doses of particular vitamins (generally B_3 and C) allow schizophrenics to recover their health naturally — without (and this is vitally important) damaging side effects. But it must be realised that it was not the lack of these vitamins which created their problem. Such remedy primarily helps the body physiologically recover its natural chemical balance after being so critically disturbed by the illness.

What induced the illness of schizophrenia is the same general factor found to induce all bodily ills — disharmony. Disharmony in one's physical habits when they conflict with the natural is a major cause of ill health. The other major cause is disharmony between one's body and psyche, erupting from emotional disturbances.

Human emotions are very real. No one has ever seen them, any more than they have ever seen electricity (we recognise its presence by lamps being lit, elements being heated, etc.). And everyone recognises emotions because they produce in our body certain reactions. It is these reactions which produce the disharmony, the out-of-phase condition between body and psyche which induces physical "dis-ease".

So we see the psyche as the non-physical (metaphysical) component of a being wherein dwell the feelings, the innate understanding which transcends mere logic, the connection with the Creator which man cannot and has not lost. All he can ever lose is his awareness of that infinite connection; and when he does suffer this ignorance, it is as a consequence of his disharmonious emotions.

Emotions must now be seen as the psyche's responses to the body's environment. They are largely reactive responses to memories of the past (usually hurts and disappointments), anxieties of the future (often based on distorted memories of the past) or present tensions created by reacting to external pressures. These emotions should be balanced (and *are* in the healthy person) by joy and happiness — the emotional responses of attuned success. Then harmony is restored and we become balanced, centred.

The psyche is normally in harmony with the body, disharmony being created not by facts but by our attitudes to them. Then, the psyche is thrown out of phase with the body, thereby unbalancing the body's nervous system, chemistry and digestion. The ill health which follows can be temporarily relieved by palliatives administered as physiological treatment, but only permanently relieved by going direct to the cause, by understanding the nature of the disharmony.

Using the Psyche

To some extent, we all possess psychic awareness. Whether it manifests through the emotions, feelings, thoughts or, most reliably, intuition. As we mature in wisdom, we learn to place more reliability upon our intuition, for it is the key to limitless understanding and maximum fulfilment in life.

Intuition is the very first impression of a situation, circumstance or person. It is the instant awareness which precedes thought. Once thought comes into play, the mind has taken charge and evaluates within the limited range of its conscious knowledge. Intuition has no such limitation, for it perceives what is, rather than what we *think* is. How the intuition is interpreted and applied must then be related to thought, but take care that thought does not rationalise to negate the intuition if the intuited message does not come within the parameters of your existing knowledge. For instance, in practice we are often guided by our intuition into the probable cause of the disease symptoms for which the patient has come to seek relief. Tests and checks might not be able to prove the intuited "hunch". But that is no reason to dismiss it — many a time we have found that to do so is to neglect the cause, resulting in a treatment which might not be the best possible.

Surprising to many within the healing professions was the publication of Dr Shafica Karagulla's fascinating and well-researched book, *Breakthrough to Creativity* (DeVorss & Co, Santa Monica, California, 1967). A qualified medical practitioner, Dr Karagulla reports her investigation of the growing application of psychic powers for diagnosing and treating within her own profession. She describes how certain medical practitioners and "sensitives" (psychic diagnosticians who work with the practitioner), see energy fields around patients. From a contraction or darkened colour in the energy field, a diagnosis of the illness can reliably be made. This can be especially valuable if surgery is required, for the "sensitive" can pin-point the exact location of the problem area, sometimes better than can an X-ray.

Some "sensitives" diagnose by finger touch, some feel sympathetic pains in their own bodies in exactly the area as that experienced by the patient. Others develop a rapid telepathic contact with their patients, thereby using the patient's own psyche to zero-in on the exact intensity and nature of the pain.

As unusual as this appears to many, especially those with orthodox scientific training, it is neither unnatural nor unscientific. No one doubts the validity of kirlian photography — the technique of obtaining regular photographs of energy fields surrounding inanimate objects, such as a leaf or piece of fruit, named after its discoverer, Semyon Davidovich Kirlian. Energy fields surrounding human hands are also regularly photographed by kirlian means. So if a camera can do it with special adaptation, why is it so unacceptable that the human eye or consciousness can be as adaptable? Certainly, such a faculty requires a range of receptivity over a wider spectrum than is normally utilised by man, but then the development of most extended faculties requires some training. (Some children are born with natural athletic ability and can easily run a mile swiftly; others have to train hard to achieve the same result.)

Those of us who have developed certain psychic abilities know how reliable they are. Others who have no such intimate experience can only accept — or not. But eventually everyone will accept that they possess some psychic ability: it is the only way they receive "hunches". And how many have realised that not to follow a hunch is to miss something very worthwhile in their life? We have all done that.

Fear of the Psychic

Let us return for a moment to Dr Karagulla's book, *Breakthrough to Creativity*. Here we uncover a perfect series of examples of the limitations placed on human understanding by humans who do not understand. We see that many eminent practitioners recognise and employ their special psychic abilities with success, yet they elect to remain anonymous. They fear both ridicule from fellow practitioners and expulsion from their profession for "unprofessional practice".

The extent to which the unknown is feared is the extent to which limitation is placed on human understanding and growth. When practitioners cannot openly discuss their proven diagnostic methods, they have no forum in which to expand their techniques. If they continue to rely solely on their personal experience, limitations must surely arise. The intent of a professional association is somewhat negated when its members are denied expression of those professional activities which do not conform to established and previously accepted patterns. In this manner, the association declines from staleness, becomes introverted, eventually losing membership and credibility. Meanwhile, other, more progressive associations emerge to cater for the sharing and development of any worthwhile professional activities of its members. This has been witnessed in Australia in the past decade with the formation and rapid growth of the Doctors Reform Society whose magazine, *The New Doctor*, even publishes worthwhile contributions from non-medical doctors.

Medical doctors, no less than any other healing professionals, constantly employ their intuition by acting upon "hunches" while diagnosing their patients' problems. Yet few are conscious of this psychic faculty in use. Religious ministers make constant use of their intuition, as well as their faith and loving concern in their parish and counselling work; but few would give credit to their psychic awareness or the psyche in action. Scientists, in every varied discipline, rely on their psyche for guidance in their research work. Investors, especially punters, are guided quite extensively by "hunches", often expressing deep faith in their intuition. This applies to virtually every profession and many occupations (unless they are of a production line nature), yet few recognise it is their psyche in action.

Perhaps the fear of the psychic is related to unpleasant experiences with people who have been reputedly psychic. Or maybe they have heard about others who had such experiences. In any profession or any type of activity will be found the occasional person who exploits it and gives it a bad name. Such people of low character do more eventual harm to themselves by their egocentric thoughtlessness, for their actions are the exception, rather than the rule.

The employment of psychic faculties is as natural as eating, talking or sleeping. Eating and talking are human activities which have to be learned and studied for best functioning. Sleeping comes naturally. It is a vital part of our lifestyle and causes us to become unconscious for up to a full third of our lifetime on this planet. Yet, although it is the most natural thing we do, sleeping is also the most psychic.

We go to bed each night and willingly allow ourselves to become unconscious. We have total faith that we will awaken next morning. This we generally do with total ease, quite automatically. We go to bed fatigued, awaken refreshed. Few people understand how we innervate during the night, how the body can lie so dormant and the psyche be sent into higher planes of existence to recharge and return to reactivate the physical vehicle through which it expresses.

Our undertakings during sleep make a more fascinating story than ever Agatha Christie has conceived and, in fact, this story will be part of my forthcoming book on life after death. For sleep is a mini-death, a vital psychic experience for everyone. It is very healthy and presents no fear.

STAGE FIVE

The Pythagorean Ideal

Carefully consider before you act.
You may not be able to retract.
Understand well all that you do
And you will have no cause to rue.

From The Golden Verses of Pythagoras

Let no man act, but that he be prepared to accept total responsibility for his action. Every leader of men, every teacher, every parent should have this golden rule of action understood until it becomes an integral part of his very being. Only then will truth supplant falseness, wisdom replace rashness and life be the ideal existence which we now only see as a distant potential. This is the promise of the New Age.

It was a promise in a bygone age that life would return to the ideal. In fact, for a few years it did, in an exercise that suggested how exciting and rewarding life could be.

The system of living developed and guided into fruition 2500 years ago by the Greek philosopher, Pythagoras, exemplified a level of perfection and idealism unsurpassed in the recorded history of man. In those pre-industrial days, emphasis on materialism and the striving for luxury and power led to no less an imbalance than it does today. All too often, such motivations have been found at the root of human action; and education is no exception. Unbalanced teaching must lead to unbalanced living.

Balance, therefore, was a part of the Pythagorean ideal. During the early part of his own education, Pythagoras discovered that the secret of success in life lay in man's ability to develop his faculties in balance with each other and in harmony with nature and his environment. Consequently, the university he founded at Crotona offered a curriculum which would today be the envy of any true educationalist.

Crotona was a Greek colony located in southern Italy. History would have probably ignored Crotona, had not Pythagoras chosen it as the location for his university. So named for the universality of its teachings, both in content and in pupil selection, this university occupies a unique place in our history of education.

Never before had such a system of learning for enlightenment been offered. Based on the new concept of progressive development by qualifying through graduated classes, Pythagoras taught that man must first attain self-command. This stage of learning he called "Preparation", for it embraced the most fundamental of all learning techniques, self-discipline. It encompassed a series of ten stages (classes) through which the student progressively graduated, at the completion of which his preparation had been deemed complete.

The second major stage in the Pythagorean educational system was called "Purification". It embraced the study of the environment and the universe, based on the laws of nature and science, especially mathematics and number. It was probably equivalent to our current secondary education levels, for it prepared the aspiring student for his final major stage of learning, called "Perfection". This brought into focus an intimate knowledge of the esoteric laws and was that stage of his development from which man never graduated.

To Pythagoras, the time factor in education was of little relevance. Personal development must be a process of natural unfoldment, he would say. It must be as the opening of the rosebud, allowed to take place naturally, slowly and in time with the growth of the stem to support it. Forced opening would only damage the bud, resulting in its premature wilting.

The axiom which guided this mode of progressive learning was: "Man, know thyself; then thou shall know the Universe and God." This is the essence of philosophy. With this guiding principle, Pythagoras chose as his pupils all who were prepared to abandon material desires for the sake of discovering the secrets of their inner selves, by which to grow in understanding and wisdom. They then learned to share these special gifts with others that they might find the true meaning in life. He drew no distinction based on race, religion or sex, requiring only that the aspirant recognised the universality, the oneness of life, and be prepared to fulfil his role in it. With the same wisdom, Pythagoras selected teachers for special training from among the rapidly growing number of students in this unique learning establishment.

Never before had women been accepted as equal to men. Here was the very beginning of co-education, for Pythagoras recognised that women had just as much capacity to grow in understanding through education as did men. Such growth depended so much upon one's individual application to the teachings. As nothing was committed to writing in the Pythagorean school, understanding and knowledge came only by application and practice, followed by more application and more practice.

Pythagoras incarnated into this world as the human mind was again being prepared for emergence from another long period of intellectual darkness. When life was still largely barbaric and its purpose appearing as little more than physical gratification, the development of the Pythagorean school 2500 years ago was to herald a distinct break by introducing a period so unparalleled in human progress that history has come to entitle it "The Golden Age of Greece". An exciting new culture began to develop, for here came a leader who neither desired to enslave man nor conquer the world, but rather to free man by teaching him to master himself, achieve independence and develop his world.

This was the first real revolution. None has since been as important to the course of human history. Its outcome has been the development of Western culture.

Nearly half a century of studying, by travel, initiation and application had prepared Pythagoras for his special purpose. In search of knowledge, his path led him to Egypt and Babylon where, during a period of thirty-four years, Pythagoras underwent ten initiations into the great mystery systems of the world's master teachers. The system he ultimately developed thus became a synthesis of Egyptian, Judaic, Hindu, Chaldean and Zoroastrian teachings, tempered with his own special understanding of life's needs.

Pythagoras was a mere youth when encouraged by his parents to sail from their home on the island of Samos in search of greater knowledge. His first port of call was the famous city of Miletus in Asia Minor, a short Aegean journey to the coast of what is now Turkey. Here, his visit with sages Thales and Anaximander gave great encouragement to Pythagoras, for they soon recognised that the genius of their student outpaced even their capacity to teach. Pherecydes became his personal tutor.

Next to Egypt, where Pythagoras spent valuable years studying under the most difficult of all teachers, the priests of the ancient mystery schools whose knowledge and wisdom was legendary in the ancient world. Although Egypt possessed the secrets of the sciences, Babylon actually became the melting pot of all leading religious teachers of the time. Most notable among these was Daniel, the Jewish prophet of Old Testament fame, under whose influence Pythagoras developed a recognition of monotheistic principles and basic dietary laws.

His return to Samos found the civilisation in its death throes, his father dead and his mother eagerly awaiting his return. In 545 BC, Pythagoras attempted to establish a school to teach those profound principles of his philosophy but, after two years, recognised the futility of attempting to inject life back into a dying culture. Reluctantly, mother and son set sail for the Greek mainland, where they spent some years while Pythagoras underwent deeper studies, simultaneously training teachers from the large group of students he soon attracted at Delphi.

But Pythagoras recognised that Delphi was not the ideal centre for his ultimate school. Now in his mid-sixties, he selected Crotona, the Greek colony in southern Italy, as the site for receiving the fruits of his studious labours. Its liberal Doric constitution encouraged the development of the Pythagorean University, once its proposer revealed, by his genuineness and eloquent knowledge, the nature of the curriculum and how valuable it would be in uplifting the culture of that city. Little did the city fathers realise, when granting the Pythagorean University its constitution about 540 BC, how influential it would be in the development of the new enlightenment to become known as Western philosophy and bring to the world a legacy for which Crotona would be forever famous.

This new school of learning created spectacular interest as its fame spread throughout the Greek world and beyond. Crotona's citizens enthusiastically embraced the concept to provide an early nucleus. This surprised even Pythagoras; those who journeyed from Greece with him were astounded. The revolutionary new system of live-in, progressive, creative education had no precedent, but the world now appeared ready for such avant-garde guidance.

The Pythagorean system of teaching offered a totally new lifestyle which, to the uninitiated, appeared quite paradoxical. It inculcated friendship through the development of individuality, freedom by the application of discipline, self-knowledge through the understanding of mathematics. Number was taught, not as an impersonal science of measurement, but as a philosophy of concepts. Numbers as symbols of qualities became recognised as keystones to the understanding of life. (For more detailed information on the science of numbers as a vital key to self-knowledge, refer to the author's *Secrets of the Inner Self*, Angus & Robertson Publishers, Sydney, 1980.)

Pythagoras saw in mathematics a system of symbols by which the unknown became understood. This was esoteric mathematics, the counterpart of which was employed to solve measurement problems on an exoteric level. Hence the famed right-angled triangle theorem by which Pythagorean mathematics became most commonly known. Although this was merely an illustration of the deeper vibrational influence of numbers on life, it induced modern scientists to discover that Pythagoras was indeed the father of mathematics, of musical theory (by developing the octave as it is known today and by relating musical notes to frequency rates), of science (by developing the deductive system of analysis) and of nutrition (by studying food and relating it to human health). These achievements, together with that of being the world's first philosopher and educationalist provide those rare qualifications that entitle a human to the distinction of "genius".

It was the development of these sciences and their interrelation with each other and with all life that formed the expression of the Pythagorean ideal. Thus was man prepared for the emergence of the then New Age, the Piscean Age, heralded by the coming of Jesus the Christ.

It is this same ideal, transformed into the present, which forms the basis for modern man's emergence into the coming New Age, the Aquarian Age, with its probable heralding by another form of Christ leadership. The mode of present preparation is essentially no different — merely an adaptation of the Pythagorean concept of preparation by self-discipline to free the mind from ignorance.

Pythagoras conceived this preparatory training as a set of "Mathematical Disciplines": an organised system of preparedness by self-mastery. The disciplines were ten in number, *viz*:

1) Silence and meditation;
2) Mnemonics — memory and awareness;
3) Temperance — moderation in all things suitable;
4) Fortitude — strength and courage;
5) Philanthropy — love, compassion and friendship;
6) Erudition — learning, especially about one's environment;
7) Music — all aspects of harmony;
8) Dietetics and fasting — the essence of health;
9) Exercise and activity — for flexibility and vitality;
10) Method, order and efficiency.

Let us now discuss each of these disciplines.

Silence and Meditation

Worse than a child's fear of the darkness is an adult's fear of "the light". This is revealed in man's avoidance of truth in his life. It is no more apparent than in his fear of what I shall call "the silence".

A man would rather run a mile or chop a ton of wood; a woman would rather cook for an army or make all the beds in a hospital than spend twenty minutes entering the silence. Yet man must learn there is nothing to fear from the void created by the absence of physical distraction, for it will soon be filled by the sounds of silence, by the psychic experience of coming face to face with himself, with reality.

The silence is the only means whereby man can reliably detach himself from imagery, reactiveness and tension, coming to a peace through which reality becomes clearly separated from its opposite. It is the natural means of leading one on the path of self-investigation, for it brings back into synchronisation the psyche and the body, returning harmony and inner peace to one's total being.

During some parts of each day, man should practise a few minutes of turning inward, of entering the inner silence. This achieves best results when undertaken in conjunction with relaxation, as described earlier, for it allows man to recover the harmony which strong materialistic forces contrive to destroy.

To enter the silence and meditate requires no effort, other than the effort of will to let go of physical desires for a brief period. For many, this creates a fear of loss; yet would they only realise it, the temporary break will actually strengthen one's control over external influences and make involvement with them all the more enjoyable and rewarding. This applies to the entire range of physical expression, from sexual intercourse to intellectual discussion.

So long as one can achieve adequate privacy, the need to exclude noise when entering the silence becomes less important as one practises this simple art. Initially, any external distraction is conflicting; but as man masters the art of self-control, he reacts less to his environment.

Exotic positions for the body are not necessary. To enter the silence one does not require a mastery of the lotus position of yoga or a specially designed bed, either of which might or might not be helpful, depending on one's structural development. Easiest and simplest for all Westerners is the chair of suitable shape which will afford all the support required by the body.

A comfortable chair is one which is designed to the body's proportions, supporting it with least muscular tension. The feet should be allowed to rest flat on the floor; the thighs should be horizontal and supported uniformly over their length on the seat of the chair with adequate clearance behind the knees. The back of the chair should be very slightly sloped so that the spine is supported in an upright position, allowing for the scapulas (shoulder blades) to protrude beyond the line of the spine. The chair should be sufficiently padded to afford comfort, but not to the extent that it creates pressure points on the body. Sitting upright in such a chair will be greatly beneficial to one's entering the silence.

Stresses in modern living are so great that man must take care not to find himself constantly reacting to circumstances over which he has no control. Not only does this play havoc with one's emotions, but it also induces deleterious effects upon the nerves, muscles, digestion and sleep. Tension will enervate the body to the point where pockets of stiffness are created. These, in turn, will impede blood and lymph circulation, induce muscle spasm, occlude nerve energy flow, produce premature tiredness and, when compounded by years of habit, bring on premature old age.

Any of the foregoing physical impediments act to restrict expression. The mind needs freedom for its fluent expression through the body; any restrictions to that freedom, be they mentally or physically induced, produce frustrations, compounding the disharmony.

Considerably more energy is required to activate a machine which is out of proper running order. A sewing machine which has not been regularly lubricated is stiff and runs with jerky motions; an automobile engine out of tune requires more gas to run, exuding unwanted noise and vibration. Likewise the human body, when out of tune by lack of exercise, improper nutrition or pockets of stiffness, performs erratically and unreliably.

Such disharmony is reflected in various habits. The presence of a high-pitched voice, jerky speech, furrowed brow, irritability and fidgeting signify some measure of disharmony and also reveal an absence of adequate self-control and unfamiliarity with the silence.

Test yourself. Right now, direct your consciousness quickly over your body. How many of the foregoing symptoms do you now possess? Any fidgeting? muscles tense anywhere? legs crossed (evidencing insecurity, creating blockages)? jaw tight or brow furrowed? All reveal tension, running counter to relaxation, harmony and self-control. If this is you in any way, here is a simple way to relief:

Put down the book for ten minutes. Sit comfortably on your chair, as described previously, and close your eyes. Place hands on thighs, palms down. Concentrate all attention on the scalp. Feel any tension and tightness gradually ease. As the jaws relax, feel tightness run down past the temples; down the back of the neck as muscles relax and the head tilts forward ever so slightly. Tightness continues to run down through the shoulders, down the arms into the hands. Now in the fingers, tightness runs to the tips, then out into the atmosphere — feel the fingers relax as all tightness "pops out" and dissipates into the air.

Back to the chest; concentrate on the breathing. Take a deep breath and feel the chest drop as you exhale. Feel the shoulders droop slightly as tension runs down the back to the waist. Abdominal muscles now slacken as the diaphragm drops a little with tightness trickling into the pelvis. Feel the pelvis slacken into the chair as tightness departs and continues its downward run to the thighs.

Thighs are horizontal, so use a little mental force and push all vestiges of tension along into the knees. You can actually feel the knee-caps slacken! Tightness now runs down the legs and, as it does, both calves slacken. Into the ankles, then along the feet, tightness now runs into the toes, then out into the atmosphere. It feels like a dam wall has given way as the fast-flowing tensions "burst out" of all ten toes into the air to be dissipated and lost forever!

At complete ease, you now float through a cool forest where everything is red. As though wafting before a gentle breeze, you pass through the red into an area of orange. Colours change through the shades of the rainbow, orange giving way to yellow, to green, blue, indigo and then you arrive at the violet. Notice that your vision no longer seems fixed onto anything, but rather is vague; things appear obscure and no longer of any interest or importance. Violet fades into nothingness; you must be entering ultraviolet now as all sight disappears, all is perfect stillness. You have entered the silence, you are now nothing — and everything!

Time matters naught in the silence. When your body feels recharged, mind again takes over and you return through the colours to the stimulation of red. You are now back to consciousness, relaxed, yet alert. You feel and look years younger!

Memory and Awareness

How often have we struggled to remember something, vital to us at the time? Try as we might, it will not come. So we relax the brain and think of something else. Suddenly, as though a book has been opened at just the right page, what we had been racking the brain for previously, jumps into consciousness. We remember. But why didn't it come to us at the moment we needed it?

When you place a precious article in a safe place, you do so with a view to going directly to it when you want it. You are completely aware of its location and how to retrieve it. This is easier with a material possession than with the memory. Yet strange as it might seem, the same rules apply — focus it in mental vision and you stand every chance of retrieving it.

Just as we needed to remember the safe place in which we stored our precious article, so do we need to recognise that the memory system which works most effectively is that of cataloguing, of storing information in a manner by which we can have instant access. To ensure this, we must test ourselves immediately after we have filed it. Once a piece of new information is acquired and stored, return promptly to that store and retrieve it for use. Then return it to its catalogued position, having confidence in knowing exactly where it is.

This is best exemplified when meeting a stranger. Once the introduction is made, use the person's name in natural conversation two or three times at least. The name is generally one of the most pleasant sounds to the ear of its bearer, so do not be reserved about offering a little pleasure. As well as using the name, associate it with a picture useful in describing it (such as Mr Walker taking great strides over a meadow); for association is a natural part of conscious awareness.

Memory is thus linked to awareness, and awareness, as we have shown previously, is intelligence in action. The smoothness of its functioning depends upon one's degree of mental control. This, in turn, depends upon an unimpeded blood circulation and nerve-energy flow to the cerebral region.

Thoughts are very real things, so if one is to develop the memory, it must be realised that the brain demands nourishment to work properly no less than the voluntary muscles do when used for physical strength. A properly balanced diet will provide the required nutrients, but these can only be adequately appropriated when harmony prevails in one's affairs.

When wisdom is exercised in discrimination towards all things, our awareness is directed towards the more important, away from the less important. The unimportant has already been discarded — that went in those experimental days, with our wild youth. As such, we recognise thoughts of negativeness, destructiveness or worry as reactions which confuse our understanding and actually demand of the brain more energy than does creativeness. For confusion never acts in a straight line; it is always running around in ever diminishing circles until it tightens into an emotional constriction. There you have the basic ingredient for an ulcer or blood clot — health impediments born of confusion, nurtured by worry.

Some people are blessed with more active memories than others. Similarly, some people are born with greater potential strength in their muscles. Unless used, neither virtue will imply any advantage. Meanwhile, those with less natural ability can readily learn to develop the requisite faculty, turning weakness into strength. That is part of the challenge of life, distinguishing the worker from the loafer, success from failure.

The power of thought is much greater than mere physical understanding can conceive. Its influence on human health and well-being is by no means fully realised yet — if it were, mental institutions would be far less crowded than they are today.

Have you ever realised why so many people land themselves in a mental institution? The answer is: worry or fear. Worry is confused thought about the past; fear is uncertainty, generally apprehension, of the future. Both worry and fear take us away from the present. And as the present moment is the only one we have, worry and fear serve to deprive us of the consciousness of this moment, leading to a considerably diminished awareness of just what is happening *now*. How can memory possibly strengthen when such distractions diminish our consciousness of the present moment and the things we do, say, read or hear have only a partial consciousness in attendance?

Contrary to the strength potential of the voluntary muscles, the brain does not naturally decline with age. No matter how active the brain might be in creative development, man never runs the risk of wearing it out. Rarely is more than 10 per cent of the brain's cells used in thinking or memory. So we have far greater reserves for the use of memory than previously imagined.

As so little of its cellular structure is used, the brain has a tremendous potential for increased use. This is always assuming that drugs, alcohol or other poisons which attack the brain's cells and irreversibly destroy them, are avoided.

The apparent decline in mentality which so often accompanies age in modern society is caused by inactivity. Once settled into the comfort of permanency, modern man generally ceases to employ his brain creatively. His interest in sports, exercise and general physical activity declines. As he does less, he tends to eat more often, due so much to spare time, physical boredom and nervous tension as his anxieties in life tend to magnify (in his mind). When he eats more, he generally snacks on junk "foods" which, in turn, fail to provide adequate nourishment for his blood and brain. When he eats more, he tends to drink less water, for the human stomach has only a limited physical capacity.

Because he does less exercise and plays less sports, man rarely gets breathless. In fact, his breathing becomes considerably more shallow. Thus he draws less oxygen into his lungs and to his brain. He also perspires less, thereby reducing his induced thirst, further diminishing his water-drinking habit.

So we find that, with his entry into the comfort zone of settled married life and a permanent job, man actually commences his accelerated rate of decline. With lowered physical activity and mental activity (having little of an intellectual challenge to stimulate him), man's brain is used less. This is compounded with his gradual dehydration from reduced water consumption, so the brain shrinks and the blood thickens. Air pockets, ever so small, develop around the brain within the skull — as these increase in size, so cerebral functioning diminishes. Senility has now set in. The longer the conditions prevail, the more the senility is compounded and the longer it will ultimately take to reverse — if indeed the sufferer or those associated with him recognise that such a condition is capable of correction.

The enviable capacity for memory in early life is rarely an indication of future success. We have all envied our peers when they have won school or college prizes for scholastic abilities. But what has become of them in later life? In my experience, many have failed to achieve success through their inability to recognise life's greater values, such as awareness by broad conceptual cognisance. Famous lives, such as those almost legendary people, Leonardo da Vinci, Einstein and Lincoln, men who fared poorly at school, illustrate that the race is never won in the first lap. Success is more the measure of control which man has mastered, plus his ability to enter "the silence" and become receptive to inspiration.

Temperance

> *Regimen is better than physic. Every one should be his own physician. We ought to assist, not to force nature. Eat with moderation what agrees with your constitution. Nothing is good for the body but what we can digest. What medicine can procure digestion?*
>
> Voltaire (1694-1778)

Temperance is the ability to apply moderation in all things suitable, but abstinence from those unsuitable. Moderation is nature's way of maintaining balance, but only when the subject is harmonious with life. If there be any degree of disharmony, balance becomes virtually impossible.

Poisonous substances are known to induce less harm when taken in small amounts than when administered in large doses. But they will cause harm, even in small amounts. Many poisons are cumulative, so their long-term effect can be almost as serious as taking a large single dose. In some instances, a large dose will cause the body to acutely rebel, maybe to throw up or convulse to remove the offending substance; whereas repeated small doses might bypass the protective mechanism and lull the addict into a false sense of security. Alcohol, tobacco and commonly used drugs offer examples of this sort of addiction.

"Moderation in *all* things" is the catch-phrase of those who would addictively ingest a constant haphazard miscellany of anything which takes their fancy. It is invariably the excuse for moderate indulgences under the guise that so long as they constitute only modest quantities, irrespective of their frequency, they will do no harm. This attitude can be applied to many components of the modern diet, revealing both ignorance and addiction, resulting in disease (the consequence of disharmony).

The intellect of man is rarely at a loss to justify habits. That is why smoking, alcoholic drinking, coffee and tea persist as part of modern living; they demonstrate the distinction between intellect and intelligence. Self-abuse, even in moderation, is intemperate and totally unacceptable to the thinking person.

However, moderation in things suitable is a fundamental part of wisdom. If you enjoy eating, then eat less at each meal; in so doing, you will live longer to ultimately eat more. It is therefore unwise to employ spices, condiments and special seasonings to stimulate the appetite and induce larger intakes of food, not to mention gastric irritations inflicted by many herbs and spices on the sensitive mucosa of the stomach. The high incidence of gastric ulcers among such people is no coincidence.

Temperance is the natural guide to man's actions. It is the discipline which guides his discrimination, first between the suitable and the unsuitable, second in the degree of suitability. It is his key to balance in all things, especially in the brain, where we need to develop both lobes (left: organisational, governing right hand and foot; right lobe: creative, governing left hand and foot).

For example, the modern tone of many advertisements stimulates sexual activity, resulting in over-indulgence if practised or unhealthy frustration if unrequited. But sexual expression, consistent with any natural action, should only be the physical portrayal of a spiritual need. Whether it be for the need to procreate, or as an expression of deep love, sexual intercourse is a very private affair which especially responds to moderation of frequency, although not of commitment to expression. So controlled, its purpose and pleasure will benefit the greater and the ability to engage in its expression will be less affected by age.

Fortitude

Life can never be a constant stream of happy events. From time to time come those periods of trial during which one's courage and endurance are tested, exercising and strengthening one's fortitude.

Courage, endurance, patience, forbearance, tenacity and intrepidity are but a few of the virtues of the discipline of fortitude, the quality whereby man becomes the equal of every vicissitude of life. Fortitude does not imply insensitivity, but it does encourage its control. It shows man that, as experience is his greatest teacher, he will never become involved in any encounter beyond his ability to endure. From experience, we learn that everything occurs for a purpose, and thus we develop our self-confidence.

Fortitude is the power by which we gain mastery over experience. It is the ability to adjust to circumstances beyond our immediate control and enables us to extract the purpose of each lesson from our involvement. This avoids the need for later involvement in a similar lesson. The power of fortitude is always greater than the demands of the lesson — that is a fundamental fact of life.

The more positive a person, the more he will grow in fortitude and the more successful he will become in life. These are the people of deep understanding, of vision, whose lives are worthy examples for those in need of moral support.

The courage to be different from the majority, to stand up for your beliefs, your feelings, your needs, is a function of fortitude. We should not fall into the trap of believing that the majority is always correct. Our ability to say "no", to decline an offer or invitation, has also become a modern demand upon one's courage, so numerous and cogent are the requests placed upon one's personal resources today. Many people are afraid to refuse for fear of embarrassment, of becoming unpopular or of having to justify their stand in some way.

Growth in fortitude, negating these restricting emotions, develops when we recognise the frailty of our self-confidence. Taking charge of our feelings helps us to protect our sensitivities by developing a high level of inner security, by recognising that no one can embarrass us unless we let them — and we give this permission whenever we default on our responsibility for developing self-control, thereby overcoming lack of confidence.

Do we realise how often we play the hiding game? Unprepared or unwilling to take charge of our feelings and confidently express our real wishes or needs, we resort to excuses. Listen to the conversations going on around you, to the frequent examples of how people hide their real feelings or expression by making excuses in statements which are not really true, by adopting a falsehood, such as: "I can't, I've got a headache." Often they haven't, or maybe they developed it as a convenient way out. "Oh, but I'm so tired." "Bored" is often the correct and honest word they should be using. "I'd like to help, but I'm so busy." So contradictory when we know that only busy people have time to help.

Other ways of hiding are encountered in the person who talks the loudest or proclaims himself the expert at a party, who resorts conveniently to anger or always wears sunglasses, who turns shyly quiet, or is always reading a book, who eats too much and gets fat, who wears drab clothes, is often in pain (for sympathy), who watches television every night, or is a workaholic. Drugs, alcohol and tobacco habits are among the most widespread ways of hiding — and so often the habits are encouraged by society and by government!

"Misfortune" is the unthinking man's epithet for experiences which prove costly in terms of losses in health, wealth or love. Yet such losses are always of a temporary nature when their purpose has been recognised and temporary suffering evolves into wisdom. Some lessons are so important as to demand significant sacrifices for their purpose to be achieved and, provided that one graduates fully from such lessons, there should be no repetition of the sacrifice. If one fails to learn properly by the experience, a later recurrence, creating greater sacrifice to more deeply impress its purpose, is inevitable.

If only our leaders and teachers were made aware of this fact, man would be trained in fortitude and lead a far happier, more balanced life. This would become immediately apparent by a significant reduction in the number of suicides, psychotics, neurotics and other unbalanced people. Fortitude would show them how to face life, attune to it and enjoy it, recognising it is not the experience creating the hurt or sadness — it is our attitude to it and the memories of past attitudes. We choose our attitudes, so we can change them just as easily.

Philanthropy as Compassion

Nearly two thousand years ago, the great Teacher from Nazareth instructed mankind: "Love thy neighbour as thyself." In so doing, He gave the perfect example of the discipline of philanthropy — the practice of love, of compassion towards all life.

But when we refer to our "neighbour", we are not restricting ourselves to the family next door or across the street — everyone and everything in life is our neighbour. Love can know no bounds if it is unconditional and totally spiritual. And for this to occur, love must commence at "home". Its foundation must lie within the very source that seeks to express it, within one's very inner being.

If man is to believe that he is made in the image and likeness of his Creator, his love for his Creator can be no less than his love for himself. Nor can it be any less than his love for his neighbour.

To love is to understand and to co-exist in harmony. It is the ultimate friendship. To love oneself is to recognise the inner divinity, and to be aware of the purpose of one's life and the potential by which this is to be achieved. There has to be harmony between one's ideals and actions, between the psyche and body. There has to be peace throughout one's entire being, one's expression and in all associations. Man's ability to love his neighbour is reflected in his degree of understanding of himself.

Jesus of Nazareth was not the first great man to teach love as the most vital of all commandments. As a reincarnation of the Divine Spirit which can be traced back to Melchizedek of the Old Testament (into whose order Jesus was born), and in the previous age to Enoch, great-grandfather of Noah, Jesus perpetuated the holy teachings, translating them for the needs of that age. For indeed, love is the central discipline around which every esoteric teaching must evolve.

Thus, when it came time for Pythagoras to develop his philosophy (love of truth and wisdom), synthesised from his experiences of many years of travel and study, the teaching of love took on a more complete meaning. He called it "philanthropy", explaining it as the love of man for man, of man for God and of God for man. He further taught that God is incarnate in all His creatures as a triangular relationship, represented symbolically by the equilateral triangle:

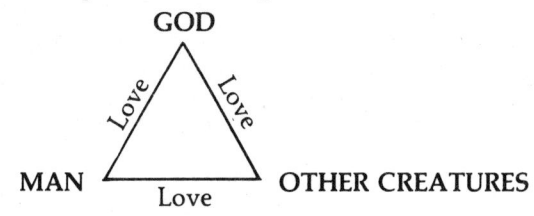

```
                    GOD
                    /\
                Love/  \Love
                  /      \
                /          \
            MAN ───────────── OTHER CREATURES
                    Love
```

This encompasses all life in a pattern of interwoven harmony.

Could it have been that Pythagoras recognised the impending coming of a Divine Master and accepted the tremendous responsibility of elevating the minds of men and women to a level of understanding by which the later teachings could be fully comprehended? If so, it is apparent that only partial success attended his efforts, but there is no disappointment when it is realised that all natural development is slow, sometimes painfully slow.

Separated by nearly 6000 kilometres of space, yet at almost the identical time in history, another great teacher was preparing himself for the fulfilment of his own mission in elevating the mind of another race of men and women. Gautama, the Buddha, employed love as a central theme of his great teachings, developing a perfect example of it in application.

History fails to reveal whether these two great teachers ever met in the flesh, yet such similarity exists in much of their teachings that it must be apparent they were not strangers to each other's basic beliefs. Variations in their teachings occur where the needs for the differing lifestyles had to be satisfied by varied expression of the same truth. The light each brought to that period of spiritual infancy is the basis upon which the world's two strongest civilisations have since evolved.

Unfortunately, the manner of that evolution cannot be regarded with very much pride. Tarnished by so much wanton bloodshed and at odds with the principles espoused by both East and West, this conflict can be traced, always, to lack of philanthropy, lack of friendship (defined as the extension of one's self into another person).

True philanthropy does not recognise biological, racial, religious or any other differences. It is an open cheque, but unlike most other offerings, will always return more to the giver. It is a natural expression of man to give and to share, not merely of his physical possessions but, more significantly, of his love, friendship, appreciation and understanding.

Erudition, Creative Learning

It has been said that life is a lesson book from which we never graduate. Such being the case, college graduates should feel less intellectually secure and begin to realise that their real education is only just beginning.

Erudition is the art of learning. It is the application of conscious awareness so that each experience can be understood for its purpose. Man is not intended to know everything in one lifetime. That is an impossibility, hence the need for many earthly lifetimes. But he is intended to know all about his own life and to apply that knowledge to the benefit of himself, his neighbour and his environment.

There is so much to learn in life. We must maintain a perspective and be able to discriminate between the more important and the less important aspects. Alternatively, life will assume a complexity which creates tension, anxiety and worry, instead of evolving as a relatively simple, natural expression of creation in harmony.

Those who are somewhat aware of this truth have invested in this book and any similar writing which purports to guide man to a happier, healthier, more purposeful existence. Those with no intent or desire to engage in anything more than mere physical gratifications will not be upset by this implication because they are not aware of what is now being explained. To them, life will appear too complex and full of secrets which, they feel, can never be known. Such is their justification for inaction — a euphemism for laziness.

There is nothing in this universe or beyond which we cannot, or will not, eventually learn. But learning is a graduated process, depending on past learning for its growth. When we stop learning, we start declining, mentally and physically. That is the pattern of life.

Everything has its purpose. Every act is part of the Grand Plan. We must learn to understand that Plan and our part in it. This implies the vastness necessary in man's learning experiences for which his school system endeavours to prepare him. But real learning experience commences when he matures to a point where wisdom guides his thoughts and actions.

Music

> *Music is the mediator between the spiritual and the sensual life. Although the spirit is not master of that which it creates through music, yet it is blessed in this creation, which, like every creation of art, is mightier than the artist.*
>
> Beethoven (1770-1827)

There is probably no better authority on the harmonising influence of music in this modern age than Beethoven. The brilliance of his prolific compositions achieves progressively greater accolades as the years since his passing increase. Yet the salient aspect of this popularity lies not in the individual melodies inherent in the compositions, as with Tchaikovsky or Grieg, but in the essence of the compositions as a whole. They are spiritual masterpieces which bring into harmony the vibrations of the psyche and the body, unifying them into one synchronised being. This is music at its peak.

The most curious aspect of Beethoven was his deafness. Perhaps were he more responsive to physical sound, his brilliance would never have been so developed. Could we accept the premise that physical hearing creates limitations by too much reliance on a very limited frequency range?

The word "music" derives from ancient Greece, where it implied "the arts of the muses". It originally embraced those harmonic arts accorded to the direction of the nine muses — singing (lyric poetry), comedy, tragedy, dancing, poetry, drama, sacred hymns, history (which includes geography) and astrology (the forerunner of astronomy, which also embraces colour).

Harmony is the common essential for each of these arts, just as it is for contentment among all living creatures. This is especially so in man, for his vibrations are the most sensitive. Therefore, external harmony is as much a food for the psyche as are fruits and vegetables for the body — each is the staple source of nutrients.

Of all the arts comprising the muses, those in which we are most interested are the visible and audible harmonies represented by colour and music, as they are commonly known. The ultra-high frequency vibrations of harmony which please the eyes are just as much harmony to the psyche as the low range of frequencies produced by a musical instrument for detection by the ears. Both are essential to human well-being and readily available in a wide variety of combinations.

By virtue of such a wide choice of music and colour, man has to be educated in selecting those aspects of each which prove the most suitable to his constitution. For this reason Pythagoras recognised the need for training in this discipline, both from a participatory and an appreciative (operative and speculative) point of view. Colour exists in everything recognised by the eyes; music prevails in everything detected by the ears. Therefore, the wise choice of each will attract benefits; unsuitable choice will inspire compounded disharmonies.

The exercise of suitable music and colour in one's life is recognised as "compensatory". Valuable in calming the emotions, aiding concentration and relaxing muscle tension is light symphonic or pastoral music. Dance and jazz rhythms aid in dispelling lethargy. Thus, suitable music can be chosen to enable the body and the psyche to achieve greater harmony and perform more suitably for whatever occasion is required.

Likewise, green shades of colour are the most relaxing, red the most stimulating, blue the most inspiring. The influences of colour and music are more than superficial; some are known to have deep psychological effects.

Soothing music prior to and during a meal will materially aid digestion. Stimulating harmonies will improve interest and inspire better sales in merchandising concerns, as well as improving output in factories. Greens and blues, suitably arranged with secondary colours, will induce better healing results in hospitals or rest centres. This has been especially noticeable in research performed recently in psychiatric centres in London and in Moscow; there may be such research going on in other centres as well.

The classic story is told of how Pythagoras saved a building from being burned to the ground by playing soothing music on his lyre. One evening, his attention was drawn to the irate manner of a youth who was feverishly stacking dried branches of trees outside the wall of his ex-girlfriend's home. Without indicating his presence, Pythagoras commenced playing soft, soothing melodies on his lyre, gradually increasing the volume so that the youth was not made unduly aware of his presence. Within moments, the youth was moving noticeably slower and in a short while stood still, looking at the pile of firewood. Suddenly, he turned his back on his actions and walked away a short distance. He soon returned and removed the evidence of his vicious intent, glancing around in the hope that nobody saw him, before quickly walking home.

The proprietor of a banana plantation located on the mid-north coast of New South Wales was referred to me when, in 1968, I began gathering supplies of organically grown foods for organised distribution throughout Australia. On visiting the plantation, one noticed occasional loudspeakers in a certain part of the producing area. Ian Hamey, the young ingenious grower, described how he had been experimenting with certain musical notes playing continuously over the amplifying system; he wished to discover what effects, if any, were registered on the fruit.

A full season after his first experiment, Ian Hamey was astounded to find that bananas from the section of the plantation with speakers were consistently larger than all others from the remainder of his plantation. Their size was between one-third and one-half larger, with a greater number of fruit on each bunch. The following season he moved his speakers to another section of the plantation and the results were repeated. All other factors — soil, humus, rainfall, etc — were consistent throughout.

Those of us sensitive enough to realise it would take little convincing of the fact that music must be harmonious to be beneficial. Discordant cacophonies of loud consecutive sounds can hardly classify as music. They are certainly not beneficial to the psyche.

Just as disharmony in sound can upset balance in the body, so will drabness in colour affect one's emotions adversely. In *Color Therapy* (The Devin-Adair Co., Connecticut, USA, 1974), Linda A. Clark, MA, records some surprising findings testifying to the effects of colour on human life. For example, when London's drab, grey Blackfriar's Bridge was repainted green, suicides dropped by one-third. Factory workers' morale improved noticeably, accompanied by a reduction in accidents, when grey machinery was repainted a light orange. There is really no end to the effects on life of colour, as colour is music made visible.

Now, if we recognise the profound influences of harmony on life, should we not be more conscious of our responsibility in selecting those external harmonies more suitable to us? Many factors in life are beyond our immediate control, but many others are within our command through which we can help rectify conflicting influences. Music, in all its range of expression, is of foremost value in this regard. Even if we ignore all its other virtues, music does provide man with enjoyment — and that is a significant measure of its success.

Dietetics and Fasting

The human body is the product of many factors, but the most abused of all is its diet. For too long, man has been eating by habit, almost completely unaware of the intimate relationship between diet and health. It is little different now to 2500 years ago, when Pythagoras attempted to correct man's eating habits by introducing the science of dietetics as an instructional course.

Although a vegetarian himself, Pythagoras did not insist that his pupils embrace abstinence from animal flesh. However, many did so. In time, all who aspired to spiritual development found there was no other way to achieve it than by embracing total compassion in all habits, especially eating. It is impossible to love life and to simultaneously condone its slaughtering.

Not only is the choice of food important, but also is its mode of preparation and the conditions under which it is eaten. Further, its method of production induces considerable influence upon man's food and its effect on his well-being.

No less dominant in the days of Pythagoras than today is the influence of parents in the determination of man's eating habits. Our modern way of living only differs to the extent that industry, with its proliferation of processed products, induces changes in dietary habit. But it must be recognised that these are far from improvements in terms of man's basic needs being satisfied.

That man should be taught responsibility for his mode of living, yet retain ignorance of his habits of eating, implies a conflict, and a very harmful one indeed.

Everyone follows a diet. "Diet" describes one's pattern of eating and does not imply a limitation to those who are careful in their choice of foodstuffs. So important is this consideration and so confused are those who seek to understand it from the endless procession of "experts" offering "advice", that it behoves us to employ some basic intelligence in throwing light on the subject of human diet. To do so involves a recognition of man's purpose in life and the part played by diet in achieving this purpose.

Whenever the purpose is frustrated, it must indicate that a wrong course has been followed. Sickness is man's most glaring and common form of frustration. The more life departs from the natural, the more it becomes confused. So with diet.

Our choice must clearly follow a selection of foods which provide pleasure to the palate and nourishment to the body. The choice is a very wide one, implying no limitation beyond man's ingenuity to adapt, conditioned by environmental circumstances of climate and geography. Knowledge and intelligent application clearly indicate the need to become as careful in the selection of one's diet as in the selection of one's spouse. Each exercises as much influence on one's happiness, health and harmony.

Just as food determines the material out of which the body is built, one's mental attitude provides the mixing agent through which actual construction takes place. The nature of one's thoughts is equally as important as the availability of nutrients from food — the former determining the efficiency by which the latter is appropriated to build, repair and energise the body.

The part played by diet in determining one's state of health is so significant that in most cases of illness, a withdrawal of diet will materially restore health. Total abstinence from food, a non-diet, is nature's way of reducing the level of toxicity in the bloodstream and bodily tissues to a more manageable quota.

Ideally, during fasting the body should be allowed a maximum of rest so as to permit it to employ its inherent detoxifying ability (a potential about which far too little is generally taught). In this way it can cleanse itself and overcome a condition of enervation by utilising its latent ability of innervation (rebuilding nerve energies).

The discipline of fasting also implies a valuable method for spiritual development, when used in conjunction with other disciplines, especially silence. Its ability to restore total harmony is the most powerful known to man. Once this condition is achieved, all manner of developments are possible. Man's level of awareness is the only limiting factor.

Exercise and Activity

Having learned temperance and balance, a man is prepared for the wise development of his body and its employment in physical pursuits of a suitable nature. His work, pleasures and sports are the more enjoyable when his body is under his command and capable of accomplishing demands made upon it.

Much of the Greek fame for sports and gymnastics derived from the cultivation of this discipline in Pythagorean education. For balanced development, man must be taught the use of his body through its full range of flexibility and control. Its efficiency in movement must be developed such that smooth, flowing motion characterises each action. The body's circulation and muscle tone must be unrestricted and adjustable to any reasonable demand. Exercise and activity are the basic disciplines for generating these conditions.

As we have already given some space to the deeper discussion of exercise and activity (Stage 3), it now only remains to indicate the importance of these in the overall development of man and his mode of self-discipline.

Having recognised that every human life has its individual purpose, we become aware that for some the emphasis should be on mental or psychic concerns; for others, on more physical pursuits. For the latter, exercise and activity become very important disciplines, essential for the physical development of these people to reach the exceptionally high level demanded by their purpose. For the former, greater emphasis is placed on the non-physical disciplines. Yet for each, balance is essential.

No matter what the physical pursuit, its success will be the greater if intelligence, rather than emotion or instinct, guides its planning. Then, as the years of life grow and the emphasis upon the physical diminishes, greater development of the mental and psychic will balance one's life, thereby avoiding a vacuum in ageing life accompanied by the acceleration of senility.

Likewise, with the greater emphasis in life directed towards mental or psychic development, a tendency to neglect the physical will induce an opposite imbalance. Adequate activity must engage the body to maintain good blood circulation and muscle tone; suitably selected exercises will improve these, enabling the body to carry out any sudden demands placed upon it without injury or strain. Muscles will tend to atrophy when not in regular use, creating an unbalanced development and inhibiting the body's physical expression. No matter how intense the mental or psychic activity, some diversification into physical expression must always be included in the balanced life. This is part of nature's plan.

Method, Order and Efficiency

As one's command of life develops, increasing possibilities are recognised. Man's expanded awareness reveals the almost limitless faculties at his command, and the manifold opportunities in which his self-expression may be demonstrated. But care must be exercised that, even in the fulfilment of his purpose, man does not exceed the steady, graduated pace of natural development. Enthusiasm should always be tempered by wisdom so that a well-regulated method prevails in all his actions, order in his choice of priorities and efficiency in his manner of expression.

It is not unnatural for man to become overly enthused by the success which comes to attend his efforts as a consequence of the growing mastery of his affairs. Such enthusiasm is itself an indication of his need to develop greater command of his actions, lest his emotions confuse method, and reaction replace action in his order of priorities.

Order is the discipline which teaches us to recognise the importance of discrimination, not between people, but in our affairs. As we grow in truth and wisdom, everything is recognised as having a measure of importance. But time is the limiting aspect of life which will not permit every experience, every pleasure to be enacted. Thus we must be prepared to follow our guidance which will always indicate the means whereby we can distinguish between the more important and the less important.

Efficiency is the time-oriented factor in one's activities, the discipline of "getting it all together", of achieving maximum results for the most economical methods. Economics of time, effort and direction allow us to undertake more experience in a given period or space. We thereby achieve greater growth, make more of the moment. Efficiency in our affairs can only be achieved when we are dynamically alert, ever conscious of the moment as a unique experience, for the only moment we can ever live is *now*. To wallow in the past or to lose consciousness by anticipating the future is to lose awareness, for awareness is essentially a function of the now.

With its great simplicity, yet dynamic potential, the Pythagorean ideal is as intensely practical now as when propounded 2500 years ago. Its inherent flexibility restricts it to no race, age or culture, but ensures that in every corner of human habitation, nothing but benefits will follow the application of its methods. *No other system propounded by man offers such complete instruction, such practical guidelines as does the Pythagorean.*

STAGE SIX

Man's Vegetarian Heritage

And God said, Behold, I have given you every herb bearing seed, which is upon the face of all the earth, and every tree, in the which is the fruit of a tree yielding seed; to you it shall be for meat.

Genesis 1:29 (King James Version)

For our present discussion, it is of little consequence whether a person upholds the King James Version of the Bible as being the source of the laws of life, whether he upholds some other version, or upholds no version. It is our present desire to ascertain facts — if they substantiate belief, all is fine; if not, wisdom dictates a reconsideration of the belief.

Science depends for its validity on factual information, free from the limitations of prejudice or the demands of sponsors. And few thinking people will deny that in matters of human diet, especially the question of vegetarianism, science has been noticeable by its absence. Instead, habit appears to be the major dietary determinant.

The resourcefulness of man often drives him to great lengths to justify his habits, especially when such habits form an intimate part of his social structure, as does eating. But here we are not really concerned with justifications, only with investigation.

Throughout the following study of the question of meat eating versus vegetarianism, it should be realised that there will be aspects applying to some people and not others. I have endeavoured to cover all major points of the argument, both theoretical and practical. For the first thirty years of my life I was an avid meat eater, but for the past nineteen years, a vegetarian; and throughout the past quarter century, a trained scientist.

Vegetarianism Defined

Vegetarianism implies a diet based wholly on foods deriving from botanical sources. This includes those crops which are commonly recognised as fruits and vegetables — the staple of the diet — plus the concentrated nuclei of crops in the form of seeds, nuts, pulses (peas, beans and lentils) and grains.

Vegetarianism also implies total abstinence from animal flesh or animal products, from fish, fowl, insect or any other living creature, either alive or dead. However, many modern vegetarians include as dietary supplements such animal products as milk, cheese, yogurt and eggs. Discussion about these will be undertaken in the section on protein foods. But no vegetarian would include in his regular diet any part of the once-living creature.

Although plant foods comprise the vegetarian diet, not all plants or their products are suitable for human consumption. Some are mildly poisonous, others dangerously so. Some are too fibrous, some too acidic. A study of basic human dietary needs will reveal those which should be included and those to be excluded.

In practice, usual components of the vegetarian diet include all commonly accepted fruits and vegetables, grains, seeds, nuts and pulses — in fact, most plant crops. Those about which special care should be taken are the herbs, spices, leaves and stalks. While many of these are quite suitable for inclusion in the human diet, others must be omitted, as generally indicated by their bitterness, coarseness or odour. Most suitable foods are, in general, recognised by their subtle sweetness, tenderness and/or delicate perfumes when ripe for eating.

Man's Genealogical Background

Anthropologists and biologists recognise man as a mammal of the primate family, the same physical classification as the great anthropoid ape, having a considerable number of common attributes.

Man's blood composition is the same in basic type as the ape. So closely akin are they, that man has been known to catch influenza from the gorilla and the chimpanzee. The question of whether or not man actually evolved from the great apes, or whether he was a separate creation, is the crux of the old Darwinian-biblical controversy. But this is beyond the intent of our immediate discussion. That is history — now we are concerned with the mystery of the present, the investigation of which commences with the point that man is structurally of the same family as the great apes.

Further certainty aiding our investigations is that archaeological discoveries have confirmed that as long as man has existed on this planet he has undergone comparatively little change in his anatomy, still resembling the anthropoidal apes in his general bodily structure and in his basic, spontaneous habits of expression.

Man's Primitive Background

Although running counter to obvious scientific evidence, many modern nutritional "authorities" assert that animal flesh is vital for human strength, health and nourishment. This notion long predates science. It actually derives from the primitive theory that if you want a strong body, you must eat one. It totally ignores the recognition that the strongest animals (the elephant, horse, ox, bullock and gorilla) are total vegetarians. These animals are also the longest living, with the greatest endurance.

This "witch-doctor conception" of flesh-for-strength appears to derive from primitive eras when man adopted the habit of hunting and killing to exert his ego and achieve an exhibitionistic glory. Otherwise, it is a paradox, for man the hunter rarely ate his kill. Even when he did, he would select the smaller, more tender portions of muscle meat and this was eaten raw.

Primitive man was first a nomad; then a subsistence farmer, producing his staple crops whenever the seasons and soil would permit. But he gradually denuded his agricultural lands, creating problems of erosion and finally deserts. Such ignorance was not confined to primitiveness, as attested by the infamous American dust bowl.

As his crops became less abundant, man tended to turn to the spoils of his hunt for sustenance, but not without increasing problems in health, both physical and mental. In spite of his gradual sophistication from the discovery of metals, wheels, etc, man grew less contented with his lot, developing an unnatural aggression. Although it did not improve his strength (but did reduce his endurance), this new "killer instinct" probably gave birth to the notion that eating animal flesh created his new "strength".

More recent scientific research has revealed the actual source of this new stimulation:

by adding animal meat to his diet, primitive man ingested those animal hormones, especially adrenalin, which induce aggressive behaviour as one of a range of psychopathic conditions.

In passing, it is consistent with the theory of muscle meat-for-strength that other animal components might be just as "beneficial" to man. Could we then expect to increase our intelligence with the consumption of animal brains? Could we strengthen our bone structure with the chewing of animal bones? Could we improve our sexual potency by ingesting animal sex organs? Such ideas could make a sensitive person celibate for life.

Historical Background

As our investigation enters the present historical period, we find that the founders of the world's leading cultural systems were usually vegetarians. They exemplified this habit by teaching their followers a reverence for all life. Pythagoras, Buddha, Christ and Gandhi rank foremost as such teachers of compassion, although the Bible does not indicate that Christ instructed His followers to embrace vegetarianism as did some of the others (perhaps because the Romans were so fond of meat).

Many leaders in Greece's Golden Age encouraged vegetarianism after the Pythagorean ideal. Socrates, Plato, Aristotle, Pericles and their followers who also embraced vegetarianism evidenced an intellectualism and wisdom unique, not only for their times, but rarely equalled today. Circumstances did not always guarantee them long lives, but the achievements of their lifespans certainly ensured their place in history.

Most famous of the pupils of Aristotle, Alexander the Great, lived only thirty-three years, but might not have been so unfortunate had not the cry from his sickbed contained so much truth: "I am being killed with the aid of too many physicians", history records as his final utterance.

Western culture is not the only system to be founded upon the ethical principles which embrace vegetarianism. Grains, legumes, vegetables and fruits have formed the staple diet of most notable ancient civilisations. From before recorded history, the Chinese, Japanese, Indians, Egyptians, Persians and Indian tribes of the Americas were basically vegetarian. Pacific islanders, African Negroes and other tropical dwellers built their basic dietary habits upon the abundance of delicious tropical fruits at their disposal.

Few of these races would have considered eating any of their precious animals. In those days, the animal populations were quite small, a far cry from today's commercially inspired overproduction and exploitation.

When most of the world's peoples lived in their natural geographic regions within the tropics and sub-tropics, abundant food was produced through the soil. Occasional supplementation with fish was the first development away from vegetarianism. As the population expanded into the colder northern (and, to a lesser extent, southern American) climates, growing seasons were considerably reduced. Occasional supplementation from animal meats thereby developed as an easier expedient than overcoming storage problems or improving the soil's diminishing fertility.

Abundant wealth in the ruling classes found the high cost of animal meats no barrier. Thus their dietary indulgences became frequent, such that meat consumption became associated with opulence; so did corpulence. White flour, white sugar, tea and coffee drinking were similarly identified. It is thus not surprising that when industry became established and wealth more widely distributed, the emerging middle class hastened to embrace those dietary symbols of wealth so envied by their forebears.

The incipient diseases which developed as a "bonus" for indulgences were never associated with dietary factors; they were blamed, rather, on aggressive germs. Only today is this position gradually changing, as understanding triumphs over thoughtless addiction.

Religious Background

The three most populous religious movements today are Hinduism, Buddhism and Christianity — in that order of antiquity. Each, at its core, was founded upon vegetarian principles, unreservedly enjoining its followers to embrace compassion and temperance as basic virtues.

Yet millions of today's adherents to these religious systems, while expressing piety toward their doctrines, are in violation of their underlying principles. Such is the nature of addiction, of the justification of entrenched habits, that many irregular interpretations have been placed on the basic religious rules pertaining to compassion and temperance. Thus are created convenient "exclusions" in attempted justification of such habits as meat eating.

The sixth of the ten commandments delivered by Moses gave the basic guideline to the Jews: "Thou shalt not kill." To the emerging Christians of twelve and a half centuries later, Christ broadened the guidance into the more positive: "Love thy neighbour as thyself."

Without wishing to dwell too much on biblical questions in this discussion, it is time to correct a few misinterpretations which have appeared over the years relating to the subject of Christ's dietary habits. Many Bible scholars persist with the theory that Christ ate animal flesh, obviously swayed in their opinions by personal habits. The desire to accede to prejudice and uphold existing tradition has been a human characteristic for many centuries, but truth appears now even more important as man exerts his independence in so many aspects of life.

Respected Bible scholar Reverend V. A. Holmes-Gore has researched the frequent use of the word "meat" in the New Testament Gospels. He traced its meaning to the original Greek.

His findings were first published in *World Forum* of autumn, 1947. He reveals that the nineteen Gospel references to "meat" should have been more accurately translated thus:

Greek	Number of References	Meaning
Broma	4	"food";
Brosis	4	"the act of eating food";
Phago	3	"to eat";
Brosimos	1	"that which may be eaten";
Trophe	6	"nourishment";
Prosphagon	1	"anything to eat".

Thus, the Authorised Version of John 21:5, "Have ye any meat?" is incorrect. It should have been translated: "Have ye anything to eat?"

"Fish" is another frequently mistranslated word in the Bible. Its reference is often not to the form of swimming life, but to the symbol by which early Christians could identify each other. It was a secret sign, needed in times of persecution, prior to the official acceptance of Christianity as a state religion.

The sign of the fish was a mystical symbol and conversational password, deriving from the Greek word for fish, "ichthus". As such, it represented an acrostic, composed of leading letters of the Greek phrase, "Iesous Christos Theou Uios Soter" — "Jesus Christ, Son of God, Saviour".

Frequent references to fish are intended as symbolic of The Christ, having nothing to do with the act of eating a dead fish. But the symbol of the fish did not meet with Roman approval. They preferred the sign of the cross, choosing to concentrate more on the death of Christ than on His brilliant life. Perhaps this is one reason only ten per cent of His life record appears in the canonical scriptures. Most of His first thirty years is omitted.

How many worshippers go home from church and sit down to a feast cut from a once proud beast in defiance of the very commandments they have just been advocating?

The dichotomy between Christ's teachings of compassion and their practice might be traceable to the exclusion from formal Christianity of much of the Master's esoteric teaching when the doctrine of the early church was welded into hard substance under direction of Emperor Constantine in early fourth century A.D.

Many early Christian teachers, early church fathers whose efforts led to eventual Roman acceptance of Christianity, upheld vegetarianism as essential to compassionate living.

Foremost for his outspokenness was Clement of Alexandria (150-217), renowned for his efforts to raise religious faith to the level of knowledge and understanding. He was quite firm in his recommendation that the consumption of flesh was anti-Christian: "Let us refrain from such food", became his famous understatement.

These simple, natural rules of good living were obviously intended to promote a happier, healthier, more purposeful life for man. Yet many act as though oblivious to these principles. While upholding their Bibles as sacred, literal testaments of perfection, they hasten to imply personal translations and interpretations to excuse their addiction to a contemporary carnivorous tradition. In so doing, they fall prey to the vice of hypocrisy. "Unto thine own self be true."

Too many religious functions condone acts of inhumanity to animals and discomfort to participants in perpetuating primitive gluttonies by gorging their bellies with beef, poultry or seafood. Such departure from otherwise high noble morals incites the alienation of sensitive, loving people. Percy Bysshe Shelley, the famous vegetarian poet, has aptly expressed such repugnance in his description of a Christmas dinner as being "a horrible process of torture which furnished brawn for the gluttonous repasts with which Christians celebrate the anniversary of their Saviour's birth".

An essay by Shelley, entitled "On The Vegetable System of Diet", was republished in 1947 by The London Vegetarian Society. In the introduction, its vice-president, Hugh I'A Fausset, wrote: "Shelley was right then in proclaiming that vegetarianism was no mere cult of eccentrics but a religious necessity for those who had awoken to the unity of life. Carnivorous Christians were as compromised and self-contradictory as Christians who approved and supported war. They perpetuated the feud between man and nature and between body and spirit which they claimed that their Saviour had come to redeem."

These points are not intended as a total discredit of Christianity, or of any other compassionate religion. Their purpose is to emphasise the errors into which addiction and misunderstanding can lead otherwise high-minded people.

More recent prominent religious reformers comprise a very respected list. Charles Wesley, with his Methodism, desired to set a vegetarian example among his followers;

but few, if any, are aware of this aspect of his teachings today. The more recent Unity School of Christianity was originally intent upon inculcating the principles of vegetarianism, but it, too, has found it expedient to compromise if the remainder of its teachings were to be of benefit to the vast majority.

Most famous of the recent vegetarian religionists was Ellen G. White. Founder of Seventh-day Adventism, she undertook a deep study of nutrition to confirm her biblical understanding that man should avoid animal foods and any others which were in any way adulterated. This, she advised, was necessary for balanced spiritual development. Today, Seventh-day Adventists are found among the most healthy people on our planet. Their Loma Linda University, at Riverside, California, has been responsible for much valuable research into human nutrition and dietetics, confirming scientifically that man is far healthier and happier as a vegetarian.

Dr Annie Besant, organiser of modern Theosophy, was a devoted vegetarian. Even today, most Theosophists follow her example. Their thoughtful, compassionate approach to life does credit to their creed: "There is no religion higher than Truth."

Emanuel Swedenborg, famous Swedish scientist, philosopher and theologian, also incorporated vegetarianism into the central theme of his metaphysical theology, although rarely does a biography make mention of this important facet. His special psychic abilities were often attributed to a development which was not hindered by coarse animal vibrations.

The Reverend Sylvester Graham attempted to introduce vegetarianism into the Presbyterian religion. In 1829, he regained health for his ailing young body by following a strict vegetarian regimen, thereby recognising these long forgotten dietary aspects of his Christianity. Although not so successful in overcoming the dogmatic habits which ignored vegetarianism in his Church, Graham's prolific writing and forceful teaching made his name famous in the field of human dietetics. The famous "Graham bread" is named after him even today, and the rapidly expanding movement of Natural Hygiene regards him as one of its founders.

Prominent Contemporary Vegetarians

As far back as the very foundation of Western culture, judges and legislators recognised that the consumption of animal flesh clouded their reasoning faculties. Today, with the increasing use of man-made chemicals, further complications are arising to distort human intelligence. Perhaps this is the reason we find so many of the world's great thinkers numbered among famous vegetarians. Leonardo da Vinci, Leo Tolstoy, Voltaire, Sir Isaac Pitman, Dr Albert Schweitzer, Ralph Waldo Emerson and George Bernard Shaw are but a few.

Benjamin Franklin was a cogent advocate of vegetarianism. It was probably as much due to his influence as that of any other person that vegetarians of the nineteenth century, both in England and America, were encouraged to form themselves into established societies to strengthen their fortitude against intimidation from those preferring to increase their addiction to animal flesh.

During the last century, a series of doctors have made their mark on the history of human health by their strong condemnation of medical practice in its almost total disregard for nutritional understanding. First among these was Dr Isaac Jennings of Connecticut; he was soon followed by Dr Russell T. Trall, famous for his revolutionary address to the Smithsonian Institution on the basic cause of disease — toxaemia.

Drs John H. Tilden and John Harvey Kellogg contributed further practical guidance to a better education of human nutrition, claiming remarkable success in their practices. Famous physical culturalist Bernard MacFadden, the founder of naturopathy in America, probably became the greatest champion of vegetarianism there, through his New York sanitorium and clinics, coupled with the vast readership of his magazines (estimated to have exceeded a million, even in those early 1900s).

The great pioneering work of these men in America was paralleled in Europe by no less a personage than Dr Rudolf Steiner. This eminent scientist and practical occultist developed the unique combination of a deep comprehension of both the physical and metaphysical, proclaiming that only by a thorough purification of his body could man ascend those heights of development whereby life revealed its secrets. Vegetarianism was a key to such purification.

More recent development in vegetarian awareness has been quite dramatic. Induced by the revulsion towards killing engendered by the Second World War, many health-oriented organisations mushroomed in the 1950s and 1960s, their central theme being adherence to vegetarian principles. These groups ranged in intensity of purpose from strictly educational to largely social, but all served to assist with the long-ignored attention to human nutrition according to man's natural needs. Included among these groups were the various vegetarian societies, natural hygiene societies and vegan societies.

Great impetus to the membership and expansion of such groups took place with a further rebellion by young people at wanton destruction of nature and human life in the Vietnam conflict. Their attention to their own living habits forcefully revealed them to be as incompassionate as that killing necessary to provide food for human consumption. Many, in consequence, embraced vegetarianism, joining such groups to understand why they had been remiss for so long.

The dean of modern vegetarianism is San Antonio, Texas practitioner, Herbert M. Shelton. Founder of the American Natural Hygiene Society, author of dozens of books on health, supervisor of over 40,000 fasts in his half-century-plus in practice, Doctor Shelton is a non-medical practitioner who may be regarded as one of the world's most dynamic reformers in human health.

The influence of Dr Shelton was probably no less than that of the famed Bircher-Benner health clinic in Zurich in developing vegetarianism in Australia in the 1940s. Even though vegetarian societies had existed here, they were little more than a gathering of older people who abandoned meat eating for ethical reasons, but replaced it with increased refined carbohydrate consumption. This also occurred in England, doing nothing to further the cause for vegetarianism, for most of its adherents were far from healthy and no closer to a natural lifestyle than if they had been eating meat.

As in all countries, a special person comes forward to take a movement out of its lethargy, correct its errors and, by example, set it on the road to dynamic growth. In Australia, it was Sydney businessman and philanthropist, L. O. Bailey. In spite of controlling a large business undertaking with hundreds of employees, L. O. Bailey dedicated his spare time, and ultimately his fortune, to the care of eighty-five fatherless infants during the Second World War and up to 1949. None of the mothers had means of support for the youngsters or, in many cases, yet-to-be-born infants whose fathers had gone to war or had deserted. The youngsters had no hope of a normal home life and were destined for all manner of illnesses.

His recognition of the importance of a natural lifestyle and vegetarianism guided L. O. Bailey to become "father" to these eighty-five children. He bought a large home at Bowral, NSW, where mothers and children lived on natural foods and in a healthy and happy environment. The children all grew up to be excellent specimens of health, with a vibrance which astounded medical and dental authorities. This gave significant impetus to a recognition of the dangers of processed foods and the virtues of natural living for children, for never before in this country had such a control group been under the watchful eye of health authorities who did not believe in vegetarianism and saw nothing wrong with sugar and white flour products.

Four years prior to his death in 1964, L. O. Bailey founded the Youth Welfare Association of Australia. It is a recognised charitable organisation, now administered by his long-time assistant, Mrs F. M. Cockburn. These two dedicated and compassionate people simultaneously founded the Natural Health Society to provide a forum for any person of any age to learn more about the natural living benefits being repeatedly proven by an ever-increasing group of people expressing preference for vegetarianism.

With its office located at 131 York Street, Sydney, the Youth Welfare Association commenced a health centre at Wallacia, on the banks of the Nepean River, west of Sydney. "Hopewood" is a delightful guest home where guests learn how to prepare and enjoy delicious vegetarian foods. The average age of its guests is thirty and it has probably been the most influential factor in Australians embracing vegetarianism and reducing their health bills. Membership of the Natural Health Society of Australia usually runs around 1500, but tens of thousands of people have moved under its influence, attended its regular meetings and continue to prove that man can live happily and comfortably without meat and processed foods. (For her dedicated and consistent work with Australian youth since 1940, Madge Cockburn was fittingly recognised by Queen Elizabeth II in 1974 by the award of an MBE. Rarely has a person deserved it more.)

Carnivore Equipment

Animals classified as natural carnivores have characteristics very different from those of man. Likewise, animals classed as omnivores are confirmed by biologists as greatly different to man. Man, biologically, has common characteristics (relevant to our discussion) only with the two-legged primates.

Carnivores are all four-footed animals with long tails, eyes which look sideways and skin without pores. Each foot has padded paws to facilitate the stalking of prey. Each paw is equipped with sharp, retractable claws for holding and killing food. Man has five toes to support his vertical movement, each with broad, flattish nails to cover the highly sensitive nerve ends in each toe, as in each finger.

To catch their prey, carnivores are capable of great bursts of speed. But they do not possess great endurance or "staying" power, they are suited more for running only over short distances. By contrast, man possesses great endurance and is able to run or walk for hours on end, covering far greater distances than carnivores. He can also work for great periods of time at gathering his food; carnivores prefer to spend that time in sleep.

The long, pointed jaws of the carnivore open very wide, but move only in an up-and-down motion. Man's mouth is flatter, framed with thicker lips and has greater flexibility in the jaw by which he can chew vegetable fibres and grind grains and nuts.

Carnivores have rough tongues, adapted to the rasping action necessary to break down tough muscle tissues of raw flesh. Man's tongue is smooth, with considerably more taste buds by which to detect unripe or poisonous plants; it is thus adapted to the far wider variety of flavours of the plant world.

Carnivore tooth formation is quite clearly designed by nature for tearing flesh.

Beside the incisor teeth, in each gum, are much larger, sharp, fang-like canine teeth. Next to these, farther along each gum, are the smaller, but equally sharp molar teeth. All of these are designed for tearing apart tough, fibrous tissue. A total number varying from thirty-six to forty-eight teeth is found in the mouths of the carnivores, whereas no more than thirty-two are found in human mouths. Human teeth are generally of similar height above the gums and flat, rather than pointed (the molars are comparatively quite broad). All are designed for a grinding motion as would be required with plant foods, nuts and grains.

With their diets comprising so many thirst-producing chemicals in the form of hormones and salts present in animal flesh, carnivores have a great need to drink. To facilitate this, their long tongues readily protrude beyond their snouts to lap up water directly from pools. Man's natural diet comprises such high percentages of water that it is usually not natural for him to require much liquid supplementation. Under pristine conditions, he would find his thirst easily satisfied by juicy fruits. But when man includes salty substances in his diet (including animal meats or preserved foods), he must include an intake of liquid, and for this he had to invent the drinking cup! Further, man's kidneys were not designed for high concentrations of acid-forming foods. Thus, when these foods (such as meat or cookies) are included in the diet, considerable quantities of water must be drunk to flush the kidneys adequately.

Animal meats are so highly acid-forming that they must be metabolised quickly. This is aided by a short gastrointestinal tract. A carnivore's tract averages three times the length of his trunk; man's averages five times his body length.

The carnivore diet contains very little carbohydrate; hence most of the catabolic action (breakdown of food into component nutrients) must take place in the stomach where the protein digestion requires a very high concentration of hydrochloric acid. Carnivore stomachs secrete proportionately ten times the concentration of hydrochloric acid secreted in the primate (and human) stomach. Such intensity of HCl is sufficient to dissolve the bones of prey and guarantees that digestion takes place before putrefaction can set in, and without the uric acid residue found in less well-equipped meat eaters.

The slower digestion of man requires food rich in protein to be retained in the stomach for many hours. If the meal is complex (containing carbohydrates and also fats), it can be held in the stomach for five to seven hours, unless pushed out by a successive intake — in which case it will not be properly catabolised and the proteins not ready for final breakdown and absorption. Long periods in the stomach can cause animal meats to putrefy, with resultant gas and toxic formations. The complex, muscular primate stomach of man will naturally reduce the transit time for protein-rich foods, retaining them for an average of four hours in preparation for the final breakdown in the duodenum and small intestine. Carnivore stomachs are simple, smooth and roundish to facilitate rapid transit with speedier digestion.

With virtually no starch content in his food, the carnivore has naturally high acidity in the saliva. Man's is slightly alkaline, containing the starch-splitting enzyme, ptyalin. Carnivore urine is highly acidic; man's should be mildly alkaline — if too acidic, it can become painful, overtaxing the kidneys until their eventual failure.

The stomach of the carnivore is the major organ of its gastrointestinal tract; with man and the primates, it is the small intestine where most nutrients are isolated for absorption. The colon of the carnivore is smooth for ease of elimination of the faeces, without the binding by fibrous cellulose as is demanded by the primate colon for proper elimination. Such cellulose only derives from plant substances and its action in binding stools together allows the colon to retain them for regular elimination after adequate water has been absorbed from them. Carnivores' colons are cleared rapidly, frequently and fluidly.

Such are the major differences between natural carnivores and man. As a carnivore can adapt to a vegetarian diet for a short time without problem, man can consume animal flesh for a short time without apparent physiological problem. But man can never properly adapt to the digestion of dead flesh, for his gastrointestinal tract just does not contain the components nor the structure necessary to extract from meat adequate nourishment without toxic residues.

World's Most Expensive Food

If the eating of animal flesh provides strength, man should be consistent in his beliefs and consume only carnivores. They have flesh built from flesh. But they are *not* the strongest animals, nor the cleanest. Man prefers cleaner meat, and thus chooses primarily the vegetarian animals for his consumption, although omnivorous scavengers are becoming more popular dietetically with the inclusion of chicken and pig — neither of which could be regarded as "clean meat".

Man's choice of animal food reflects some measure of wisdom. Cattle and sheep provide most meats for man, yet these animals produced their prized offering from a diet consisting only of plant foods; but at great expense to man. Far greater wisdom would be reflected in man's choice if he recognised that his body, too, can obtain first-class nourishment from plant foods exclusively.

With nothing more important to do than eat and procreate, sheep and cattle can spend all their days munching pasture. Man has higher objectives. He also has a smaller stomach capacity, and therefore must choose suitable concentrates (nuts, seeds, pulses and grains) for inclusion in his diet.

Man requires only small servings of nuts and seeds for his major source of protein intake, although some proteins are available in every type of plant food. Cattle and sheep do not require concentrated sources of protein, obtaining all their needs from pasture, principally tender, fresh sprouted greens. There is surely a lesson for man in all this!

Plant protein molecules are simpler and smaller than those of flesh proteins. They are thus easier to digest and have no inherent toxic wastes. So man has the choice of consuming first-hand proteins, produced directly by nature, or of second-hand proteins, manufactured from primary plant sources, by the animal whose flesh is highly prized. Yet for every pound of this flesh produced on the animal, at least ten pounds of pasture had to be consumed, a loss factor of 90 per cent.

Man's educated sense of efficiency would never allow him to tolerate a machine which showed only a 10 per cent efficiency. It would be regarded as an intolerable waste of energy and much too uneconomical to maintain. It should be just as unacceptable in the production of his food.

Such gross inefficiency is rarely considered by the advocates of animal food for man. Yet these same people lament the rapid increase of our world's population (a doubling in the last forty-four years to its present four billion), primarily because we are "running out of food and resources". Conservationists often fail to realise how wasteful our eating habits have become — far more so than our transport methods.

In spite of the United Nations' warnings that actual availability of arable land is diminishing, man persists, with the same United Nations' encouragement, in devoting so much of this precious resource to grossly inefficient animal feeding and breeding. The present proportion of fertile land to each person is less than half a hectare — and diminishing. If some two-thirds of the world's population were not vegetarians, we would all be starving.

Compare these reliable estimates of the area of land required for food production for human needs:

Total vegetarians require about a quarter of a hectare for food per person; part vegetarians, about half a hectare; most Westerners, about three-quarters of a hectare; eaters of three meat meals a day nearly one hectare. ("Part vegetarians" include cheese, milk and eggs in their diets; "most Westerners" consume the conventional diet centred around meat, but including some vegetable foods.)

It is reliably estimated that only one-twelfth (around 8 per cent) of the total cultivated crops, including pastures, provide direct food for man. Livestock gets the huge majority, returning only 10 per cent to man for his consumption or use. When we realise that in most countries, livestock outnumbers man by 5 to 1 (in Australia, nearly 16 to 1), we can gauge somewhat the huge waste of resources being perpetuated by the prolific artificial breeding of herds.

If, by the turn of the century, an anticipated eight billion people inhabit the earth, there is no possible way to feed them except by a significant reversion to vegetarianism. Even then, man will need to exercise greater discipline of moderation towards the quantity of his intake. We will also need to avoid such foodless indulgences as teas, coffee, cocoa, tobacco, alcohols, etc. which require huge tracts of valuable arable land for their production, yet offer no nourishment, but contribute to world health problems.

Unbelievable Savings

Even among people set in their ways and unmoved by humanitarian needs, there is one argument so forceful and immediate that it never fails to get attention: What family would refuse a new car every three years, absolutely *free*?

Let us suppose that the only condition to being awarded such a gift is a diet change involving the major source of concentrated proteins. It necessitates replacing animal meats with plant proteins. The savings to a family of four are astounding.

The following simple exercise in economics proves the point. Prices quoted were prevailing in Australia in 1981. With the average cost of animal foods (meats, poultry, seafood, cheese and eggs) at $4.96 per kilogram, we multiply by the government estimate of the average Australian consumption (not including infants) at 520 grams per day. This brings us to an average daily cost of animal foods at $2.58 per person. Total weekly cost of animal protein concentrates, then, for a family of four is $72.24 ($18.06 per person).

The same family can adequately replace the above animal-derived protein foods with vegetarian protein concentrates. A suitable weekly selection covers quite a variety of costs. Thus, to suitably analyse these for a valid comparison, we shall list them below, taking into account such quantities of each as will provide adequate protein concentrates for the average person on a daily basis:

	Cost per kg	Cost per meal
85 g raw almond or cashew kernels	$10.00	85c
70 g raw sunflower kernels	4.10	29c
70 g brown lentils, cooked or sprouted	2.30	16c
85 g sesame seed kernels, ground	3.15	27c
85 g raw Brazil kernels	5.25	45c
60 g raw pepitas (pumpkin kernels)	6.30	38c
70 g soya beans, cooked	1.35	9c

Totalling these daily costs, we arrive at a week's basic protein needs of $2.49 per person — $9.96 for a family of four. Compared to meat costs for the same family, an almost unbelievable weekly saving of $62.28 is offered in direct food expenses (not to mention the savings accruing from improved health, lower medical and dental bills and longer life).

This huge weekly saving multiplies to an annual amount of $3238.56. Over a three-year period, the total saving on this one aspect of the family's diet is enough to buy a brand new family car (nearly $10,000). And every three years thereafter, another new car is obtained free simply by applying the savings from replacing animal foods in the diet with vegetarian protein sources. Is there any reason for poverty in this land of opportunity, high wages and ample fresh food? Poverty only prevails when people fail to take care of their health or fail to accept opportunities life always has on offer.

Often we have heard the foundationless argument that vegetarians eat more fruit and vegetables than others so their living costs are higher. When you consider that for a person to become a vegetarian, concern is felt for their general health; when you reason that they generally do not smoke or drink alcoholic liquors; do not munch on cakes, cookies or candies between meals (if they do eat between meals, it is usually fruit or dried fruits), then it becomes clear that the general vegetarian bill for living expenses is less than for non-vegetarians.

A further important area of saving can arise from a substantial reduction in health care costs. The cost of health insurance will more than pay for the cost of insuring the family's new car each year!

Why refuse such an offer — free car, even free insurance? Surely this must warrant discarding old addictions!

Promotional Frauds and Misunderstandings

A combination of two powerful influences do much to condition man's dependence on meat. First, those industries which have developed into multi-million dollar ventures based on the use of meat cannot afford declining patronage. By retaining skilled promoters and lobbyists, they guarantee their investments.

The second influence is the force of habit. This is a downhill slide all the way, for a majority of people generally accept meat and its products as an essential part of their diet. The promoters only have to keep people thinking that way and encouraging them to increase their meat consumption. The strong desire to avoid a change offers a powerful basis for conformity.

But, as Henrik Ibsen's play *An Enemy of the People* proved, the majority is often wrong where vested interests prevail, although not easily convinced of it. Fortunately, as youth rebels against man's inhumanity towards man, it inquires further and questions many of our hitherto unquestioned habits.

Many industries seek to justify their existence and promote their sales by means that invite questioning. Let us examine the meat industry to see the fast pace it has set, both by direct advertising and promotional falsehoods.

1. "Meat Provides the Only Complete Protein"

Not only do nuts and seeds provide all essential amino acids, but their molecular structure is far simpler than that of animal meats. So, too, is the physical structure of nuts and seeds easier for man to chew, for they are most nutritious and convenient when raw — raw meat does not attract man's appetite. For example, methionine, an essential growth amino acid, has its richest source in Brazil nuts. The ease with which protein from nuts and seeds is catabolised is evidenced by the lower concentration of hydrochloric acid demanded by them, as compared with animal protein and the heavy concentration of HCl it demands of the stomach.

2. "Meat Provides Body Warmth and Strength"

Here we have a further serving of primitive superstition. We earlier looked into the "strength" aspect, noting that the strongest animals are vegetarian, and dismissing as gross superstition the notion that by consuming strong tissue, man can absorb its strength. Likewise, the animal's ability to withstand greater temperature extremes than man is non-transferable. The rich, red blood of an animal is of no use to man — he must manufacture his own from basic nutrients. The mineral iron is essential for this, but iron is more abundant in almonds and sunflower kernels than in beef (see the following table). Animals do not wear clothes compelled by the vanity and self-consciousness of man — thus their skins are tougher. They also exercise more and their blood circulation is not as restricted by poor diet as is man's. These are the real requirements for body warmth.

3. "Meat Is Not Fattening Like Nuts and Seeds"

True, meat is lower in calories by analysis, but inside the human body a different picture emerges. Man cannot store protein in excess of his requirements; hence excess amino acids are broken down by the liver into carbohydrates and fats. One of the habits in meat eating is overindulgence, with the obvious consequences of greater calorie intake. Nuts and seeds are fattening when eaten as snacks, between meals — especially since they are usually roasted and salted to induce greater consumption. Anything can be fattening when eaten in excess — and snacking is just that. Nuts and seeds are intended for meals, to be eaten raw and unsalted. As such, in correct quantities, they are definitely not fattening. Instead, they provide man with excellent sources of most nutrients, as may be seen in the table on page 77. These figures were provided by the CSIRO and the Commonwealth Department of Health for my food analysis book, *Guidebook to Nutritional Factors in Edible Foods* (Pythagorean Press, Sydney, 1977 and Woodbridge Press, California, USA, 1979).

It is important to note that, on average, calorie content of animal meats is half that of nuts and seeds. But let us not forget that those people who depend on animal meat as the crux of their dietary habits consume at least four times as much (on average) as do vegetarians who depend on nuts and seeds. The meat eaters, therefore, are consuming twice as many calories from their protein concentrate as are vegetarians.

Please also note the absence of cholesterol from the analyses of almonds and sunflower seeds — in fact, from all vegetable protein sources. The bodies of animals and humans require cholesterol to perform properly, so nature has endowed each with the ability to manufacture its own in accordance with its needs. Foreign cholesterol is thus unneeded and undesirable. In man, it can precipitate dangerous health problems which are avoided completely when animal foods are absent from the diet.

This section should not be concluded before we also take a look at the fat situation. Nuts and seeds contain up to twice as much fat, by analysis, as does beef. This again implies that, with four times the amount of beef being consumed on average, the meat eater is swallowing twice as much fat by weight. But what makes this consideration far worse is that animal fats are largely saturated fatty acids — fats in nuts and seeds are largely polyunsaturated and therefore more readily digested and utilised by the body.

Also note that animal foods are totally devoid of dietary fibre. This is a significant factor in modern man's pre-occupation with constipation and bowel problems. No other animal suffers this way, for they eat foods which instinct tells them are natural to

Nutrients in Various Protein Foods

Protein Source	A	B	C	D	E	F
Water — %	59	74	36	79	5	5
Protein — g	22	13	26	18	20	24
Fat — g	19	12	33	4	54	47
Carbohydrate — g	0	1	0	3	19	20
Fibre — g	0	0	0	0	2.6	3.8
Calories	258	160	402	91	598	560
Calcium — mg	16	54	860	93	245	120
Phosphorus — mg	209	218	506	182	473	837
Iron — mg	3	2	1	3	4	7
Sodium — mg	82	122	610	290	4	30
Potassium — mg	377	129	100	72	773	920
Magnesium — mg	21	11	45	45	270	38
Carotene (A) — mg	0.01	0.28	0.42	T	0	T
Thiamine (B_1) — mg	0.06	0.1	0.04	0.02	0.2	2
Riboflavin (B_2) — mg	0.16	0.3	0.5	0.3	0.8	0.2
Niacin (B_3) — mg	4	0.1	0.1	0.1	4	5
Cholesterol — mg	70	550	100	15	0	0

g indicates number of grams;
mg indicates number of milligrams;
all referring to 100 g of edible portion.
A is choice rump beef, "rare";
B is whole, raw eggs;
C is cheese — natural cheddar;
D is cheese — cottage, uncreamed;
E is almonds — raw, unsalted;
F is sunflower kernels — raw, unsalted;
T indicates that only a trace exists.

their needs. For man, nuts and seeds provide significant contributions to his fibre requirements — they also provide abundant alkalising minerals, whereas animal proteins contain higher concentrations of acid-forming minerals than alkaline.

The table of comparisons seems to reveal that, of all the animal protein sources, soft cheeses prevail as the most nutritionally desirable for man, but they are regarded as inferior to the plant proteins of nuts and seeds which are more easily digested.

Most vegetarians today include cheese, eggs and milk in their diet. Occasional meals including cheese and eggs can be easily handled by the body, but not milk (discussion to follow). These vegetarians have come to be known as ovo-lacto-vegetarians.

The Menace of Milk

The use of certain milk products to supplement the natural vegetarian diet has become a modern habit in response to skilful promotion, rather than in answer to man's need. If prepared from raw, fresh milk, some cheeses, yogurt and the like are reasonably acceptable as occasional substitutes for superior plant protein sources; but it is not easy to obtain these products from healthy animals or free from chemicals. And great care should be exercised in choosing the commercial varieties.

Most animals encourage their infant progeny to suckle mother's milk until old enough to take solid food. Man, the glaring exception, appears to believe that his offspring are never weaned. Not only do humans accept the general habit of milk drinking as natural, but they compound ignorance by willingly drinking copious quantities of "foreign" milk.

All infant mammals have the need for mother's milk and nature has seen to it that every female mammal has the natural ability of providing this whitish lymph secretion through her mammary glands. The suckling infant possesses suitable digestive enzymes to extract necessary nutrients from its mother's milk, each animal requiring varied dietary components to satisfy its natural growth needs. It is therefore of fundamental importance to realise that milks from different mammals are not interchangeable, some being richer in certain nutrients, inadequate in others.

No more pertinent comparison can be made than to examine the suitability of cow's milk for the needs of the infant human. Human milk has more than twice the lecithin content of cow's milk, although other proteins are much richer in cow's milk. In fact, the total protein content of cow's milk is nearly three times that recorded in human milk. This reveals how imbalanced is cow's milk in terms of satisfying human infant needs for minimal protein in the early months.

Vitamin A, niacin and ascorbic acid are richer in human milk than in cow's, by factors of up to three. Yet cow's milk contains some three times more calcium and phosphorus, the bone-forming mineral elements, than human milk. Furthermore, these minerals are combined in different compounds (more complex and concentrated) than are found in human milk, a factor not readily recognisable from superficial analysis. The comparison can be continued for every nutrient so far known to man, and in every instance considerable differences will be recorded. Goat's milk is also considerably different in composition to human's, but the combining of the elements into compounds in goat's milk results in simpler chemicals, somewhat more suited to infant human needs than cow's milk.

The natural growth pattern of the infant human is the reverse of that of the other animals. Human life demands far greater powers of mental aptitude than physical; hence the brain must develop faster than the body. The reverse applies to animals. By age five, the human child has learned, basically, as much as will be learned during the remainder of life, so psychologists tell us. This indicates how much nourishment is required by the brain and nerves of the infant human.

However, physical growth of the infant human is very slow compared to other animals. Calves are running around a day after being born. After a year, a calf is at least ten times its birth weight. Human infants need one to two years to develop sufficient strength in their legs to walk; one year after birth, their average weight is only a little over three times birth weight. And it requires another dozen or so years before they are able to produce offspring — animals can do so in a fraction of the time.

At this point, it is appropriate to consider the food manufacturers' alternative to mother's milk: infant feeding formulae. This laboratory-conceived concoction might appear similar to breast milk in general formulation but the variations are far more discernible to the body of the infant. Whereas 60 per cent of the protein in mother's milk is in the form of whey and 40 per cent as caseinogen, formulae provide 100 per cent caseinogen. Whereas breast milk provides saturated fat and high cholesterol to satisfy the infant's particular needs in these preliminary years, formulae are almost entirely unsaturated fats and low cholesterol. Hence, formula babies become fatter — a condition which is aggravated by the formula baby's intake being controlled by the mother, whereas the breast-fed baby regulates its own intake. Perhaps obesity begins here with the production of too many fat cells! This is exacerbated by introducing solid foods too early — they must be introduced slowly and singly and certainly not before six months.

A further problem with bottle feeding relates to the teeth. There is some considered opinion that the development of protruding upper teeth can be traced to bottle feeding. But whatever diversion of opinion greets this proposition, it is swept aside by the general agreement that the bottle-popping baby dribbles far more than does the breast-fed infant. With the saliva containing so much lactose (milk sugar) during and immediately after feeding, a potentially devastating development of dental caries can commence at this early age.

The final problem associated with bottle feeding relates to both the cellular and emotional benefits of breast feeding. Antibodies from the mother are communicated to the infant from the first suckle upon mother's breast, continuing for the duration of breast feeding involvement. This conveys vital assistance to the baby by which its own auto-immune system is speedily developed; meanwhile, that of the mother provides support. This implies the mother's need to avoid smoking, drinking alcohol, or any other self-destructive habits which reduce her own auto-immunity. In the area of emotions, there is nothing to compare with the intimate communion between mother and babe such as takes place during breast feeding — bottle feeding so totally denies this intimacy that it can induce the subtle feeling of separation in the infant and give rise to conditions underlying future insecurity.

To enable the complex protein of milk to be digestible, the human stomach is equipped with a special enzyme, rennin, designed to coagulate caseinogen, the principal protein in milk. This is the essential initial step in its effective digestion. However, once infant teeth commence to form, rennin is found to diminish and has completely dried up by the time the second teeth are cut. Milk protein thereafter is only partially utilised, and can be harmful.

To many a mother whose anxious nights have been spent watching her asthmatic child gasping for breath while its mucus-filled respiratory passages react to a predominantly milk diet, little further proof is necessary as to the menace of milk. Within a week of eradicating all milk and milk products from their diet, 50 per cent of all asthmatics show remarkable recoveries. (If removal from disharmonious surroundings could also be achieved, the other 50 per cent would recover.) Try it — there is no better way to prove for yourself. Remember, no other animal suffers from asthma.

(When infants feed on mother's milk, they should not have any other food in their stomach for the duration of milk's gastric digestion — milk impedes the digestion of any other food — see Stage 9.)

Cheeses and yogurts derived from most commercially produced milk bypass the body's rennin limitations by providing the milk protein in a far more usable form, having been chemically coagulated. But care should be taken to choose those coagulated dairy foods which are freshest and made with the least chemicals. Raw milk cheeses and yogurts are to be preferred.

"Vegetarians Are Too Sensitive"

This might be totally correct, explaining my reason for considering the criticism of vegetarianism by ex-vegetarian people. There has been a noticeable refinement of sensitivity since our family converted from meat eating in 1965. But this has taught us that, instead of hiding one's sensitivities, we must mature to develop proper control over them. Sensitivities are our reliable guides to intuitive knowledge and are intended to guide us through uncertainty as a cat's whiskers guide it through the darkness.

When on a lecture and research tour through South America in 1969, my contact with leading archaeologist and philosopher, Gene Savoy, provided rare insights into the ancient Inca civilisations and culture. He had undertaken many exploratory treks to the headwaters of the Amazon Basin region of eastern Peru where he found himself exposed to witchcraft and such negative vibrations that he had to take up meat eating to protect his sensitivities. As he told me this, I was enjoying my avocado salad while he enthusiastically tucked into baby lamb chops in the dining-room of the Hotel Carillon, Lima, Peru. Such excuses for addiction!

As a delegate to the 1980 National Nutrition Foods Association Convention at the Hyatt Regency, Chicago, Illinois, I had the opportunity to meet and listen to one of the founders of the modern health food industry, Gayelord Hauser. Now in his eighties, Hauser explained from the platform that he is not a vegetarian "because vegetarians are too sensitive". He added that he drinks lots of milk which he blends from powdered and skim, "whips into a cream which is delicious atop my coffee". For lunch, he eats leftover meats in his salad; for breakfast, eggs and cereal; for dinner three to four ounces of meat, a cheese omelette, a salad, a potato and fresh fruit — defying all rules of food combining! But, unfortunately, he is a rather insensitive egocentric.

One has to be careful not to appear critical, especially when evaluating information provided by one's elders — and more especially if they are famous people. But when one is sensitive, one learns to discriminate between fact and habit. Meat is one of the many addictions to which one can become so attached that it determines one's line of reasoning, for habit often demands justification. There is no justification to a belief that meat improves one's outlook on life, but it certainly does reduce one's sensitivity by its own heavier vibrations (from dead substances), the heavier feeling it leaves in the stomach and the way it clouds the reasoning faculties.

It does make one wonder why anyone would choose to reduce the level of their awareness when most people seek to sharpen it! Anyone with acute sensitivity is fully aware that it is an endowment which must be understood and channelled, rather than curtailed. To develop and utilise sensitivity is to become more attuned to life, happier by the improved emotional control. For this reason, we rarely find people with balanced sensitivity eating meat.

"Vegetarians Rob Life"

One amusing, though erroneous, argument has developed over recent years, arising from the vegetarian's argument that the eating of meat robs the animal of life in a cruel, murderous way. No-one in his logical mind can refute this, but to counter it, the argument has been concocted that the eating of plant foods also robs life. Does it?

Animals must be killed. Once dead, decay sets into animal flesh to such an extent that it must be very thoroughly cooked to kill the numerous bacteria which take up residence in degenerating tissue. Prior to being killed the animal usually has vigorously resisted the death it senses approaching, having as much desire to perpetuate its life as does man.

The resistance in the animal is always stimulated by the pumping of adrenalin into its bloodstream. This natural hormone (precipitating a fight-or-flight attitude), incites aggressiveness in the animal, transmitted to people who insensitively bury the dead flesh in their stomach after cremating it on their kitchen funeral pyre. Although adrenalin is a natural drug, its presence will often induce a build-up of mild hostility which is itself intensified by the copious chemical compounds fed to animals raised for human consumption. In fact, the biggest drug users in the world are not humans but animals reared for human consumption. (Wild animals, upon which man originally fed when in need, were not only chemical-free, except for adrenalin, but were far richer in muscle meat and lower in flabby, fatty tissue than today's artificially fed herds.)

The bounty of plant life is very different in its action. Plants produce perfumes to attract the picking of their fruits when ripe. They offer bright colours and create tempting flavours so that man takes the fruit at the stage of its maximum maturity, releasing the seed for further propagation, absorbing the life force into his own (dead animals have none to give!)

Scientists now know that plants have feelings. Highly sensitive electronic equipment has been used in many experiments to prove what students of metaphysics have always known. Animals also have feelings — much more forcefully expressed than those of the plant, far nearer those of man. So for those who respect feelings and revere life, for the conservationists who work so diligently to preserve our environment, for those people who would elevate their awareness, for all who seek freedom from illness, the vegetarian way of life has everything to recommend it.

STAGE SEVEN

Not by Bread Alone

So prone are men and women to regard their own ingrained prejudices as established first principles, that it is difficult to attack and expose old errors without offending those who hold to these. For men usually regard such an attack upon their inherited beliefs and prepossessions as an attack upon their persons.

— Herbert M. Shelton, Ph.D.

Every person is entitled to his beliefs, but if he is to become identified with them, would it not be best that they be worthy of possessing? If such beliefs induce misery, sickness, disharmony and failure of any kind, they should be discarded as offensive to life and replaced by those with proven virtues. There should be no allegiance to stupidity.

Nature has endowed all life with adequate intelligence for its purpose. Man's potential for intelligence is virtually unlimited. Any limitation is imposed by man himself in ignorance of his Creator's endowments upon him.

We are often told that man cannot live by bread alone. This holds true in so many ways — implying that any limitation is unnatural, creating barriers both physical and metaphysical. Barriers to the digestion of foods create indigestion, a name no less applicable to the more subtle barriers constricting understanding, for many people suffer from mental indigestion — a condition known to humorous practitioners as "psychosclerosis" (hardening of the attitude).

Dietary Indigestion

The two basic purposes of food are to derive nourishment for the body and enjoyment for the senses. It is impossible to fully satisfy only one of these requirements, for when either is dissatisfied, indigestion occurs.

Indigestion implies disorder, difficulty, disharmony, displeasure. It is invariably caused by some form of blockage and, more often than not, such blockage is mental. The very best food will give the body no nourishment if the emotions are in conflict. By contrast, even a hamburger — "America's most dangerous missile", said Ralph Nader — will give some form of nourishment if one is at ease, at peace and happy. This example only serves to illustrate how important are one's emotions in nutrition, but it is perhaps not the most suitable choice of example — for the peaceful person will not be long in that harmonious state once the effects of his hamburger have been inflicted upon his digestive tract!

But, all too often, ingenious man discovers potions and cures for his rebelling intestines just as readily as he finds excuses and justifications for his emotional peculiarities and mental limitations. By wilfully avoiding causes, man allows himself to dwell in a sort of fool's paradise which offers nothing but delusion. He becomes his own confidence trickster.

Common belching, stomach rumbling, distension, flatulence and the like are certain indicators of indigestion. Their purpose is to give acute warning that unless the condition is corrected, more serious and chronic distress will follow.

These symptoms of indigestion are craving to have their causes removed. The ingesting of antacids only compounds an already complex chemical problem within the body. For best immediate relief, a short visit to the toilet is the first call, followed by a cup of alfalfa mint herb tea and a long rest. Then one should learn what went wrong, recognising that either the "good food" was not so good after all, or the emotions were in a state of disharmony — must probably, a combination of both.

Indigestion and its colonic companion, constipation, share similar origins and together effectively induce more physical discomfort than anything contrived since the Inquisition. Man has been coaxed away from his pristine lifestyle, offering him long years of abundant health, by an "industrial Eve" tempting him with processed "apples", dulling his sense of awareness of their uselessness with powerful drugs and, finally, offering him death in the most comfortable style since hospitals were first invented to house the offenders of nature.

Food for Confinement

Neither an expectant mother about to give a long-awaited birth, nor a hardened criminal about to be placed in solitary confinement as a maximum level of punishment, will derive any nutritional benefit from the common food for confinement (regarded as "the staple food of man") — white bread. Nor will any other person between these two extremes of human achievement be able to live on bread alone. It would eventually kill him.

Whether served as hot toast to the new mother after giving birth, or thrown into the criminal's cell — no matter how the eyes accept it — the body just can't. Whether spread with melted butter and sweet jam to be washed down by a cup of cocoa, or sitting lonely upon a cracked, dirty plate beside a glass of water — white bread is dangerous. If a slow death is intended by the offerer, white bread is certain to contribute, but this is no fitting reward for a new mother, nor a just punishment for the criminal unless capital punishment is intended as compensation for his crime.

When man became discontented with his natural, ideal environment in the tropics and moved into colder climates, not only did his skin change colour, but also his diet became surprisingly restricted. No longer did he have unlimited growing seasons. Thus, grains became the most popular foods.

It was soon learned that grains could be easily grown, conveniently stored and cheaply prepared into foods which, although not as nourishing as tropical fruits and nuts, compensated by filling the stomach with plenty of bulk. When these grains were ground into a coarse flour and mixed with water, a dough formed. This could be baked to provide a basic stomach filling. Gradually breads were produced in a variety of shapes and sizes, flavours and fillings, so that they took on an unusual measure of importance in daily affairs.

Thus, when the religious leaders prepared their holy books, the importance of bread was reflected in its use as the symbol of life. Jesus, too, chose the use of this symbolism in occasional discussions with His followers. Hence, bread became symbolic of the body of Christ, as well as "the staff of life".

In those pre-industrial days, bread was far more nutritive and sustaining than its modern counterpart. Made from whole grains which were organically grown in fertile soils, early breads were the centre of a working man's meal, his true "staff of life".

These breads were baked fresh each day from flour milled only as required; they contained no chemicals and provided both flavour and nourishment.

Any comparison between that bread and today's innutritive replica exists only in the imagination of the advertisers. The modern basic ingredient is so denatured that even weevils find it impossible to live on white flour. Additions of salt, chemical preservatives, aerators, binders and the like, render today's bread both non-nutritive and indigestible. It is more suitable as a bouncing ball for children than as a staple in their diet. In fact, it is quite easy to convert a loaf of white bread into a bouncing ball — simply withdraw a handful of doughy innards and squeeze it into a ball. It will almost have the bouncing properties of a tennis ball — and just about as much nourishment.

This section cannot be completed without commenting on the favourite promotional gimmick of modern bread manufacturers: "enriched bread". To admit that their bread was so deficient as to need enriching should make any thinking person suspicious, but the whole concept of enriching is itself fraudulent. It is comparable to being accosted by a robber who makes you hand over all your possessions and also takes all your clothes. As you stand in the nude, he takes pity on you and hands back your underwear. Certainly, you feel a little warmer — enriched, even, compared to when you had nothing. But you are far less endowed than when you had all your clothes and possessions.

The analogy is true for milled wheat. Instead of grinding the whole grain to make bread, millers now remove the germ, then the bran, thus effectively retaining only the endosperm, the doughy substance which is mostly carbohydrate. The original grain is robbed of its major protein and fibre components. Then it is bleached and further processed until it possesses virtually no nutrients — it will certainly have a longer shelf-life this way, but that only benefits the shop-owner, while constituting a great loss for the consumer.

So then the bread manufacturer takes pity on the consumer and restores a minimum, a token of the original nutrients as a form of apology and appeasement.

The relative cheapness of modern bread camouflages its tastelessness. For this reason, it is always served adorned with some fatty spread, topped with another spread of sweeter composition, generally the product of refined sugar and salt with boiled fruit. With any other food, this combination would prove troublesome to the digestion; by itself it offers little in the way of nourishment, yet fills the stomach so that the appetite for nourishing food is diminished.

Women of today rarely devote time to the preparation of wholesome food for their families. "Convenience" foods are preferred, in spite of their later inconvenience when it is found that illness has developed. Not at any time can bread be considered a primary source of nourishment, irrespective of how "wholesome" its ingredients may be. But if people elect to eat bread, they should be encouraged to consume freshly made, home baked, whole grain bread, rather than the commercial white substance bearing that name.

Under no circumstances should bread be regarded as the staple of man's diet. It is the staple of no diet — no animal, bird or fish could live on it; yet man sometimes thinks that his body is in such great variance to all of nature, so "superior" that he can defy nature and live on inferior substances. Increasing hospital admissions attest to this gross error.

Not by Bread Alone

Man cannot live by bread alone because bread is not his staple food. To be so classified, food has to provide a balance of nutrients covering the five major groups — proteins, carbohydrates, fats, minerals and vitamins. This type of food must then occupy the bulk of the diet. It must be enjoyable to consume and easy to prepare.

Man's staple food should thus be nothing other than the products of plants — fruits and vegetables.

So simple to obtain, to produce with most normal soils, to eat and to digest, fresh fruits and vegetables should comprise 75 per cent by weight of man's food intake. They are not intended to be employed as snacks, decorations upon the table, or "something to make you go to the toilet", but should be recognised for their vital place in man's world, the basic source of his nutrition.

As such, fresh fruits and vegetables offer a splendid variety of flavours and textures. As living organisms, they abound in a life force which charges their high moisture content with a special quality, much of which is lost when the food is cooked. The older fruits and vegetables become after picking, the greater the loss of nourishment — if cooked or processed, this loss becomes quite considerable. To some extent, the loss can be arrested or somewhat averted if the crop is either promptly frozen or sun-dried, depending on its nature. Carrots and sweet corn, for instance, respond to snap freezing without any prior cooking and they retain most of their nutrients. Fruits generally respond better to sun-drying if their preservation is sought.

It is not always possible for man to produce his own fruit when living in cities. With a relatively small garden he can produce most of his vegetable needs, but he depends on modern transportation for a wide range of fresh fruits. Such fruits must be picked somewhat unripe, although mature, allowing ripeness to take place slowly, away from the plant. This allows for most of the optimum nutrients to be made available, although it is obviously not as ideal as if the fruits were allowed to ripen on the plant. Yet, if that were the only compromise to health emanating from city life, we would indeed be blessed.

Fresh fruits offer a vast variety of shapes, sizes, tastes, colours and perfumes. The greatest range is produced in sub-tropical and temperate climates; although modern transportation now guarantees that within a few days of picking, fruits can be airfreighted anywhere around the world. Thus, from the twenty or thirty different fruits which mature at any given time of the year, man may select his menu from a wide variety. It is obviously best to consume those fruits which are grown locally, but even more important is the manner by which they are cultivated. Preference should always be given to those produced by the organic or biodynamic methods, for they are the most nutritious and the tastiest.

A Garden for Every Kitchen

In some of the closely settled countries of Europe, those people who have learned the vital importance of obtaining fresh fruits and vegetables have employed commendable resourcefulness in acquiring a small plot of arable land on the outskirts of their cities. Each weekend, it is a common sight to see these city dwellers cycling or motoring to their own intensive gardens where they will probably spend the entire weekend engaged in producing their own food.

This is an example of which every apartment dweller should take particular notice. Not only does it guarantee one the very best food, but it allows a vital "unwinding" from the oppressiveness of the city, thereby providing subtle food for the nerves.

Unfortunately, this "radical" suggestion is invariably met with any number of reasons for not being undertaken. Rarely does one hear a confession of having not considered it previously, and advice sought as to how it can best be done. To own one's own small segment of producing land, devoted primarily to the raising of the family's food, plus a few flowers for the home or apartment, is to invest in the most beneficial insurance man's health has received since he took to city dwelling.

To accept the idea of city dwellers producing their own food is to recognise the importance of real independence. And it should be remembered that there are always more ways of being able to do a thing than of excusing its omission.

An excellent start towards the goal of an out-of-town food plot is to develop one's tiny kitchen garden for the sprouting of seeds, pulses or grains at home.

An essential ingredient of all salads should be fresh sprouts. Alfalfa, as the name (in Arabic) implies, is the king of all sprouts — grown as a plant, its roots are known to burrow as much as twelve metres into subsoil to bring up valuable trace minerals of which manganese is especially important to health and digestion (it is a vital component of human insulin). No day should pass without our including a sprout salad as a vital component of the meal, if not the entire meal.

Of all vegetables available to the human diet, sprouts have been proven to rank as the freshest and most nutritious. By a process of natural transmutation, sprouted food has greatly improved digestibility and nutritional qualities when compared to the non-sprouted embryo from which it derives (whether it be seed, pea, bean, lentil or grain).

For thousands of years, sprouted foods have been part of the diets of many ancient races. Even to this day, Chinese people retain a fame for their delicious mung bean sprouts and bamboo shoots, well known to those Westerners fond of Chinese cooking. Herbivorous animals roam the pastures in search of the choicest grass sprouts, to the benefit of their health and vitality. The same animals fed on silage or processed stock feeds evidence marked reductions in health, as witnessed by the increasing occurrence of such diseases as foot-and-mouth.

If only they could talk to man, every animal would rave about how much it enjoys eating tender, young sprouts. If the sprouts could talk, they would have man realise just how much nourishment they offer, how they provide all those essential vitamins and minerals, how they "enjoy" being eaten and appreciated and converted into the higher "vibrations" of man's healthy living tissue! Not a man nor woman should consider their education complete until they learn how to include a range of delicious sprouts in their diet, and how to produce these sprouts in tiny gardens in their very own kitchens. No kitchen should be without at least one sprouting tube, trough or bowl.

Sprouting requires no constant care, no soil and only an occasional sprinkling of water. Many varieties of seeds, pulses and grains are easily sprouted whenever desired; until such time, they can be stored in their dried state for years without decline in potential food value, provided the place of storage is dry, clean and cool.

The Simple Science of Sprouting

By far the tastiest and speediest way to grow sprouts is in a double-ended tube known as a "Sprout Ease" or "The Tube". This is recommended by the world's leading sprout expert, Dr Ann Wigmore of Boston, Massachusetts, whose health clinic, responsible for so many recoveries, features sprouts as the primary food.

Sprouting tubes permit thorough daily washing in just a few moments. They are generally sold with four different end caps — one solid and three with a variety of mesh openings designed to suit different types of sprouts. They always look attractive on the kitchen shelf, especially if you have a few of them with different varieties of sprouts growing simultaneously. They carry an instruction leaflet, but for those who seek general guidance or prefer to use a kitchen jar with coarse cloth over the opening, here are the easy steps to follow:

1) Ensure that the seed, pulse or grain selected is a sproutable type. Soya beans do not sprout well, often souring; wheat has to be grown in soil; watercress in water, etc.
2) Soak overnight in a cup of pure water (chemicals, especially fluoride, will slow the rate of sprouting — even halt it). Select a suitable quantity to sprout — usually two tablespoons per tube.
3) Allow to soak for up to twenty-four hours.
4) After securing the solid cap to the end of the sprouting tube, place the sprouts inside. Screw on the appropriate mesh to the other end (smallest mesh for alfalfa seeds, medium for most other sprouts). Rinse sprouts under running water in the tube; allow to drain.
5) Place tube in a dark cupboard (the oven is a good place, so long as it is not being used for cooking) for another twenty-four hours. This gives an early stimulus to the sprouts. Take care they do not get too hot (this causes souring) or too cold (the cause of stagnation).
6) Remove from dark place and rinse again. Allow to drain and leave draining in the light (be sure to avoid direct sunlight since this causes souring). Rinse under running water and drain once each twenty-four hours — if the weather is hot and dry, rinse each morning and evening. Ensure proper draining by standing the tube so that water will drain from the mesh at the lower end.

If using an open trough for sprouting, regular sprinkling a few times each day will be necessary. These troughs are a convenient means of sprouting and are cheaper than the tubes, but they do not produce as much, nor do the sprouts grow with the lushness provided by the more controlled humidity inside the tube.

Sprouts should be ready for use within four to six days from commencement of soaking, depending on temperature and humidity. Always take care not to allow the sprouts to lie in water — they should be kept well drained to prevent souring.

Sprouts are at their optimum level of flavour and tenderness when tiny green leaves appear at the tips. Their nutritional value will also be optimum and can be retained if care is taken to avoid souring. To retain freshness when sprouts have reached suitable maturity and cannot be immediately eaten, place in the refrigerator; but the temperature should not drop below 5°C, otherwise the sprouts might tend to freeze and wilt. Rinse each day and return to the refrigerator — sprouts can be kept for weeks this way.

Sprouting in soil can be undertaken in much the same manner as seedlings are nurtured for cultivation. Dr Ann Wigmore made her Hippocrates Health Institute famous for its meals of varied sprouts, all raised in soil, and for the "miraculous" recoveries of health experienced by so many who followed her natural living programme.

Dr Wigmore's method is the most suitable when sprouts are required for a large number of people. She and her associate, Viktoras Kulvinskas, would take great delight in watching those amazing sprouts absorb nourishment from the atmosphere and convert it into vitamins and minerals for human consumption. Each has written some excellent books on the health advantages offered by including such living, vital foods in the diet, especially valuable to people living in cold climates which cannot support fresh outdoor cultivation in winter.

Irrespective of the season, no salad is complete without fresh sprouts. Few people realise the amazing increases in nutrients in sprouted foods when compared to their dried embryos. During the transition, the vitamin, mineral and protein contents increase measurably, with corresponding decreases in calorie and carbohydrate contents.

These comparisons must be based on an equivalent water content in each of the foods measured. Analysis of dried seeds, grains and pulses reveals a very low water content; but this increases up to ten-fold as the same food converts into sprouts. Thus, to obtain accurate comparisons, each must be brought to a common denominator of equal water content to measure the exact changes which occur in nutritional value.

For a typical example of recognising the increased nutritional properties of sprouts, let us compare the "before" and "after" figures for mung beans as provided in the *Guidebook to Nutritional Factors in Edible Foods*.

Mung beans sprouted have an 8.3 increase in water content over the dried bean. So that we could compare nutritional values of sprouted and dried beans, it was necessary to multiply the analysed nutrients of sprouted mung beans by the factor of 8.3. Comparing this with the analysis of the dried mung bean, we recorded a percentage increase or decrease in the particular nutrient. These are the changes found in the sprouted mung bean when compared with the figures for the bean in its dried state:

energy content — calories	down 15%
total carbohydrate content	down 9%
protein availability	up 30%*
calcium content	up 34%
potassium content	up 80%
sodium content	up 690%**
iron content	up 40%
phosphorus content	up 56%
vitamin A content	up 208%
thiamine (vitamin B_1) content	up 285%
riboflavin (vitamin B_2) content	up 515%
niacin (vitamin B_3) content	up 256%
ascorbic acid (vitamin C) content	an infinite increase.***

* The high increase in protein availability is of special significance. While not as dramatic as the increases recorded for vitamins, it is a most important indicator of the improved nutritional value of a food when sprouted. The simultaneous reduction in carbohydrate content tends to indicate that many carbohydrate molecules are broken down during sprouting to allow an absorption of atmospheric nitrogen and a re-forming into amino acids (protein). This is a most important transition, an aspect of the chemical process known as autolysis which has hitherto been ignored in relation to improved human nutrition and the provision of protein-rich foods for the world's underprivileged. The resultant protein is the most easily digestible of all proteins available in foods.

** This dramatic increase in sodium content supports the contention that sprouts offer superior nutritional properties. Sodium is a mineral vital to the digestive processes within the gastrointestinal tract and also to the elimination of carbon dioxide. Together with the dramatic vitamin increases, sodium materially contributes to the easy digestibility of sprouts.

*** Dried seeds, grains and pulses contain no discernible traces of ascorbic acid, yet, when sprouted, they reveal quite significant quantities which are eminently significant in the body's ability to metabolise proteins. The infinite increase in ascorbic acid (as available vitamin C) in sprouts derives from their absorption of atmospheric elements during growth.

In light of the foregoing, it must appear an unfortunate omission in the general study of human nutrition that the vital nutritional advantages of sprouted foods are neglected. Especially so when this neglect is compounded by so much concentration on the minimal nutritional properties of processed, refined foods — "foodless" by comparison.

STAGE EIGHT

Our Nutritional Needs

Reason should direct, and appetite obey.

Cicero (106-43 B.C.)

But it does not follow that way! After all these years, after the greatest teachings of the world have been given us, man keeps getting sicker and sicker. Appetite still directs and reason remains at bay.

Not only with food, but with almost every activity involving mankind — it is far more a case of what do I want, than what do I need. Yet, when reason prevails, we find that our needs provide far more fully than our wants. All we have to do is be able to recognise them.

In terms of human nutrition this is not difficult, provided that man will act in reasonable honesty and that he is guided by his intelligence rather than misguided by his prejudices. Modern technology has been very generous in providing man with a greater depth of understanding about his nutritional needs than any previous generation has been privileged to receive. All we need now is to use this knowledge. It is time to realise that a basic general knowledge of human nutrition is a vital fundamental to life.

To many, nutrition is a complex science, largely because they have had little familiarity with it during their formative years. Actually, its basic rules are comparatively simple. Each group of nutrients has characteristic functions when allowed to perform naturally, unimpeded by interfering artificial chemicals such as abound in many processed "foods". The major nutrient groups are: proteins, carbohydrates, lipids (fats and oils), minerals and vitamins.

If you do not take care of your body, where are you going to live? So let us look into each of the five basic groups of food nutrients, and observe how they are handled by the body to its greatest advantage.

Proteins

Of all nutrients, proteins are recognised as primary to the body's needs for living. They constitute the basic structure of every living cell, representing a group of complex chemical compounds which are constantly subject to wear, growth and replacement.

The name "protein" indicates the importance of this nutrient. It derives from "primary", being so named from the German word used to describe its function in the human body.

Proteins are the most complex chemicals in the study of nutrition, yet their activities in the body are relatively easy to understand. As with carbohydrates and fats, proteins include carbon, hydrogen and oxygen; however, proteins also contain nitrogen and sometimes sulphur or iodine, essential elements in body maintenance.

All plants and animals contain protein and all proteins are composed of amino acids.

Whereas plants feed upon simple inorganic chemicals from which they synthesise their amino acid requirements, animals do not possess this ability.

For all animal bodies to build protein, they must eat either plants or other animals which have lived on plants. However, animal proteins are more complex; they demand very high concentrations of hydrochloric acid in the stomach to initiate the chemical breakdown which will finally isolate the component amino acids. Human stomachs do not possess such high concentrations of hydrochloric acid; they are designed by nature to handle simpler plant proteins more efficiently. Thus animal proteins usually do not undergo thorough gastric breakdown in the human stomach. By the time they reach the duodenum and small intestine for final breakdown, there has been insufficient preparatory digestive work. This suggests that not all of the amino acids are isolated, implying a wastage factor when some are eliminated from the body before becoming usable.

Since protein was scientifically recognised a little over a century go, man has tended to focus concern more on the quantity of available protein in a food, rather than its quality. He relies more on chemical analysis than a knowledge of his body's ability to digest, even though there is often a great divergence between theory and practice. This is especially evident in the study of protein in human nutrition. Let us endeavour to exemplify with the general, although not entirely accurate, analogy of fuelling a car.

Semi-crude petroleum contains enough essential chemicals to run a car. But to use this complex ingredient in the fuel tank, even with selected additives, would place a heavy burden on the engine, which does not have the ability to fully break down the semi-crude into totally usable petrol. The car will run ever so much better if simpler fuel is fed into its engine.

The human stomach, likewise, does not possess the ability to sufficiently "refine" complex nutrients for total breakdown. The stomach is vital in preparing proteins for final breakdown, but its limitations are exceeded when the protein intake is too great or too complex. This demands extra energy of the body as the stomach works hard to fulfil its purpose, but is not always totally successful. This energy drain is felt by the body, which registers tiredness after a huge meal. At least a period of relaxation would aid the gastric juices in their heroic efforts, but it must be obvious that greater wisdom lies in not eating huge or complex meals.

A penalty which follows the incomplete catabolism of food proteins is that they tend to become absorbed into the bloodstream in an unusable state. There has been insufficient isolation of component amino acids to allow the process of anabolism (build-up of food nutrients into protoplasm and cell tissue) to be properly performed. Being unusable and undesirable passengers in the bloodstream, these proteins are rejected in the most expedient way — either through the normal organs of dietary elimination or through the skin. This latter condition gives rise to many uncomfortable allergies so prevalent in human society today.

The total quantity of protein required in man's daily diet is determined by the size of his body, the amount of work in which it is involved and the climate in which it lives. An average daily requirement of around 50 g of usable protein concentrate per day is generally accepted — more for a hard-working person, less for an inactive one. This implies that a food containing 20 per cent protein would provide the body's daily needs if 250 g were eaten each day, and if all of this protein were totally usable.

All foods should be considered relative to their protein content and amino acid composition. As all foods contain protein, it is obvious that the body does not have to be fed huge quantities of concentrated protein sources to obtain its basic protein requirements. However, remember that the body cannot store protein as such.

Intake of protein greatly in excess of the body's needs creates extra work for the liver. Its job includes the deamination of excess proteins, the process which removes the amino (NH_2) group of chemicals. The remainder is converted to carbohydrates or fat, with some of it being oxidised to carbon dioxide and water. The type of protein determines the manner of the reaction.

Excessive protein intake also creates extra work for the kidneys. Ideally, it is their job to remove excess acids, the deaminated group of chemicals being most conveniently eliminated from the body when excreted as urea.

Protein-rich foods, especially of animal origin, are usually the most expensive components of the diet. With increasing affluence in our society, protein-rich foods occupy a higher proportion of the average person's daily food intake. This, in turn, places an increased burden on the kidneys and is a major factor in the pandemic prevalence of kidney failure throughout the Western world today — the general protein intake having risen out of all proportion to the body's needs.

With animal protein foods being consumed from habit, induced by taste stimulation and with little or no recognition of the body's protein-handling abilities, it is of little wonder that modern man has so much uric acid in his bloodstream, so often leading to gout and arthritis. It is true that protein requirements might vary considerably from person to person — some might find 60 g of protein-rich food provides an adequate nitrogen balance in their body; others might need up to 400 g per day. Variations can be created by the person's age, nature of work, the climate, amount of exercise undertaken, body weight, etc. Experience and observation will indicate actual protein needs, but the usual amount of protein-rich foods is as indicated on page 74 (meat-eaters require an average of 150 g — far less than actual consumption indicates).

Insufficient protein is rarely encountered in Western man's dietary intake. But in the "underdeveloped" countries, inadequate dietary protein is a common problem. It is registered in the prevalence of such diseases as anaemia, kwashiorkor, pellagra, various liver problems, etc. However, it is the quality of the protein in the food which determines whether the body's needs are satisfied, rather than the quantity. For instance, 80 g of raw nuts, such as cashew and Brazil nuts (found growing prolifically in Africa, India and Brazil), would provide more usable protein than 300 g of beef, a kilogram of milk powder or of high-protein wheat. The United Nations would do well to consider the natural alternative, for it would also be far less expensive in direct food costs, as well as in the saving accruing from reduced medical and dental care costs.

I was very disappointed to see countless tonnes of valuable cashew nuts rotting in the forests of Tanzania during my visit in 1972. While many natives were being trained to fight in "wars of liberation", others who were at home were often not encouraged to collect the nuts for shelling, or even for shipment to India, where most cashew nuts are shelled. That government's priorities seemed so out of order, yet no one was venturesome enough to say anything. The result of that neglect (which was paralleled in neighbouring Mozambique) meant that the world's two largest producers of cashews created a serious shortage which prevails even to this day, forcing the price of cashews up into the luxury class. This is where the United Nations' guidance is lacking and people's health is suffering.

To moderate one's protein intake by adjusting to the body's needs does not imply a monotonous diet, as many people tend to fear. Instead, there is more room in the planning of the diet and in the capacity of the stomach for the inclusion of suitable and tasty combinations of fresh fruits and vegetables. Their added vitamin and mineral abundance will also materially aid the digestion of proteins. As will be detailed in Stage 10, when we discuss man's ideal diet, no monotony exists once man realises how bountiful nature can be with a little encouragement from your own garden.

It is a widely held view among conventional nutritionalists that man's primary protein foods are meat, eggs, cheese and milk. This is a view influenced by habit, but it runs counter to opinion expressed by other students of nutritional science. There we learn that plant foods provide man's primary sources of protein, just as they do for all animals which do not possess claws and fangs.

The argument that plant proteins are not complete proteins is equally false. Man can synthesise twenty different amino acids in his liver by the process of transamination, in which molecules are exchanged under the influence of a special enzyme, transaminase. This allows the diet to be deficient in some of these twenty amino acids without the body suffering loss. However, eight or ten additional amino acids (children need two more than adults) cannot be synthesised by the body. These are known as the essential amino acids.

A protein-concentrated food is accepted as a complete protein when it contains all essential amino acids. This category includes most proteins derived from animals and plants. Nuts and seeds are just as much complete proteins as are meat and fish. But we do not need only the proteins that come from concentrated foods — they also need to be provided from plant foods, such as vegetables and grains. Vegetables are especially important as supportive aspects of a meal. Rarely is a meal complete without a salad, even if cooked vegetables are included (the one exception is a fruit meal, for then the fruit provides some basic protein).

There has been a misconception for years that each meal must provide a complete range of essential amino acids for the body to function properly. Responsibility for such an error is due in part to successful propaganda by meat promotional organisations (usually governments whose vested interests are not so much in suggesting a suitable diet as in selling more meat). The second factor behind this error can be traced to studies made between 1929 and 1950 on rats and other animals. As reported by Dr John Scharffenberg to the American Association for the Advancement of Science (see his book, *Problems with Meat*, Woodbridge Press, Santa Barbara, California, 1979), these studies were based on the use of purified amino acids. Now the human diet does not include purified amino acids in isolation, but rather many amino acids in whatever food we consider.

Recent studies have convincingly proved that if any essential amino acid is missing from a meal, it can be provided in the next meal, or the one after that, and still be as effective in facilitating an adequate balance in the protein intake.

The proper test for a food's protein usefulness is based on its amino acid content — its variety, concentration and degree of complexity. Up to thirty amino acids are known to be required by man, the smaller quantity of essential ones being necessarily present in the food. The degree of concentration of total amino acid content is an important guide to the quantity of food desirable, but not as important as the nature of the amino acids available. The more complex they are, the less efficiently the body can handle them. Thus, plant proteins are obviously to be regarded as primary proteins by virtue of their simpler molecular structure. Animal proteins are secondary because they have undergone concentration of simpler plant proteins in the animal's gastrointestinal tract. Deriving from plants, they have actually become second-hand proteins.

Plant proteins require less digestive time than animal proteins. Demanding a lower concentration of hydrochloric acid, they are more in tune with the ability of the human stomach, thereby creating much less strain than do animal proteins.

As the building stones of cellular protoplasm and, eventually, vital tissue, amino acids deserve more attention than any other food nutrient. Therefore, we shall present a brief resumé of each of the most important amino acids, commencing with the ten essential ones. To assist in understanding their composition, the simple chemical formula for each is given, by which the component elements are shown in proportion to their occurrence in each acid: C = carbon; H = hydrogen; N = nitrogen; O = oxygen; S = sulphur. In addition, the vegetarian sources of each amino acid are listed.

Arginine ($C_6H_{14}N_4O_2$) Essential to the growth of infants; not essential in adult diets from which sufficient can be synthesised for the body's needs. Vital to the elimination of nitrogen from the liver, to the contracting of muscles and to the control of body cell degeneration. Found in most vegetables, especially green and root vegetables.

Histidine ($C_6H_9N_3O_2$) The second essential for the growth of infants. Vital to the formation of glycogen in the liver, the means by which carbohydrates are stored for future energy requirements. Used in HCl production and in mucus control; component of haemoglobin in the blood and semen. Found in root vegetables and all green vegetables.

Isoleucine ($C_6H_{13}NO_2$) Another essential growth amino acid, but one which adults cannot synthesise. It maintains bodily nitrogen equilibrium and regulates metabolism and the thymus, spleen and pituitary glands. Richest in sunflower seeds, all nuts except cashews (where it is only moderately present), avocados, olives and pawpaw.

Leucine ($C_6H_{13}NO_2$) Also essential to growth; the complement of isoleucine, with a similar chemical composition although in different arrangement. Its functions and sources are also similar.

Lysine ($C_6H_{14}N_2O_2$) Essential to the metabolism of fats and the functioning of the gall bladder. Regulates many glandular functions. Rich in most nuts, seeds, vegetables and fruits classified as "sub-acid" (see Stage 9); deficient in grains and yeast.

Methionine ($C_5H_{11}NO_2S$) Essential to the metabolism of fats and cellular growth; a vital sulphur-bearing compound required by haemoglobin (red blood cells), the pancreas, lymph and spleen; works with choline (a B-vitamin) in liver to detoxify amines (by-products of protein catabolism). Richest source of methionine is Brazil nuts, then hazelnuts and other nuts; also found in Brussels sprouts, cabbage, cauliflower, pineapples and apples.

Phenylalanine ($C_9H_{11}NO_2$) Essential to the production of the hormone, adrenalin; to the production of the thyroid secretion, thyroxine, and the skin and hair pigment, melanin. It is also essential for the efficient functioning of kidneys and bladder. Major sources are nuts, seeds, carrots, beetroot, parsley and tomatoes. An important recently discovered therapeutic use for Phenylalanine is in its ability to overcome most conditions of lethargy through the stimulation of adrenalin.

Threonine ($C_4H_9NO_3$) Essential to the formation of many non-essential amino acids in the liver, as well as for the growth of infants. Major sources are nuts, seeds, carrots and green vegetables.

Tryptophan ($C_{11}H_{12}N_2O_2$) Essential to blood clotting, digestive juices and the optic system; vital to the manufacture of vitamin B_3 (niacin), but only if other B-vitamins are present. It is used by the brain to synthesise serotonin, vital neuro-transmitter chemical for carrying messages between nerve cells and to the brain — as well as being one of the biochemical mechanisms of sleep. Hence, tryptophan is now used therapeutically to overcome insomnia and to non-addictively induce normal sleep and dream cycles. Major sources are nuts, seeds and most vegetables.

Valine ($C_5H_{11}NO_2$) An essential body growth factor, particularly for the mammary glands and ovaries. Major sources are almonds, apples and most vegetables.

The following list includes some of the amino acids not regarded as "essential", being capable of synthesis by the liver. Similar to the foregoing essential amino acids, their natural (non-animal) sources can be found in nuts, seeds, vegetables (especially sprouts and green salad vegetables), and some fruits. Fruits, in general, have a very low protein content. This is observable by the protein deficiencies which manifest in such conditions as tropical ulcers and irritability, characteristic of people who do not secure adequate dietary protein (generally seen in fruitarians living in the tropics).

Alanine ($C_3H_7NO_2$) Used in skin and adrenal glands. Richest in almonds.

Aspartic Acid ($C_4H_7NO_4$) Used in bone and teeth strengthening, respiratory functions and blood vessel growth. Richest in almonds.

Cysteine ($C_3H_7NO_2S$) A principal source of sulphur for the body; transaminated from methionine; a general growth factor.

Cystine ($C_6H_{12}N_2O_4S_2$) Although varying in formula, possesses similar properties to cysteine; also a derivative of methionine.

Glutamic Acid ($C_5H_9NO_4$) Used to assist secretion of digestive juices; aids ready availability of glycogen conversion to energy sugar. Predominates in wheat protein, giving the toughness characteristic of dough. In purified form, has a strong "meaty" flavour, implying commercial value in meat-substitute foods; dangerous for coeliacs.

Glycine ($C_2H_5NO_2$) The simplest and lightest amino acid, it has manifold uses in man, such as cartilage and muscle fibre formation and sex hormone control. Demanded in huge quantities by animals and birds during periods of rapid growth, such as for the young chicken.

Hydroxyglutamic Acid ($C_5H_9NO_5$) Assists in controlling generation of gastric juice; works in conjunction with glutamic acid.

Hydroxyproline ($C_5H_9NO_3$) Used by the liver and gall bladder to emulsify fats and in the formation of red blood corpuscles.

Iodogorgoic Acid ($C_9H_9NO_3I_2$) One of the two complex amino acids containing iodine, vital to all glands, especially the thyroid. Abundant in dulse and kelp.

Norleucine ($C_6H_{13}NO_2$) Derives from leucine, working with it to balance its functions.

Proline ($C_5H_9NO_2$) Balances functions of hydroxyproline; it also has a part in the manufacturing of white corpuscles.

Serine ($C_3H_7NO_3$) Works to maintain efficiency and cleansing of respiratory passages.

Thyroxine ($C_{15}H_{11}NO_4I_4$) The second complex iodine-carrying amino acid. It is the heaviest of all known amino acids, with similar functions as iodogorgoic acid; it also assists in the regulation of metabolism.

Tyrosine ($C_9H_{11}NO_3$) Active in the functioning of glands, development of blood protoplasm and the hair.

This is by no means an exhaustive study of amino acids, but rather a guide to their composition, their essential or synthesisable nature and their function within the human body. Again it should be stressed that when man lived in a pristine state, on natural foods free from foreign chemicals, he had no bother in obtaining adequate nourishment for his body from a balanced diet. It is much easier today, with greatly improved transportation. But man must realise the extent to which foreign chemicals interfere with his metabolic processes, and his diet should therefore consist almost entirely of fresh, natural foods.

Carbohydrates

The most prolific nutrients in nature are the carbohydrates. They constitute the bulk of every plant, being synthesised from water and carbon dioxide in the presence of sunlight. Carbohydrates are thus composed of various proportions of carbon, hydrogen and oxygen, appearing in the form of starches, sugars, fibres, gums, etc.

It is not surprising that carbohydrates form the major part of the human diet, varying from as low as 40 per cent of the diet of highly affluent people (who consume large amounts of proteins and fats), to as high as 90 per cent of the poor man's diet. Their relatively low cost and ease of storage makes for the unduly high percentage of carbohydrates in the diet of poorer people. With these are often associated protein deficiencies.

In the natural diet of man, around 60 per cent carbohydrate content is the optimum. Lower percentages often imply a lack of dietary fibre (cellulose), predisposing towards constipation, a characteristic complaint of wealthier people. Compounding this complaint, as well as inducing the bases for others of a more serious nature, is the high intake of refined sugar and flour products which form part of the diet of today's affluent society.

It is important here to distinguish between the refined product of the sugar cane or beet, commercially named "sugar", and the chemical group of saccharides which are fruit sugars. The former is sucrose ($C_{12}H_{22}O_{11}$). Rather than being a food, sucrose offers no nourishment whatsoever. Instead it leaches from the body its valuable stores of alkaline minerals, especially calcium, in the body's effort to handle it. Fruit sugar, on the other hand, is known as fructose ($C_6H_{12}O_6$). It provides the natural sweetness in fresh fruits and some vegetables. This is a natural source of energy, is easily metabolised by the body and does not rob its mineral reserves, nor its insulin.

a) Dietary Fibre

Man need not concern himself over whether he is obtaining adequate carbohydrate if he includes one large salad meal in his daily diet. Salad vegetables provide essential starches and fibre, as well as vitamins and minerals, for which reason they are a vital component of the daily diet. Without salads, the chances are that man is not obtaining sufficient fibre, unless he deliberately includes whole grains or bran in his diet.

A best-selling book has recently caught the imagination of English-speaking people. It offers what it considers the ideal remedy for "saving your life" — eating bran. Written by an eminent medical practitioner, this book certainly succeeds in drawing attention to the omission of fibre from the modern diet, but its method of remedying the omission is not the ideal one.

Bran, the outer husk of wheat and rice grains, contains in addition to fibre, many valuable nutrients, including alkalinising minerals, phosphorus and B vitamins; but it is not a natural food in terms of its low water content. It is difficult to digest without added liquid. As this is generally milk, the eating of bran implies the inclusion of an unsuitable substance in the diet. If people will not learn to eat a daily salad, then the intake of daily bran will be better than developing constipation and its attendant problems. However, it should be realised that bran is only a cheap substitute for a salad, being devoid of adequate moisture and the balanced vitamin and mineral content which is available from a fresh salad of celery, lettuce, cucumbers, capsicums, tomatoes, carrots, beetroots and fresh sprouts.

Being so high in fibrous carbohydrate and low in sugars, bran must be chewed long and thoroughly. It must be remembered that the stomach has no teeth! Bran demands the thorough breaking down of its fibres to allow digestion to work towards extracting its nutrients. With this breaking down by chewing, ptyalin, the starch-splitting enzyme in the saliva, works on reducing starches into sugars for easier digestion. However, when such a dry substance as bran is consumed, it is necessarily saturated in milk or, preferably, fruit juice. The human tendency is then to semi-drink it, swallowing much too prematurely. Consequently, its digestive time is prolonged by the omission of ptyalin's preparatory work.

Fresh fruits and vegetables contain abundant quantities of moisture. As such, they are easily chewed and consumed. Further, their delightful flavours induce them to be retained in the mouth longer for their enjoyment and more thorough mastication; whereas bran tends to possess a semi-bitterness which many people find unpleasant, inducing that premature swallowing.

Fresh fruits and vegetables offer a full range of carbohydrate nutrients — sugars, starches and fibres. In general, fruits are richer in sugars, vegetables in starches; but if one meal each day is devoted to fresh fruits, and one to fresh vegetables, abundant carbohydrate intake (plus vitamin and mineral intake) will be assured.

b) Ripening

The conversion of starches to sugars in fruits occurs during the process of natural ripening. This develops both the delicious sweetness of fruits and their ease of digestion, for fruits are the easiest of all foods in terms of digestive demands on the body. For this reason, fruits pass from the stomach in less time than any other class of food, allowing speedier availability of their nutrients for energy.

If fruits are forced into premature maturity or ripening by chemical gases, they do not develop a proper sugar content and become deficient in their optimum general nutrient levels. Modern marketing techniques demand uniform ripening of fruits, but nature has other ideas.

When we observe the natural maturing and ripening of fruits, we notice that this occurs irregularly over the crop area and even on the one plant. Bananas ripen on their palms in staggered disarray. This is nature's way of allowing them to be eaten consecutively, as they ripen — if they all ripened together, many would be wasted before being eaten. Nature did not organise itself for large-scale marketing, so man has to use his intelligence and adapt to the needs of non-farm dwellers while still allowing maximum nutritional properties to develop in the food.

Bananas, as with all fruits, mature before ripening. Thus, if picked in the mature state, natural ripening will continue away from the plant. It will be slower, but it does continue, even though just a little of the natural sweetness fails to develop. Thus, if living in the city, it is wise to buy mature bananas green; allow them to ripen slowly at home, rather than having a forced "ripeness" such as fruit merchants demand.

When bananas are artificially ripened by gas, their skins are yellowed and the fruit softened to resemble natural ripening. However, the core remains hard and often turns black. Because natural sugars have not had time to develop from the mature starch, gas-ripened bananas have little flavour when compared with natural ripening. They often turn black before this sugar balance has had time to develop and their relative indigestibility is such that unless they are very thoroughly chewed, they will ferment in the stomach, creating distension and gas.

Artificial ripening by chemicals is also often performed on other fruits and vegetables. Oranges, tomatoes and grapefruits are frequent victims, especially very early in their season, in an effort to obtain higher prices in the market. Thus, special care should be taken when buying fresh foods, to ensure that they are properly grown and ripened, or at least allowed to mature naturally before picking. This can take a little more time than merely selecting food by its appearance alone, but it creates no problem once a good source of fresh foods has been found. Is it really any more trouble than a search to obtain well-made furniture for the home or clothes for the body? Everything worthwhile requires a little effort, especially in selecting a suitable, balanced diet.

c) Fattening Carbohydrates

Of the concentrated carbohydrates, dried fruits and grains offer most nutritional properties, followed by beans and sweet potatoes. All possess a reasonable concentration of protein in balanced form, which is an added bonus to their vitamin and mineral benefits. Dried fruits and potatoes have the advantage of a better balance of minerals than grains, conferring the important and beneficial alkaline reaction after digestion. Grains, when ground or cooked, create an acid reaction; but when sprouted they become alkaline, together with the development of an improved balance of amino acids and vitamins.

These foods will be discussed in more detail, with particular regard to their most suitable style of preparation, in my forthcoming *Australian Health Food Recipe Book*. For carbohydrates do form an important part of man's ideal diet. Too often they are regarded as "fattening" and are assiduously avoided by anyone with a tendency to accumulate body weight. Certainly, if you are one of those who are inclined to an overweight condition, concentrated carbohydrate foods should be carefully chosen and minimised. But the problem lies farther afield than in the food alone.

Factors which contribute to overweight can generally be traced to overeating. Often, the total quantity is more than required; the combinations of foods are unsuitable; or insufficient exercise and over-sensitive emotions are to blame. Rarely is overweight related to "gland problems", lest it be the salivary glands!

People will generally suffer from overweight when they consume more food than their bodies require. Many deny this habit, but if a total of their daily intake were made, it would prove the point. Often, the problem is compounded by habitual snacking between meals, even if only of small portions of foods (or, more likely, sweets). Such items that are prepared from refined grains and/or sugar are known contributors to the problem, generating the reputation they now carry of "weight producers".

But carbohydrates will not induce an increase in body weight if they are eaten wisely. Grains should be sprouted, not ground into flour and baked; dried fruits should be eaten with suitable fresh fruits, not baked into cookies or confections; refined sugar, the most concentrated form of carbohydrate, should at all times be avoided.

Few people realise the dangers associated with the consumption of refined sugar. For this reason, it has to be classified as one of man's poisonous "foods" — not as acutely poisonous as some strong drugs, of course, but by virtue of its subtle chemical danger to the body, the false sense of pleasure it creates marks it for special attention. Raw sugar, brown or black sugar are almost as dangerous and as highly acid-forming.

d) Selecting Carbohydrates

With their high carbohydrate content, significant protein content (8–14 per cent) and high content of B-complex vitamins, grains can be included in the diet as a valuable source of nutrients. However, their value is somewhat lost when they are ground into flour, refined or roasted. Sprouting grains not only preserves their nutrients, but actually increases them (as proved previously with mung beans) — especially vitamins A and C, neither of which is found in dry grains. This significantly improves their digestibility. If they are required to be cooked or made into bread, sprouting first will greatly improve nutrient content and flavour. However, it must be remembered that the more foods are cooked, the less beneficial are these two qualities.

To cook grains for serving hot, steaming will cause less nutrient loss and will require less time if the grains are first sprouted. Buckwheat, rice and corn can be made into reasonably nutritious meals in this manner. Buckwheat is a grain which is often overlooked by most people who tend to regard rice in preference.

Nutritionally, buckwheat is superior to rice in all aspects. Its further advantages are to be found in its ability to grow in poorer soils with less rainfall than rice demands. Its only limitation is the hard husk which must be mechanically removed to expose the softer, irregular-shaped kernel which offers more flavour than rice. So, too, does corn, which also possesses more nourishment potential than rice, and consequently is a far more suitable food for man.

Fats and Oils

"Lipid" is the correct chemical name to describe all fats and oils found in the human diet. They are known as "fats" when appearing as solids; "oils" when in liquid form. Chemically, lipids are complex molecules known to be insoluble in water, yet digestible in the gastrointestinal tract when of plant or animal origin.

Digestible lipids are found in nature in the cells of all living plants and in the fatty tissues of animals. This does not include such indigestible oils as mineral hydrocarbons with their recognised poisonous effects on the body, whether drunk accidentally (as gasoline or kerosene) or intentionally as a drug (usually as a laxative).

"Vegetable oils" describes lipid extracts from plant substances, which include fruits, nuts, seeds, grains and generally vegetables. These oils are used primarily in cooking or salads. They can also be skilfully employed in freezing foods, such as in the making of ice cream — the inclusion of a good quality vegetable oil will give a smoother taste, reduce crystallising and allow it to be refrozen after thawing by binding the other ingredients together (see recipe in *The Australian Health Food Recipe Book*, to be published in 1983 by Bay Books).

Oils derived from plant substances are also used in cosmetic applications. They are far superior to mineral oils, which are injurious to the skin. However, the application of any oil to the skin should be tempered with care so as to avoid clogging the pores, thereby reducing the action of perspiration and the skin's efficiency as an organ of elimination.

Digestible lipids are an essential part of man's diet. Their concentration in natural foods can vary from less than 1 per cent (in most fresh fruits and vegetables) to as high as 71.2 per cent in pecan nuts and 71.6 per cent in macadamia nuts. All nuts, seeds, grains and pulses contain significant concentrations of natural fat, nuts registering the highest percentages. Much smaller concentrations are found in fruits, with the exception of olives (21 per cent) and avocados (up to 17 per cent). Over the range of fresh vegetables, sweet corn (1 per cent) has the highest fat content by analysis.

Extracted oils and fats will generally register 100 per cent fat concentration in the refined state and a little less if unrefined, due to the presence of residue nutrients.

In foodstuffs, it is not so much the concentration of fats which is of vital concern as the nature of their composition and other nutrients or chemicals with which they might be associated. Basically, three types of fatty acids occur in nature:

a) saturated fatty acids — the "unmarriageables";
b) mono-unsaturated fatty acids — the "once-only marrieds";
c) polyunsaturated fatty acids — the "polygamists" with two or more partners.

Dietary fats generally include some proportion of each of the three groups. The predominating degree of saturation determines the ability of the body to digest and use them, and also determines the physical nature of the fat.

a) Saturated Fatty Acids

Saturated fatty acids are the most complex and difficult to digest. They are found in relatively small proportions in plant foods, with the exception of the coconut, in which they comprise almost a third of the total edible portion. Quite high concentrations of saturated fatty acids (triglycerides) are found in all animal fats, a factor significant in their reduced ease of digestibility when compared with vegetable oils, most of which contain predominantly polyunsaturated fatty acids. Fats dominantly composed of saturated fatty acids are found to be solid at room temperature, as obvious in lard, butter, etc.

b) Mono-unsaturated Fatty Acids

Molecularly, mono-unsaturated fatty acids possess one double bond (a chemical link), allowing them to chemically combine with another element or compound. This is in contrast to the saturated fatty acids which cannot so combine. This ability of combination improves their potential digestibility.

By far the most common mono-unsaturated fatty acid is oleic acid, for it represents at least 30 per cent of the fatty acid content in most common fats. Oleic acid is richest in olive oil (76 per cent) and constitutes 45 per cent of macadamia and pecan nuts. While mono-unsaturated fatty acids are the most prolific in nuts, polyunsaturated fatty acids predominate in seeds.

c) Polyunsaturated Fatty Acids

Polyunsaturated fatty acids possess two or more double bonds. They are thus the easiest fatty acids to digest and constitute the largest group of fatty acids in plant foods. Three acids within this group are regarded as "essential fatty acids", due to their important role in body growth and energy supply. These are linoleic, linolenic and arachidonic acids, found in greatest concentration in edible seeds — safflower, sunflower, sesame and pumpkin as well as in walnuts and wheatgerm. Linoleic acid is favourably regarded by many researchers as being of particular value in reducing foreign cholesterol in the body, probably by virtue of its ease of digestion and ability to combine with other chemicals. It is most abundant (72 per cent) in safflower oil, making it the most desirable for those who include meat in their diet.

d) Cholesterol

Although a lipid, cholesterol should not be confused with fatty acids. The term "lipid" embraces not only all fatty acids (triglycerides) such as we have been discussing, but also includes phospholipids (the fats forming part of cell membrane structure) and sterols (a group of solid alcohols). Cholesterol is a sterol. Its presence in the blood is necessary to fulfil the vital role of transporting fats around the body. Cholesterol has the property of forming compounds (esters) with fatty acids and other organic chemicals in acid form, especially important in delivering energy to the muscles as well as positioning fatty acids in suitable locations around the body.

A derivative of cholesterol (cholic acid) also plays a vital role in the body. It combines with the amino acids glycine and taurine to form bile salts. These are concentrated by the liver for excretion through the bile duct to initiate the digestion of fatty acids by emulsifying them in the duodenum.

Cholesterol is not an essential ingredient in the diet — rather, it can be an encumbrance. All mammals are capable of synthesising cholesterol from a diet of basic nutrients; thus foreign cholesterol is of no benefit. Foods containing it should be consumed only in moderate amounts, if at all! This applies especially to meat and eggs.

Let us return, for a moment, to the consideration of the basic function of fat in the body. Body fat serves two vital roles — it provides a convenient and concentrated form of potential energy and, as adipose tissue, forms soft pads of protection for the organs and bones. It also creates the smooth curves and contours which shape the body's physical beauty. In determining the body's shape, it is apparent that careful moderation in the amount of accumulated body fat is essential. It is even more important that the internal organs are not encumbered by excessive fatty tissue.

Although the quantity of dietary fat is important, even more vital is the nature of the fat. This is especially critical when the source of fat is animal. As cholesterol is already formed in animal bodies, it is apparent that when one animal eats another, foreign cholesterol will be ingested from the victim. (So, too, will foreign toxins and other chemicals, many of which can be definitely unsuitable to the eater.)

When man consumes animal flesh, organs, offal or eggs, he finds that he can appropriate moderate amounts of the fat, but the foreign cholesterol he just cannot handle. Since it occasions no pain, man is unaware of the difficulties created by foreign cholesterol until its presence is registered by a dangerous accumulation. By then, it is often too late.

Foreign cholesterol acts in much the same way as the body's natural cholesterol, making itself available in the bloodstream. There it tends to accumulate until excesses have to be removed. This is done by the blood depositing excess cholesterol in out-of-the-way places. The favourite one is behind the valves of the arteries.

From its discarded position, cholesterol makes its presence felt by attracting to it more of its own kind. This accumulation gradually restricts the free flow of blood by inhibiting the proper opening of the arterial valves. In time, a valve might become so blocked as to be forced into the closed position, thereby occluding the blood flow. Should this artery service a major organ of the body, such as the heart or brain, it is to be hoped that one's will has been properly drawn up and signed!

This problem will not overly concern vegetarians, even though the fat content of certain plant foods is higher than animal foods. It illustrates the importance of recognising the difference between fatty acids and cholesterol. It also explains why some fat people, living on a high-meat diet to lose weight, can reflect a high cholesterol count in their bloodstreams and thus become contenders for premature heart disease.

e) Body Fat

It must be clearly recognised that the amount of body fat accumulated is not necessarily directly related to the intake of dietary fat. Conditioned by a long history of intermittent deprivation of adequate nutrients, the human body has adapted by developing an ability to accumulate reserves against future shortages. These are stored around the frame as fatty tissue and, in times of continued affluence, this storage is inclined to swell the body into discomfort and disproportionate ugliness.

When the body consistently fails to use all food fed to it and fails to eliminate all excess, additional internal storage space must be sought. Fatty tissue will continue to accumulate as long as food intake exceeds the energy expended. This urgently dictates a need to reduce the intake or increase the body's activity.

Modern living habits are characterised by reduced activity and increased food consumption, reflected in a general rise in average weight statistics. This is especially apparent in cities and in highly mechanised rural areas. By contrast, remote rural areas generally produce slimmer people. Those engaged in intensive sports are also characterised by a slim figure, yet their retirement from such activity is invariably accompanied by an increase in body fat as they fail to reduce their food intake proportionally.

The general tendency is for people to accumulate body fat as they age and especially after marriage. It is as though the chase is over and less activity, compounded by an increased food intake of richer ingredients, is at fault. By middle age, this accumulation often becomes so severe as to precipitate serious health problems, which are really no more than the body's anguished appeal to be allowed to fast and restore its correct proportions. In affluent countries, up to 60 per cent of total body weight is often found to constitute fat — medically evaluated by measuring serum triglyceride count; yet it is widely recognised that the human body functions best when its fat content is in the order of only 10 per cent. This is best achieved by the regulation of the diet to suitable proportions of weight-producing concentrated foods, especially carbohydrates and fats.

The refined carbohydrates and the extracted fats are the ones which offend most diets. Whole carbohydrate foods, complete with balanced fibre, starch and sugar, are generally so filling as to naturally regulate their intake; whole fat-concentrated foods likewise. But it is the biscuits, breads, sweets, spreads and oil products which cause problems. Minimise these (even better, eliminate them) and your avoirdupois problem is solved.

f) Dietary Oils

The role of extracted oils in the diet and their method of extraction are often subjects of divergent opinions. There is limitless evidence to prove that vegetable-type oils are dietetically far superior to animal or fish oils, especially in the light of the latter's undesirable loading of foreign cholesterol, toxins and saturated fats. Even so, vegetable oils should only be used minimally and chosen with care as to their method of extraction and type.

Today, edible oils are generally obtained by either the solvent-extraction or expeller-extraction methods. The former will be referred to here as the "commercial" method and the latter as the "cold pressed" method — the general names by which they are recognised.

Both methods once had certain common factors: each first required the oil-bearing source to be crushed, then fed into an expeller extractor in which some 30 per cent of available oil was extracted. This is the cold-pressing method, which leaves a residue of mashed meal containing fibres, gums, phosphotides, etc., together with the majority of oil still locked in the mash.

The oil obtained from this first pressing is obviously of superior quality and it is this which is termed "cold pressed" or "cold processed", the latter term being used to appease the American Food and Drug Administration. Being thus free from impurities, "cold pressed" oils are often free from the need for refining and deodorising. Instead, they generally retain some of the flavour and perfume of their original sources. However, because this method fails to extract so much potential oil, it is necessarily the most costly in terms of discarded raw material; thus cold-pressed oils cost more to buy. But when quality is sought, it must be paid for!

"Commercial" edible oils were obtained from the mashed meal residue left after expeller extraction. The general method was to feed this meal into a multi-chambered tank where it was "washed" with a chemical solvent — hexane (C_6H_{14}) being the favourite. This dissolved the remainder of the oil, taking with it some of the phosphotides and gums, until the discarded pulp was fit for nothing more than stock feed (and poor quality feed at that). The next step was to remove the solvent to render the oil edible.

With the greatly increased demands on commercially extracted vegetable oils, most processors no longer bother with the preliminary process of extracting a first pressing in the expeller. Instead, they cook the oil seeds or beans, then immediately apply the solvent as described in the foregoing paragraph.

Hexane is chosen as the principal solvent for its inert properties and its low boiling point (69°C). Vacuum evaporators have been developed to drive off the solvent, which is recycled for further use. However, the processors will never guarantee that all solvent is evaporated. The processes of deodorising and refining which must follow in the production of "commercial" oils fail to remove the residual solvent. Thus, the resultant product will be found to contain traces of chemical solvent. The final product becomes a bland, tasteless liquid which offers only one advantage — the dubious one of low cost, consistent with mass production.

If post-extraction treatments were not employed on "commercial" oils, their shelf-life would be very short, due to their susceptibility to rancidity. The natural purity of "cold pressed" oils allows them a long natural life, provided they are not subjected to external heat or air flow. For this reason, when their bottles are opened they should be stored in the refrigerator during summer heat, to avoid possible rancidity.

Oils should always be shielded from heat, but they are not troubled by light. The concept that they require storage in opaque bottles bears no logical relation to chemical fact. All glass is a filter of ultraviolet light, opaque glass filtering only visible light which has no effect whatsover on edible oils. However, opaque glass does hide visual recognition of the viscosity and colour of the oil. Incidentally, there is no evidence that ultraviolet light has any effect on oils, but higher up the vibratory spectrum, we know that very high frequency radiation will cause some molecular change and chemical instability.

Cooking can also induce molecular restructuring of the fatty acids. The higher the temperature, the more danger of carcinogens being formed in the oil. Therefore, deep-frying of foods in oils or fats can be seen to attract definite dangers to health. Thus, if cooking with oil, one should choose an oil with a high boiling point (sesame being best) and limit the cooking temperature to the minimum. It is my researched opinion that general avoidance of cooking with oil is a step towards better health. If foods are desired cooked, steaming is by far the best method.

Minerals

Fourth in the classification of major food nutrients are minerals, those relatively simple chemical compounds which form the essential structure and vitally assist in the physiological functioning of the body. Minerals are required by the body in far smaller quantities than any of the foregoing groups of nutrients. But lack of quantity does not diminish the importance of dietary minerals in maintaining good health and well-being.

Actually, the entire composition of the living body can be analysed into its component chemical elements. Minerals supply some of these elements in compound form through the diet. Dr Wilhelm H. Schuessler, the reputed founder of biochemistry, was first to draw attention to the chemical composition of the blood and its component "cell salts". His system was somewhat improved by Dr George W. Carey, his contemporary, also living in the last century. They taught that the body consisted of water, plus organic and inorganic chemicals; but Carey went further by relating the inorganic chemicals to the personality in a manner which is not yet generally accepted, although proved by those who have studied and applied it.*

Discovery and isolation of the chemical factors of the human body are still unfolding. While their study continues to occupy the mind of man in specialised research, its expense appears to be far outweighing the benefits. Too much specialised study tends to fragment life, especially in the field of human nutrition, to the extent that man sees the tree, but is blind to the forest.

The mistake made by so many academics is to limit their research to the material alone, overlooking the vital part played by the paraphysical or metaphysical factors which distinguish the human being from the sum of his chemical components. The total human being is always more than his component physical chemicals.

We can perpetuate that modern academic trend and intimately investigate each mineral, listing its sources and composition, its functions within the body and factors relating to its deficiency, but with what benefits? Your time and mine are more valuably employed in understanding how to acquire and maintain perfect health than in seeking to fragment it. As long as one's diet includes the balance of natural foods, as discussed in this book, all nutrients required for perfect health will be provided without a fanatical preoccupation with fragmented factors. Isolating nutrients to provide an explanation for health and disease can, *per se*, never give the total picture any more than the breaking down of a musical composition into its component notes will uncover its meaning.

There is, of course, a basic need to know something of the chemical substance of the body, just as a composer needs to understand the properties of each musical note in order to compose a piece of music. For this reason, the following capsule summary of each mineral of the body (later followed by each vitamin) has been prepared. The mineral list includes gaseous elements, as well as the solid chemical elements known as minerals. All chemical symbols are also shown.

Oxygen (O) The most abundant element, comprising an average of 61 per cent of the body's weight. Its sources are through the lungs from fresh air and through the mouth from food nutrients. It is a component of every function of the body and in constant demand by the blood.

---

* I have used it successfully in my practice and have expounded the system in my book, *Secrets of the Inner Self* (Angus & Robertson Publishers, Sydney, 1980).

Carbon (C) Next in quantity, comprising 23 per cent of average body weight, it is a vital component of all proteins, fats, carbohydrates and vitamins. After serving its purpose, it is oxidised and freely eliminated through the lungs as carbon dioxide.

Hydrogen (H) Combines with oxygen and carbon in all vital nutrients; is the third most abundant element in the body, occupying an average of 10 per cent of body weight, primarily in the body's most vital compound — water.

Nitrogen (N) Fourth of the gaseous elements, it occupies an average body weight of 3 per cent, is a vital component of protein and essential to body growth.

The foregoing four elements are the major components of the physical body and although usually found in nature in their gaseous states, the human body ingests them from their solid states in foodstuffs, for they are the intrinsic components of the major nutrient groups, protein, fat and carbohydrate. These elements are chemically classified as the "organic four" in the body.

The following elements are chemically classified as inorganic macro-nutrients. They are needed by the body in far smaller quantities than the organic four, yet are no less essential. They will now be investigated in descending order of their presence in the body.

Calcium (Ca) This most abundant mineral in the body contributes about one kilogram of the weight of the average adult male (about 1.4 per cent of body weight). Most of this is found in the skeleton where it is in salt form with phosphorus (where it must be in a ratio of 2:1). This combination provides the basic hardness of bones and teeth. Calcium also combines with magnesium to nourish the cardiovascular system. Its source must be dietary, being richest in most protein foods — cheeses (especially Swiss and cheddar), dietary yeast, carob powder, soya milk (such as "Soyvita"), parsley (an especially important source for the many other vital minerals it contains), nuts and dried figs. Calcium is alkaline-forming and important to nerve, muscle and metabolic functions, as well as blood coagulation. Its absorption is inhibited by oxalic acid (from tea, coffee, meat, cocoa and rhubarb) and sucrose. Absorption is facilitated by essential quantities of vitamin D. Recommended dietary allowance (RDA), based on average dietary requirements of calcium is 800–2000 mg (milligrams) daily, depending on age, sex and occupation.

Phosphorus (P) Comprises an average 1 per cent (650 g) of body weight, with functions similar to calcium. It also works with cellular function, assists with the transportation of fatty acids for energy, influences heart regularity, kidney function, transfer of nerve impulses to the brain, and physical endurance. Richest sources are dietary yeast, bran, pumpkin and sunflower seeds, nuts (especially Brazil), soya milk and egg yolk. It is acid-forming, acting as a chemical balance to calcium. RDA is very similar to that of calcium.

Potassium (K) Comprises approximately 0.3 per cent (200 g) of body weight and is alkaline-forming. Its primary role in health is working within the body's cells to regulate water balance and normalise heart rhythms. In these duties, as well as in nerve and muscle functioning, the potassium-sodium balance is vital. Stress is a major factor in creating potassium deficiency and non-absorption. Primary sources are dietary yeasts, soya beans and soya products, other beans, dried fruits, bran, sunflower seed kernels, parsley, nuts and fresh green olives. RDA is 2000 mg daily.

Sulphur (S) Comprises approximately 0.2 per cent (130 g) of body weight and is acid-forming. It is essential for maintaining correct brain functioning through the regulation of the body's oxygen balance, for balanced functioning of liver and bile secretion and for maintaining healthy skin, hair and nails. Care must be exercised not to ingest too much inorganic sulphur, such as from sulphur-dried fruits (the bright-coloured apricots, peaches and nectarins), for the sulphurous acid (H_2SO_3) will impair the kidneys. Richest food sources of assimilable sulphur are protein foods rich in the amino acid methionine. These include Brazil and most other nuts, meat and fish, eggs, watercress, beans and green leafy vegetables. RDA is 850 mg daily, although this figure is one suggested by Dr Henry Schroeder, leading American nutritional scientist and founder of the low-sodium diet for heart problems (no official government figures have yet been suggested). Diets containing adequate protein foods will provide more than sufficient sulphur.

Sodium (Na) Comprises 0.2 per cent (130 g) of body weight and is alkaline-forming. It was discovered with potassium, with which it works very closely in regulating cellular water balance — sodium works outside the cells, potassium inside. Sodium also works with other minerals in the blood to maintain their solubility, but high intakes of it can be dangerous to the health, especially from common salt (sodium chloride) — cardiovascular problems, from cramps to heart attacks, are the usual problems. Best natural sources are eggs, meat and celery. Problem sources are bacon, ham, soya sauce, margarine and butter, breakfast cereals, kelp, canned foods (especially fish), fresh fish, bread and cheese — all of these should be avoided by anyone with a sodium problem; daily intake of over 12 g can produce toxic effects. There is no RDA, so prevalent is sodium in foods.

Chlorine (Cl) Comprises 0.14 per cent (90 g) of body weight and is acid-forming. It works with sodium and potassium in extracellular fluids, and helps to cleanse the body of toxicity, especially in the region of the liver. High intakes of chlorine, however, can create toxicity, as can sodium, so care should be taken to avoid common salt wherever possible — over 15 g daily is regarded as high and is easily achieved since chlorine is also present in town drinking water supplies. Too much chlorine can destroy intestinal bacteria and vitamin E and can have a detrimental effect on the skin. Its sources are similar to sodium, so care should be taken to avoid those "problem sources". Natural sources are tomato (1.8 per cent by weight — 1.8 g per 100 g), celery, lettuce, cabbage, spinach and parsnip. No RDA has been recommended, but around 500 mg daily is suggested.

Magnesium (Mg) Comprises 0.03 per cent (20 g) of body weight and is alkaline-forming. It is found in the bones, soft tissue cells and blood plasma. It is also necessary for calcium metabolism, with which it is present in the bones in compounds with phosphate and bicarbonate. Magnesium is vital for efficient nerve and muscle functioning, as well as for converting blood sugar into energy. There is very little chance of magnesium being deficient in the diet, for it is an essential component of chlorophyll, therefore present in foods of vegetable origin. Its major sources are wheat bran and germ, nuts, buckwheat, dietary yeasts, beans, grains, dried fruits and vegetables, especially the greens. RDA is 350 mg daily.

Silicon (Si) Comprises 0.025 per cent (16 g) of body weight and is acid-forming. It is a mineral into which too little research has been undertaken, for it was only in 1973 that significant research into its usefulness in maintaining good health was scientifically reported. Some nutritionists have been claiming, far earlier than that, important nutritional benefits for silicon, especially for the skin. It has, in fact, been proved in practice that silicon has valuable healing properties in cases of acne, psoriasis and most skin diseases. Therapeutically, silicon is best administered orally in the form of rice bran syrup. Connective tissues and cartilages are also found to be rich in silicon when good health prevails, especially in the trachea, aorta, skin and eyes. In ageing, significant decreases in silicon have been observed in the aorta and the skin and thymus. Although some 28 per cent of the earth's surface is composed of silicon, the body's requirements are very small, around 30 mg daily (no RDA has yet been established). Best sources are lettuce (a few leaves will supply minimum daily needs), parsnip, asparagus, rice bran (best therapeutic source) and all fruits and vegetables.

This completes the list of major mineral nutrients. It is interesting to note that each mineral listed alternates between alkaline and acidic. As this list is in descending order of bodily quantity, we recognise how perfectly the body maintains the balance between the two. All we need to do is provide the balanced diet. The following list is comprised of those essential minerals that the body requires in smaller quantities and whose presence in the body is also smaller; they are known as "trace minerals".

Iron (Fe) Comprises 0.006 per cent total body weight (about 4 g in a 65 kg person). This is a very low percentage, yet iron heads the list of trace elements and is, without a doubt, the most important because of its vital role in haemoglobin of the blood. Its presence in muscle tissue allows rapid utilisation of energy in expansion and contraction of the muscles by the rapid transfer of oxygen. A deficiency of iron is a common cause of varying degrees of anaemia — this is twice as prevalent in women as in men, due to their reproductive capacities and menstruation. Although the RDA for iron is 10–16 mg daily, only a small percentage of dietary iron is actually absorbed into the bloodstream — from 5 per cent to 15 per cent. One important cause of lowered absorption is nervous tension; another is inadequate vitamin C. Best sources of dietary iron are yeasts, rice bran, liver (but this also contains so much of the animal's toxicity that it is not recommended), wheat bran, pepitas (Mexican pumpkin seed kernels — the best whole food source), beans, seeds, nuts, eggs and parsley (the best vegetable source and a must in every salad). Iron is an alkaline-forming mineral.

Fluorine (F) Comprises 0.004 per cent of body weight. This is a most misunderstood chemical. It is soluble in water in the form of sodium fluoride and regarded as poisonous if 5 g or more are present in the body (see Stage 3). In its natural form as calcium fluoride (available from almonds and other nuts, plus green vegetables), it strengthens bones, teeth, nails and eyes. However, with so many city water authorities uncritically accepting the fluoride concept, it is not surprising that the quantity found in modern man is close to toxic level. It has an affinity for bones and tooth enamel and is often absorbed within a few hours of ingestion. There is no established RDA and no problems associated with its deficiency (any more than there is with a deficiency of arsenic!). The belief (for it is only a theory which is being progressively disproved) that it offsets tooth decay and hardens bones is invalid (this is calcium fluoride). Another theory is that it will delay tooth decay for a few years, but then the onset in middle teen years becomes serious, for sodium fluoride not only weakens the bones, but also the teeth at their core.

Zinc (Zn) Comprises 0.003 per cent (2 g) of body weight. Its essential role in maintaining good health is currently being unfolded. To date, zinc is known to be vital to the body's enzyme systems and is found most abundantly in the Islets of Langerhans (where insulin is manufactured and stored for secretion through the pancreas) and in the male genitals. Deficiency of zinc is now considered to induce prostate problems in older men and to contribute towards diabetes. Zinc deficiencies are easily created — poor soils in which foods are grown, food processing, diarrhoea and excessive perspiring are the frequent causes. Zinc deficiency has also been found in many cases of schizophrenia. Although meat and oysters are among the richest sources of zinc, their abundance of oxalic acid and adrenalin (in meat) tends to negate the body's ability to absorb it. Pumpkin seed kernels, nuts, egg yolk, rye, wheat germ and brewer's yeast are actually the best nutritional sources. (It is important to always look for nutritional sources, rather than mere analytical figures, as this proves.) RDA is presently regarded as 15 mg, but this is certain to be increased as more research reveals other vital roles for zinc.

Copper (Cu) Comprises 0.0015 per cent of body weight — about 80 mg. It is the lesser brother (in terms of required quantities) of iron in many of the body's reactions. But unlike iron, copper is rarely deficient in the body; when deficiency occurs, it is found only in the more primitive areas, for traces of copper are found in most reticulated water supplies. Copper is required by the body to convert iron into blood haemoglobin, for oxidising ascorbic acid and converting it to vitamin C and for oxidising the protein, tyrosine, by which its work on the pigmentation of skin and hair is accomplished. Most suitable sources of copper are nuts, legumes, grains and prunes; animal livers and seafood can also be included for those whose diets normally include such. There is no RDA, but average suitable intake appears to be around 2 mg daily. Toxicity from copper is rarely from dietary sources — if it does occur, it will usually be from the use of excessive copper sulphate as a bactericide (especially in swimming pools).

Manganese (Mn) Comprises 0.00002 per cent of body weight — only 13 mg. It is important in bile production and in some hormone and enzyme functions. Its particular importance lies in the formation of the thyroid hormone, thyroxin, as well as in the manufacture of insulin. Deficiencies of these factors (primarily from refining of foods) can be corrected by taking therapeutic doses of manganese, or by increasing the intake of those foods rich in this trace mineral, such as alfalfa sprouts, nuts, parsley and other green vegetables, carrots, beetroot, egg yolk and grains. Alfalfa tablets and liquid chlorophyll are two of the best sources of therapeutic manganese. No RDA has been set, but at least 6 mg and up to 10 mg is considered to be the range.

Iodine (I) Comprises about 13 mg of body weight; the same as manganese. Most of this is concentrated in the thyroid gland from where it is released in controlled amounts in the form of thyroxin and other related hormones. These hormones are determinants of the level of metabolism in many of the body's cells. If iodine is deficient, thyroid secretions are low, metabolism slows, the circulation is reduced, resulting in lack of energy, underweight and mental lethargy. It is as though iodine governs the tempo of life. With the output of thyroid hormones controlled by another hormone from the pituitary gland, a deficiency of iodine tends to induce the thyroid gland to work hard at producing its hormones when triggered by the thyrtropic hormone from the pituitary. This causes the production of colloid cells which accumulate in the thyroid, in turn inducing progressive swelling and the characteristic appearance of goitre, which can become so large in the neck as to interfere with breathing. Goitre is more common in women than in men, because iodine is used by the reproductive organs during puberty and pregnancy. Best sources of iodine are sea foods, kelp, pineapple, eggs, cheddar cheese, onions and vegetables grown in iodine-rich soils (most of the earth's soils are normally low in iodine). The elemental iodine is extracted by the body from potassium iodide and it is this salt which, when added to table salt produces the iodised salt many people now use as a food supplement. However, its problem is the large intake of common salt necessary to obtain the small quantity of iodine. Kelp is a far better form of supplementation, but this is only required if insufficient green vegetables (or seafood) are included in the diet. RDA is 80–150 µg (micrograms) — 0.08–0.15 mg.

Selenium (Se) Its component of body weight is about the same as each of manganese and iodine, yet this is a much rarer mineral, being no more prevalent in the earth than is gold. Selenium was discovered as a dietary nutrient in 1957 by German-born physician, Klaus Schwarz, but it was not until 1973 that Dr Rotruck and his team at the University of Wisconsin identified it as a vital component of the enzyme glutathione peroxidase. In this role, it is a protector of cell membranes and, as Dr Richard Passwater expands in his book, *Selenium as Food and Medicine* (Keats Publishing, Connecticut, 1980), it also helps to prevent cardiovascular disease, reduce the incidence of cancer, suppress arthritis, reduce ageing and generally contribute towards better health. Many other roles are considered to be attributable to selenium, such as preventing cataracts, detoxifying pollutants and radiation dangers, preventing liver necrosis and, in concert with vitamin E, muscular dystrophy. Selenium's role in averting vitamin E deficiency is perhaps its most vital and for this its natural food sources supply adequate quantities. Best natural sources are whole grains, wheat germ, Brazil nuts, alfalfa sprouts, mushrooms and most other vegetables, traces in most fruits. Other sources are organ meat, seafood, other meat and garlic, but sufficient will be available from the natural foods diet, analyses varying with soil fertility. Much research has yet to be done on this mineral; so much so that an RDA was established only as recently as 1980 and is given as 50–200 µg, although some authorities appear to regard 200 µg as approaching the toxic level. Most natural selenium is destroyed by cooking and modern processing.

Cobalt (Co) This is a very rare mineral in the body, in which its total quantity might only be 2 g; however its presence is vital to the red blood cells. In 1948, it was discovered that vitamin B_{12} (the anti-pernicious anaemia factor) contained 4 per cent cobalt, but to date, no supplementary sources have been formulated, nor has any RDA been set. Therefore, sources of supply must be foodstuffs. Traces are present in most foods, especially whole grains, alfalfa and other green vegetables. No dietary supplementation is available in Australia for this mineral, nor for selenium.

This completes the list of twenty minerals deemed most essential in the body to maintain optimum health. But this is not an exhaustive list, for other trace minerals are gaining recognition as vital to human needs, guaranteeing them inclusion on the expanding list of essential trace minerals. These now include: rubidium, strontium, boron, bromine, barium, chromium, molybdenum, arsenic and vanadium. Other trace minerals known to reside within the human body, and thus far deemed "non essential" are: zirconium, lead, niobium, aluminium, cadmium, tellurium, titanium, tin, nickel, gold, lithium, antimony, bismuth, mercury, silver, caesium, uranium, beryllium, radium, and probably many more so far too rare to have been recognised.

Vitamins

The chemistry of human metabolic processes is an amazingly complex study, yet one which continually fascinates many scientists. Considerable light has been thrown onto the scene by discoveries, within this century, of the role of the fifth group of dietary nutrients, vitamins.

The group of organic compounds termed "vitamins" embraces an ever-increasing number of unrelated chemicals with differing physiological reactions within the body. Yet, with their common purpose of facilitating metabolism, this general grouping is justified.

As a result of its comparative newness, interest in vitamin study has captured the imagination of the academic world to such an extent that many "miraculous" properties are accorded to particular vitamins, while the total concept of balanced natural nutrition is all too frequently relegated to a minor position.

At first the medical profession, in its characteristic conservatism, refused to accept the role of vitamins in nutrition and for years actively denounced them as of no consequence. Now, the reverse applies. In many countries, the medical profession has become so interested in vitamin therapy that it seeks to acquire a total franchise on their prescription and in some instances has been so successful as to limit the availability of vitamins from one of their primary established sources — the health food stores. Perhaps the huge potential market for vitamin sales has now been realised! But, vitamins are not medicines; they are distinctly food nutrients, intended as non-toxic therapeutic aids.

Unfortunately, the truth of the vitamin concept lies somewhere between the two opinions of the medical profession, the old and the new. Vitamins are neither useless, nor miraculous. They have an essential role in human nutrition and health, but only when they are ingested as components of a balanced natural diet. Otherwise, their isolated application and its often-attested remedied benefits will be short lived. Alternatively, other diseases will manifest as a result of nutritional deficiencies, because the cause of the original disease was not remedied — the total dietary habits were not corrected. For this reason, vitamin therapy has the same limitations as any other form of therapeutic method, be it physical or spiritual. Unless the cause is found and rectified, any indicated benefits from the therapy will be only temporary; and they will invariably distract the patient's attention from pursuing a proper corrective course.

The role of vitamins in the nutritional picture is almost in homoeopathic proportion to the total quantity of food nourishment consumed by man. Vitamins are organic compounds, required for health, especially by the metabolic processes to facilitate the most efficient digestion of the major nutrients. They are required in very small quantities and, with few exceptions, cannot be stored in the body. Vitamins should therefore be generally available in foods daily.

All fresh fruits and vegetables possess varying amounts of vitamins so that with sunshine, fresh air and a balanced natural diet, man acquires adequate quantities of essential vitamins for his daily use. Were it not so, it would presuppose that some grave error had occurred in the divine creative plan which only modern scientific intervention could remedy! All that laboratory-formulated vitamins can do is to show man something of what is lacking and afford temporary relief to the symptoms of deficiency. But to continue with their dosages is to perpetuate ignorance of the real cause of disease, thereby predisposing towards its symptoms erupting elsewhere.

Vitamins offer a nutritionally oriented approach to the maintenance of health by remedying many disease symptoms without causing any iatrogenic (drug-induced) complications in the body. By so doing, they indicate to the patient that food nutrients are directly related to the health of body and mind, thereby inducing the patient to correct his or her dietary intake, selecting foods with known nutritional benefits in place of those known to be nutritionally deficient. Thus, vitamin therapy provides the bridge between the modern junk-food, highly processed, convenience-oriented eating habits and the natural-foods, health-promoting, fresh-food diet.

Another advantage of vitamin therapy is that informative guidelines are so readily available through hundreds of inexpensive books, from health food stores and nutritional specialists (naturopaths) who do not demand referrals and who do not charge an arm and a leg for a consultation. Costs of vitamins to the patient are far less than drugs — certainly prescription drugs are often highly subsidised by the government, but it creates a heavy tax burden. Yet drugs do not promote health — at best they only temporarily relieve symptoms. Often the iatrogenic effects of drugs are unknown and the patient becomes the guinea pig, whereas vitamin action on the patient is highly predictable. On those rare occasions when your naturopath makes a misdiagnosis, his recommendation of vitamins will cause you no harm and will provide a little extra nourishment, even if they do not correct the symptom. Drugs, on the other hand, can (and often do) cause added discomfort if incorrectly prescribed; they certainly increase taxes!

Vitamin therapy is comparatively new in the field of health treatment. Their presence in foods has been suspected for centuries, but it was not until the latter part of the last century that vitamins were brought into research focus in chemical laboratories. Their discovery, isolation and property recognition is possibly the most valuable contribution by chemists in the food arena, especially in these days of so many congenital weaknesses induced by so many unnatural living habits.

It was not until 1912 that the naming, analysing and isolating of vitamins really commenced. Polish-born biochemist, Casimir Funk, was not the first researcher into vitamins, but he was the first to set forth the vitamin hypothesis that many diseases were not the result of infection, but of vitamin deficiency. He identified many vitamins and was responsible for choosing the generic name, for he erroneously thought them all to be amines (compounds containing nitrogen). Thus he chose the name "vitamine" — "life-amine". Dr Funk was by no means a medical hero; in fact he was regarded with derision and suspicion until, little by little, medical authorities were forced to admit that vitamins were "somewhat" connected with health. Even today, with irrefutable evidence confirming the vital role of vitamins in health, some medical practitioners refuse to consider them as anything but "sources of expensive urine". In fact, there is currently a move afoot in the United States to discredit vitamins as "potentially toxic substances", a claim for which there is not an iota of evidence (intimidation is often used when science and logic are exhausted).

By the time the Second World War had begun, most of the vitamins had been isolated and named. Many researchers, working independently or in small groups, could not accept the germ theory and recognised specific deficiencies when experimenting with certain diseases, especially beriberi and scurvy.

Further vitamins have been discovered since the Second World War and research continues to occasionally uncover new vitamin compounds, although these are not always related to human nutrition. Some are connected with the growth of guinea pigs, others with chickens, etc. As vitamins are isolated, they need to be coded with letters of the alphabet until their precise chemical formulation and name are established. This is the manner by which vitamins have been traditionally identified and explains why they are widely known by both systems today.

A list of all major vitamins connected with human nutrition is given below. The simplified chemical formula of each is given, together with their roles in human nutrition, sources of supply in foods and consequences to expect in cases of deficiency:

VITAMIN A — RETINOL ($C_{20}H_{30}O$)

Characteristics: Insoluble in water, soluble in fats, a sterol (solid alcohol), retinol enters the body in two different forms: from animal foods, it comes direct from the fat of the animal (which also contains toxic factors and some of the animal's cholesterol); from plant foods, as carotene, the red or yellow colour of fruits and vegetables. Carotene is also found in green vegetables, where it is in association with chlorophyll.

Absorption: Retinol is synthesised within the walls of the small intestine soon after absorption. Its rate of absorption from the diet varies in accordance with the source and the state of the gastrointestinal tract. A relaxed person whose diet includes abundant fresh green vegetables, plus red and yellow fruits and vegetables, will probably absorb over 50 per cent of available carotene. A largely meat-eating person might only absorb 25 per cent. Retinol functions in conjunction with bile salts and can be stored in the liver in comparatively large amounts, thus avoiding the need for ingestion each day. Tests have shown that healthy people can store as much as 150 mg retinol in their livers with no risk of toxicity, sufficient for some months without any further dietary intake.

Loss Factors: Residual retinol and carotene, unabsorbed from the small intestine, are lost to the body through the faeces. However, there is more chance of retinol being lost than carotene, for the former can easily become rancid, unless vitamin E is present in the fat. Rancidity is due to oxidation of the fat and this can also be induced by over-cooking. Vegetables and fruits which are highly cooked will evidence a retinol loss, yet retinol and carotene are both stable when frozen.

Deficiency Symptoms: One of the most obvious indications of vitamin A deficiency is night blindness. Others are acne, impetigo, boils, skin ulcers (for which it should be taken orally as well as applied externally as an ointment with vitamin E). Most other skin abnormalities, emphysema and chronic nephritis also respond to oral vitamin A.

Benefits: Known to directly support all cellular growth, especially of the eyes (counteracting weak eyesight as well as night blindness), the organs, outer tissues of the body (skin, hair and gums), and the bones and teeth. This is probably the most sensitive vitamin in terms of minor toxicity from over-dosage, due to its ease of internal storage. For this reason, care should be exercised in the amounts taken. If too much is ingested, the liver will overflow and induce a yellowishness in the skin and the eyes, with a possible feeling of nausea.

Food Sources: Best sources of carotene are parsley, carrots, yellow sweet potatoes, silverbeet and all green, yellow and red fruits and vegetables. Best sources of retinol are cod liver oil, animal livers, butter, egg yolk, margarine, milk and its products but — care must be exercised with these items in the diet. The highest absorption of carotene comes from the green leafy vegetables, for the body enjoys the enzymic action of the accompanying chlorophyll to improve digestibility.

Dosages: RDA for adults is from 1.2 mg to 1.8 mg daily; proportionately less for children and infants. Pregnant and lactating women require 2.4 mg daily. Some authorities still give vitamin A measurements in international units (i.u.), for which the conversion rate to milligrams is: 3333 i.u. = 1 mg. Recommended maximum daily therapeutic dosage for adults is considered very safe at 9 mg or 30,000 i.u., although for extreme deficiency conditions, up to four times this amount can be prescribed (one-third this for children), taking care to check the liver's capacity to store and the body's to utilise.

VITAMIN B-COMPLEX GROUP

Although chemically unrelated, this group of water-soluble compounds is generally found to occur in the same food sources, but to have dissimilar reactions to heat, light, etc. Their sources and interrelation in nutrition qualify them for classification within the B-group. All B-vitamins are synergistic, being more potent together than when used separately, even though they have many diverse chemical factors in their individual formulations. It is as though they are really fond of each other and do not enjoy being separated.

VITAMIN B_1 — THIAMINE ($C_{12}H_{17}ClN_4OS \cdot HCl$)

Characteristics: A white, crystalline compound, thiamine is stable in dry form or in an acid up to 120°C. It is highly water soluble, indicating it can be easily leached from its natural sources if care is not taken in handling.

Absorption: Thiamine cannot be stored in the body to any degree, so it must be ingested daily. Factors aborting its absorption include caffeine, alcohol, sulphur drugs, oestrogen and food processing (especially the removing of rice bran from its husk).

Loss factors: Heat, water and oxidation are major causes of thiamine loss from foods. For this reason, frying, boiling and grilling thiamine-rich foods are guarantees of intake deficiencies. Wherever possible, these foods should be eaten raw, always stored covered and in a cool place — if they are to be cooked, they should be steamed at a low temperature in stainless steel cookware. Women should be especially careful to obtain a little extra vitamin B_1 if they are nursing, pregnant, or on the contraceptive pill.

Deficiency symptoms: Many of the symptoms of thiamine deficiency reflect modern living. They relate to poor quality foods and to stress. Processing and chemical fertilisation of soils are major causes of poor quality in foods, thereby inducing an unbalanced diet. For instance, removal of the bran from rice results in an extremely deficient product and is one of the primary causes of beriberi, the antidote for which originally put thiamine on the vitamin map. Enervation, a leading consequence of stress, worry and anxiety, can also indicate a thiamine deficiency.

Benefits: Many physical and emotional symptoms, not themselves deficiencies of thiamine, respond to its therapeutic application. Depression, depleted nervous system, tired muscles and heart, multiple sclerosis, myasthenia gravis, air and sea sickness, herpes and alcoholism come within the range. When treating alcoholism, care must be taken to keep the patient away from alcohol while thiamine is being given, for it is lost to the body in the presence of alcohol. Remember, thiamine should be taken in suitable combination with other B-vitamins for synergistic benefits, especially in the treatment of stress conditions.

Food sources: Significant therapeutic benefits can be derived from the inclusion of dietary yeasts, rice and wheat brans in the daily intake. Best whole food sources are sunflower seed kernels, nuts, soya beans and whole grains. Soya milk, soya grits and soya flour are also highly beneficial sources. Meats, seafoods, dairy products and eggs are low in the thiamine food lists.

Dosages: RDA for adults varies from 1.3 mg to 2.0 mg, but it is 1.8 mg for youths, since their rapid growth rate must be adequately fed. For children it is 0.5 mg to 1.0 mg and for infants it is only 0.2 mg, ideally obtained from green vegetables and soya milk. Therapeutic dosages for youths and adults varies from 50 mg to as high as 500 mg for severe deficiency symptoms. Thiamine was once considered to be the most effective of the B-vitamins, but recent research with megadoses appears to favour B_3 and B_6 with this distinction. There is no toxicity problem, for any excess is excreted in the urine and not stored.

VITAMIN B$_2$ — RIBOFLAVIN (C$_{17}$H$_{20}$N$_4$O$_6$)

Characteristics: Riboflavin is a yellow crystalline compound occurring in smaller quantities than thiamine in most foods. This implies a guide to the relative relationship of these two in general therapeutic dosages. It is water soluble and easily absorbed.

Absorption: The human body cannot store B$_2$, readily excreting any excess to its immediate need with a characteristic bright yellow tinge to the urine. This will indicate the rate at which therapeutic preparations containing B$_2$ have been disintegrated and made available to the body. As with thiamine, daily food intakes of riboflavin are essential.

Loss factors: Unlike thiamine, riboflavin is not destroyed by oxidation, heat or acids, but is lost when subjected to strong light, especially ultraviolet. Alkalis are also detrimental. Storage of therapeutic preparations containing B$_2$ must always be in opaque or light-resistant containers.

Deficiency symptoms: Decline of vision and inflammation around the eyes are perhaps the most common, although the series of symptoms designated ariboflavinosis (recurring mouth, lips and tongue soreness) was originally the more recognised deficiency problem area.

Benefits: In its general role of aiding growth and reproduction, riboflavin works in conjunction with other vitamins in the metabolising of major nutrients and in promoting healthy skin, nails, hair and eye tissues. It is also an important aid to the respiratory system and can be especially beneficial to people suffering diminished vision, particularly the elderly. Recent research has found riboflavin in megadoses beneficial in overcoming an addiction to sugar.

Food sources: Major food sources of riboflavin are similar to those of thiamine, although higher concentrations of riboflavin are to be found in cheeses, meats, and parsley.

Dosages: Recommended RDA for riboflavin averages 20 per cent higher than for thiamine, being 1.8 mg to 2.7 mg for adults, 2.5 mg for youths and up to 1.2 mg for children. I do not agree with government sources placing riboflavin higher than thiamine for daily allowances; not only does the body handle thiamine in larger quantities than riboflavin, but natural foods generally possess higher counts of thiamine. One is inclined to conclude the Creator knows best. Recommended therapeutic dosages are less than thiamine, in the range 5 mg to 250 mg, with the most common requirement around 15 mg to 30 mg daily. Rarely is toxicity a problem, but over 500 mg daily could cause unusual irritability over the skin and/or numbness.

VITAMIN B$_3$ — NIACIN (C$_6$H$_5$NO$_2$) or NIACINAMIDE (C$_6$H$_6$N$_2$O)

Characteristics: Here we have two vitamins with B$_3$ properties, the former an acid with the chemical name of nicotinic acid, the latter a nitrogenous alkaline compound with the chemical name of nicotinamide. Their common names are niacin and niacinamide, respectively. Although researchers have known of nicotinic acid since the 1860s, it was not until 1913 that Dr Funk isolated and attempted to use it against beriberi. Because of its ineffectiveness in such experiments with pigeons, it was neglected until 1935. It was then "discovered" and identified as the third of the B-vitamins, due to its amide being a component of the respiratory co-enzyme, NAD (nicotinamide adenine dinucleotide). Vitamin B$_3$ is stable when exposed to heat, oxygen and light. It is found in foods in far greater quantities than either of the previous B-vitamins, indicative of a higher daily requirement.

Absorption: Vitamin B_3 differs from thiamine and riboflavin in its ability to be synthesised in the liver from the essential amino acid, tryptophan, implying that the diet can be temporarily deficient in B_3 without the body suffering. But for this conversion to occur, vitamins B_1, B_2 and B_6 must be present in that day's food intake. In nature, both forms of B_3 are often bound to other nutrients, thereby rendering them somewhat difficult to absorb in the body. This tends to make B_3 less prevalent in the diet, even though its analyses show it to be often abundant.

Loss factors: As a water-soluble vitamin, B_3 is easily leached by water, especially boiling water, if it is freely available and not bound to other nutrients. It is also lost to human absorption if in the presence of alcohol, sleeping tablets, oestrogen or sulphur drugs. Most of it is lost in food processing techniques and refining.

Deficiency symptoms: Three major areas of deficiency symptoms have come to be attributable to inadequate B_3, two on the physical level and one on the mental. The original pathological condition for which B_3 was recognised as directly corrective was pellagra. It was a deficiency problem occurring largely in populations where corn occupied the role of staple food (this prevalence has considerably decreased since wheat has become more universally utilised). Pellagra is characterised by dermatitis with light-sensitive inflammations on the skin, plus diarrhoea, depression and sometimes psychotic disorders indicated by mental confusion, these mental conditions developing in the more chronic sufferers. As the B_3 in corn is so tightly bound to other nutrients, normal cooking does not release it — limestone must be added to the cooking water, by which its calcium acts as a releasing enzyme.

The second area of deficiency manifests in the subnormal synthesis of some hormones within the body — primarily the sex hormones, plus cortisone, thyroxine and insulin. The area of mental and emotional correction for which B_3 is especially effective relates to a range of symptoms manifesting in unstable nervousness (acute worrying and anxiety), varying in intensity from apprehensive moodiness to causeless depression to schizophrenia to suicidal tendencies. These symptoms are jointly related to a negative attitude by the sufferer and nutritional deficiencies, being probably initiated by the latter, caused by "junk-foods" in the diet. Vitamin B_3 is most effective (usually in conjunction with B_6 and C) in massive doses under appropriate supervision, accompanied by wise counselling when mental problems are also present.

Benefits: The recent use of B_3 in the treatment of schizophrenic problems has succeeded in countless thousands of cases, many of which were previously under conventional treatment for some years. Such therapies even included shock treatment which, as usual, proved so ineffective that the sufferers were still patients, but with added iatrogenic problems. Vitamin B_3 has no equal in its therapeutic role with schizophrenia, so it would have been expected to attract excited support from the psychiatric fraternity — here was a nutrient providing highly effective correction for a baffling problem which hitherto had only occasionally been responsive to savage electronic and drug treatments. But this was not to be. From the moment this therapy was introduced in 1952 by eminent practitioners, Drs Hoffer and Osmond, in Canada, it was (and they were) subjected to aggressive intimidation by the "medical establishment" (see Dr Abram Hoffer's, *Orthomolecular Nutrition*, Keats Publishing, Connecticut, 1980). But, gradually, more and more modern, open-minded practitioners are attaining rapidly responsive benefits from this treatment, with Dr Hoffer still in the vanguard of research through his practice in Victoria, B.C., Canada. Other regions of benefit in the use of B_3 include arthritis, digestion and ageing syndromes. During the 1940s, B_3 was found to provide an effective nutrient against the pain and physical deterioration caused by arthritis and rheumatism. But at that time, cortisone was also discovered for the same relief and, since it was a drug, was greatly preferred. Experience has found that cortisone falls far short of expectations and often compounds the suffering by creating iatrogenic problems. Many practitioners now turn to B_3, preferring a therapeutic nutrient to a drug, with eminently better results (which are further improved if the patient is at the same time on a highly alkaline diet — see Stage 13). More recently, B_3 (as nicotinic acid) has been recognised as a vital co-enzyme in fat metabolism within the body, where it aids in the control of triglyceride and cholesterol levels. It also assists in relieving canker sores in the mouth (small, painful ulcers) and halitosis (bad breath from indigestion). In treating the ageing diseases, Ménière's and vertigo, B_3 has also been found highly effective in reducing symptom discomforts. Finally, as a therapeutic aid to sufferers of senility, B_3 constitutes a vital role in the treatment programme (see Dr Hoffer's most recent book, *Nutrients to Age Without Senility*, Keats Publishing, 1980).

Food sources: Best food sources for B_3 are similar to those for B_1, with the addition of animal livers, tuna fish, plus most other meats and seafoods for those who would include these items in their diet. For people on a natural-food diet, additional food sources of B_3 atop the list already recommended for B_1 are peanuts, mushrooms and dried fruits. It is important to note that, although corn has a reasonably high analysis of B_3, it is not a good source, as previously explained — whole wheat, buckwheat and unpolished rice are far richer sources in the grain category.

Dosages: RDA is given as 15 mg–22 mg for adults, 6 mg upwards for children, but only 2 mg for infants. Therapeutic doses can vary from 50 mg to 3000 mg daily in either form of B_3. Great care should be taken in administering high doses and should be done only under the direction of a competent practitioner. Niacin is the most effective form for therapeutic use, but it increases blood pressure and produces facial flushes when taken in megadoses. This may be advantageous for arthritic and rheumatic sufferers, but can cause anxiety and discomfort for other patients. Currently being developed are slow-release niacin tablets which also have the advantage of not producing flushes. Niacinamide does not produce flushing, either, nor is it as effective as niacin.

VITAMIN B_5 — PANTOTHENIC ACID ($C_9H_{17}NO_5$)

Characteristics: This is another water-soluble vitamin, unstable in the presence of heat, acids and alkalis. It was discovered in the 1940s by the eminent biochemist Dr Roger J. Williams at the University of Texas, who recognised it as a vital component of body cells and of nutrition. Pantothenic acid is part of co-enzyme A, where it is involved in releasing energy from carbohydrate utilisation and necessary to the synthesis and breakdown of fatty acids, sterols and hormones.

Absorption: Care must be taken with the selection and preparation of foods to ensure sufficient pantothenic acid is available for digestive absorption. Being a component of every cell in the body, B_5 deficiency will induce a biochemic imbalance which could unleash a variety of deficiency symptoms. Although some B_5 can be synthesised in the body in the presence of intestinal flora, this is not always reliable, for many people have intestinal deficiencies, so daily dietary sources should be ensured.

Loss factors: Possible causes of nutritional losses of B_5 are generally similar to B_3 — the boiling of foods when cooking (steaming reduces loss potential), alcohol, sleeping tablets, oestrogen (in medicines, especially oral contraceptives), sulphur drugs and in food processing and refining. The presence of caffeine (found in tea as well as coffee) also induces dietary losses of B_5.

Deficiency symptoms: With Dr Williams's original experiments on B_5 related to the origin of individual life, it is not surprising that we still regard the major deficiency problems as being related to birth defects. Stillbirths, premature births, malformed and mentally retarded babies are all often due to lack of B_5 during and prior to pregnancy. Failure of the body's auto-immune system to produce sufficient antibodies can also be traced to inadequate vitamin B_5, as can nerve degeneration, resulting in muscle weaknesses, often indicated by pins-and-needles in the body's extremities. Loss of memory and greying hair can both be benefited by B_5 in conjunction with PABA and choline. Lack of adequate co-enzyme A will create a lack of energy and possible hypoglycaemia, due to insufficient conversion of fats and sugars to energy. Cellular deficiencies can manifest in sterility or gastrointestinal ulcers (jointly induced by stress), as well as dermatitis.

Benefits: As every cell of the body benefits from pantothenic acid, both before and after birth, it is unnecessary to list areas of specific usefulness. It should be regarded as a general growth, repair and maintenance vitamin, providing some special benefits in the area of combating stress, allergies, constipation and transmittable illnesses. Tests have revealed sufferers from arthritis and rheumatism to be deficient in B_5 by as much as 50 per cent below average, but this does not imply that these conditions are induced by this lack, only that B_5 is of benefit in relieving the symptoms temporarily. Its nutritional benefits against stress are related to the value of B_5 in nourishing the adrenal glands and maintaining good blood circulation by aiding the assimilation of fats and cholesterol from dietary sources. In combination with other B-vitamins and vitamin E, it is also beneficial in the treatment of post-operative shock.

Food sources: Vitamin B_5 is found in many of the same foods as other B-vitamins — in smaller quantities than B_3, but larger than B_2. Best natural food sources are the dietary yeasts, nuts and seeds, mushrooms, soya beans, oatmeal, broccoli and avocados. Animal foods sources are organ meats, seafoods and eggs. But the richest source of natural B_5 comes from Royal Jelly, larval food of the queen bee. For infant needs, mother's milk is a far better source than animal milks.

Dosages: RDA has only recently been established for B_5 from 3 mg to 6 mg for children; 8 mg to 12 mg for youths and adults. However, Dr Williams recommends up to 25 mg per day for best performance. Therapeutic dosages are generally taken in the form of the salt of pantothenic acid and calcium, calcium pantothenate — $(C_5H_{16}NO_5)_2Ca$. In this form, it is usually found as a component of B-complex formulae in varying potencies from 25 mg to 150 mg. As the major component for specific use, it can be obtained up to 500 mg and administered orally up to 10,000 mg daily for severe stress conditions. For remedying possible reproductive failures, regular dosage of 100 mg daily is usual. To combat senility, dosage should increase to 500 mg daily, plus adequate components of vitamins B_1, B_3, C and E.

VITAMIN B_6 — PYRIDOXINE ($C_8H_{11}NO_3$)

Characteristics: This water-soluble vitamin currently shares the honour with B_3 as the most significant of the important B-group for nutrition and therapeutic usefulness. As it is excreted if not utilised within eight to ten hours after ingestion, B_6 needs to comprise a regular part of one's diet. The name pyridoxine is actually a group name referring to naturally occurring pyridine derivatives having B_6 activity, essential in the metabolic processes of all animals, especially the catabolism of proteins, fats and carbohydrates.

Absorption: The enzyme activity by which the major nutrients are assimilated is dependent on effective B_6 assistance, especially the desulphurisation of amino acids. The assimilation and conversion of tryptophan to vitamin B_3 can only take place in the presence of B_6. Pyridoxine is also required for the adequate absorption of vitamin B_{12}, for the production of antibodies and of red blood cells. Some authorities claim that B_6 can be produced in small quantities by synthesis as a function of intestinal bacteria, but this is not yet totally accepted. Due to its rapid absorption or excretion, therapeutic dosages are now available in time-release formulae to provide gradual disintegration within the body.

Loss factors: In common with all B-vitamins, pyridoxine is destroyed by boiling water, food processing and refining, by alcohol and by certain drugs. One of the most destructive of these drugs is oestrogen, especially in oral contraceptives. Many nutritionists (this author included) have long suggested the incorporation of B_6 in the formulation of all oral contraceptives — this would avoid the high deficiency factor of B_6 among women on the pill. Long-term storage of foods containing B_6 or of B_6 therapeutic tablets can also considerably reduce the potency of this vitamin.

Deficiency symptoms: Kidney disorders and stones which fail to respond to other treatment can leach B_6 from the body, thereby robbing it of its important functions. These include diminished health, evidencing some critical deficiencies of B_6 in infancy, adolescence and adulthood. Overprocessing of baby foods is known to destroy B_6, symptomised by irritability and convulsions which, if not corrected, can lead to permanent brain damage. Other indications of B_6 deficiencies in infants are excessively dry or oily skin, and occasionally autism and anaemia (especially if the mother has been in the habit of consuming alcohol during pregnancy or lactation). Nervousness in all age groups can also be a deficiency symptom of B_6 and, when combined with irritability, induces pre-menstrual tension, acne and/or depression in women. In men, it can lead to stress and to skin problems, especially scales around eyes and ear lobes, dandruff (which accompanies poor scalp circulation and tight follicles), aggressiveness and sometimes acne. Hands which are inflamed, unusually dry and cracked also reveal a deficiency of B_6, as does numbness or cramps in the arms or legs. Hypoglycaemia can sometimes be traced to the same deficiency.

Benefits: The role of B_6 in alleviating nausea is one of the most common benefits recognised by health practitioners. It is very successful in combating morning sickness during pregnancy, nausea caused by X-rays and inadequate assimilation of fats, especially the morning after a heavy meal of mixed proteins, fats and carbohydrate foods. Vitamin B_6 works within the gastrointestinal tract as an enzyme aiding catabolism of these major nutrients, as well as working in the stomach wall to produce hydrochloric acid for protein catabolism in the stomach. The more protein-rich foods are eaten, the more B_6 the body demands. When tea, coffee and/or cocoa are also consumed, B_6 is kept really busy, for these items, as well as animal foods and seafoods, greatly contribute to the formation of kidney stones and gravel. These can be averted by adequate doses of B_6 with magnesium. Here B_6 is of great benefit because it aids in the conversion of oxalates to glycine, an amino aicd. Its role in overcoming anaemia (not caused by iron deficiency) is another important benefit of B_6, where dietary deficiencies, tension or alcohol have been responsible. Another of the metabolic roles of B_6 is sometimes so heavily demanded that therapeutic supplementation of it is necessary — that is, in fat metabolism causing obesity. For this reason, B_6 is combined with apple cider vinegar, kelp and lecithin in helpful formulations (such as KLB6) for the control of overweight problems. Increased B_6 intake is also of benefit during pregnancy and when fevers occur, where it should be combined with vitamin C. Physiologically, B_6 participates in the body's manufacturing of hormones histamine and adrenalin, as well as aiding the activity of the pituitary gland to stimulate body functions. Some researchers have used B_6 with success in the presence of other B-vitamins for the control of Parkinson's disease, which in some cases has proved quite successful.

Food sources: Naturally, B_6 is not found as abundantly in foods as most of the other B-vitamins, for the body does not need it in such high concentrations, even though it is a most versatile vitamin. Best natural sources are dietary yeasts, sunflower seed kernels, wheat germ, beans and lentils, buckwheat, brown rice, hazel nuts, bananas and avocados. Other rich sources are seafoods and organ meats.

Dosages: RDA is set rather low, at 0.4 mg for infants, less than 2 mg for children and 3 mg to 5 mg for adults. Therapeutic doses are normally given in the form of pyridoxine hydrochloride, for this is the more assimilable form and the easiest to prepare and store. The great variation in these dosages implies that professional guidance in their prescribing should be obtained, especially for infants. In cases of infant convulsions, the preventative dosage is usually 5 mg to 10 mg daily, but the therapeutic dosage for established symptoms can be up to 100 mg by injection. This can be increased to twice daily by injection if anaemia is also prevalent for either infants or adults. However, adults can take these larger doses in tablet form, together with vitamin B_{12} and folic acid (another B-vitamin). For kidney stone correction, B_6 with magnesium oxide (10 mg and 300 mg respectively) has been of benefit to four out of five chronic sufferers by dissolving the stones. Nausea, obesity and pre-menstrual problems are generally treated with tablets of 25 mg or 50 mg daily in a B-complex or multivitamin formulation. While some serious symptoms are known to require up to 1000 mg daily under supervision, the occasional patient has been prescribed up to six times this amount, for B_6 has virtually no toxicity, other than perhaps swelling or numbness in the feet or too vivid a recall of dreams (these are often regarded as important indicators by the patient of possible maximum dosages).

VITAMIN B_{12} — CYANOCOBALAMIN ($C_{63}H_{88}CoN_{14}O_{14}P$)

Characteristics: This is the most active form of the vitamin B_{12}, component of a co-enzyme which influences human fat metabolism, the conversion of carbohydrates to fat and the catabolism of protein amino acids. It is in the form of red crystals or powder, is soluble in water, resistant to boiling and unstable with alkalis. It is the only vitamin known to contain essential minerals as part of its structure — phosphorus and cobalt. It was, in fact, the cobalt which gave the ultimate clue to the discovery of B_{12} in 1948. Since the 1920s, research had been undertaken to isolate the cause of a wasting disease in sheep and cattle in Australia. Many scientists in other countries were involved in the research and it was finally discovered in England that a red vitamin, containing cobalt, was an inherent component of animal livers. Although required in exceedingly small quantities, this vitamin (B_{12}) proved to be essential to human and animal survival and became known as the "anti-pernicious anaemia" vitamin.

Absorption: This is a vitamin which is very effective in minute doses, but its absorption does depend on a substance called the "intrinsic factor" being present in the healthy stomach. Correct functioning of the thyroid gland and of the liver are also necessary for the satisfactory absorption of B_{12}. As this is such a new vitamin in the annals of human nutrition, much is yet unknown of its properties. Some authorities state that its absorption is facilitated by combining with calcium (which should present no problem since calcium is one of the most abundant minerals in the body). Others are convinced that humans cannot emulate the feat of animals and synthesise B_{12} in their livers, deducing that total vegetarians will be deficient in this vitamin if they do not add animal foods to their diet or take B_{12} supplements. This flies in the face of the fact that man is, by nature, a vegetarian and can metabolise his nutritional needs from plant foods and synthesise any deficiencies within his body *if* he has maintained his body in the state of optimum health.

Loss factors: Those same chemicals which have been shown as destructive of other B-vitamins are also the enemies of B_{12}. Such commonly ingested tablets as the oral contraceptive and sleeping pills are the worst offenders. Both will negate the absorption of B_{12} and induce the possibility of mild anaemia which, if not corrected early, can deteriorate to pernicious anaemia. As the trace mineral cobalt is essential to the effectiveness and structure of B_{12}, any inhibitor to the absorption of cobalt will simultaneously create a loss of B_{12} availability. Alcohol is just one of these inhibitors, for it also impedes the normal functioning of the liver, thereby reducing its effectiveness in the protein digestion chain, as well as interfering with the functioning of B_{12}.

Deficiency symptoms: The most important role of vitamin B_{12} is in averting pernicious anaemia or therapeutically working to overcome the condition if it has prevailed. A problem with B_{12} deficiency is that its symptoms may not become apparent for some time. Anaemia is one of those slowly manifesting conditions resulting from a variety of nutritionally deficient possibilities. It can also be induced by stress-related deficiencies of B-complex vitamins. Anaemia symptoms include lethargy, impatience, incipient memory loss, etc. — but it is often many years before the anaemic condition has been diagnosed. And until recently, it has taken even longer to recognise the symptom as being related to a deficiency of B_{12}. The symptoms were often attributed to deficiencies of iron and other B-vitamins, but now most practitioners direct early attention to the possible deficiency of B_{12} — so much so that B_{12} is now often prescribed in tablet or injection form at the first sign of a possible anaemic condition. Such treatment will, of course, rarely induce any toxic effects, even if it is not the primary solution; but such hasty prescribing might detract from discovering the primary cause, which could be stress, schizophrenia, disharmonious attitudes, or any number of other causes. In this way, B_{12} could be a mask and not provide the best cure. Many commercial brewers now use cobalt to increase the frothing of their beer, which in turn can provide an increase of dietary cobalt for the drinkers. But such people generally have a deficiency of thiamine and high-protein foods in their diet, thereby inducing a potentially toxic condition from the cobalt. Again, a high regular alcohol intake will adversely affect the liver, reducing its effectiveness in the handling of B_{12}.

Benefits: Best known for its essential role in the development and regeneration of red blood cells, B_{12} has also been found to produce other important benefits in human and animal health. These include the correct metabolising of major nutrients, in turn promoting normal growth, increasing appetite of the young, increasing expressed energy, nourishing the nervous system, thereby averting reactiveness and irritability, improving brain functioning and mental balance. As most of these factors have only recently been discovered, it is reasonable to assume that many more will gradually be unfolded as research continues.

Food sources: It is interesting to note that most authorities regard only animal foods as possessing adequate vitamin B_{12} for human consumption. Sources listed are organ meats, seafoods, egg yolks, lean beef, cheeses and whey powder. This is to imply that total vegetarians all suffer from pernicious anaemia. But experience has shown the opposite to be true. Most vegetarians not only have a suitable blood count, but also have a lower than average blood pressure. In fact, many meat eaters who have converted to a vegetarian diet have found, to their surprise (and that of their medicos), that a prior condition of anaemia has been overcome without therapeutic assistance. As we know B_{12} to be vital in this regard, could it be that the human body, counter to many meat-eating researchers, can actually synthesise its own B_{12} in the liver with the aid of balanced food nutrients from plant foods? Indeed it is so. As B_{12} is required in such small amounts and the nutrients which comprise it in even smaller quantities, it is not surprising that, with a healthy body, plant foods known to be rich in B-complex vitamins are not devoid of minimal B_{12} plus cobalt to assist the body in synthesising additional quantities if needed. Such plant foods are already listed, but those of special benefit are the whole grains, alfalfa sprouts and other green vegetables. After all, that is how the ruminant animals do it, for they are non-carnivorous and one can be assured that the Creator did not give them something that mankind lacks, when such a faculty is just as vital to the highest form of creation!

Dosages: The unit by which vitamin B_{12} is measured is the microgram (μg). This is one-thousandth of a milligram; one-millionth of a gram. It is one of the few vitamins measured in these minute units, indicating its almost-homoeopathic need in the body. RDA varies from 2 μg to 4 μg for infants and children, 5 μg to 7 μg for adults, increasing to 8 μg for pregnant or lactating women. Therapeutic dosages can vary from 10 μg to 100 μg in tablet form. But the stomach does not always readily receive and prepare for absorption such quantities of B_{12}. Thus, higher dosages must be given by injection and these can be anything up to 2000 μg. It should be remembered, however, that if the nutritional deficiencies or emotional excesses negating the body's absorption of B_{12} from food sources are allowed to go untreated, the large therapeutic dosages will only have temporary benefit.

VITAMIN B_{13} — OROTIC ACID ($C_5H_4N_2O_4$)

Very little research has been undertaken to date on this remote member of the B-complex group. It is known to have similar characteristics to other B-vitamins insofar as its water solubility is concerned and it is also known to assist in the metabolising of vitamin B_{12} and folic acid. Its primary use is to facilitate a better absorption of essential minerals, by combining with them chemically to form salts such as calcium orotate, magnesium orotate, etc. These are found to be especially beneficial wherever calcium and magnesium are required by the body. Some practitioners also use orotic acid for the treatment of multiple sclerosis, although insufficient case histories are yet available to provide established guidelines. Therapeutic sources of orotic acid are not yet available in Australia or the USA, but are in Europe. Dietary sources are whey liquid and powder, as well as root vegetables. No RDA has been established.

VITAMIN B$_{15}$ — PANGAMIC ACID (C$_{14}$H$_{27}$NO$_8$)

This is another rather remote B-vitamin on which comparatively little research has been undertaken. Pangamic acid was discovered when it was isolated from apricot kernels and rice bran in the Californian laboratory of Krebs and Krebs. This father-and-son team (of laetrile fame) patented their discovery in 1949. In 1966, Ernst T. Krebs, Jr edited a 217-page publication in conjunction with the McNaughton Foundation in California of extensive Russian studies entitled, "Vitamin B$_{15}$ — Properties, Functions and Use". The Russian monographs were translated in Israel, where a considerable interest is developing in the usefulness of this vitamin. So it would appear that although Russia, Israel and many European countries consider it an important step towards greater nutritional and health knowledge, American governmental authorities as yet do not. Nor do the health departments in most Australian states. Although the sale and prescribing of B$_{15}$ in Queensland is now permitted, it is illegal in most Australian states and in the USA.

Characteristics: Rather than present a lengthy treatise on this largely unavailable vitamin, here is a brief summary of its properties. As part of the B-complex, it is water soluble and found to work most effectively with other B-vitamins, particularly B$_{12}$. Interestingly, this vitamin works something like vitamin E, in that it acts as an antioxidant. When the Krebs were developing and experimenting with B$_{15}$, they produced its calcium salt, calcium pangamate, as well as the sodium salt, which was obviously not suitable to people on a low-sodium diet.

Absorption: In its salt forms, B$_{15}$ is more readily absorbed by the body. Vitamins A and E also facilitate both absorption and effectiveness of B$_{15}$, especially in its role as an important antioxidant.

Loss factors: Exposure to sunlight and boiling water will greatly diminish the usefulness of B$_{15}$. Other loss factors are not yet on record due to its comparative newness.

Deficiency symptoms and benefits: Pangamic acid is known to offer very valid benefits to human health and longevity, but it is not yet certain whether its deficiency in any of these conditions has actually precipitated or contributed to the development of the condition. This acid is known to improve heart conditions by working to overcome atherosclerosis of the coronary blood vessels and other cardiovascular diseases, thereby improving blood circulation and the more rapid recovery from stress, exercise and fatigue. It also works to remedy the symptoms of angina pectoris and to lower serum cholesterol levels. The liver is another organ to benefit from pangamic acid by overcoming the effects of alcoholism and the condition of cirrhosis (in conjunction with the permanent removal of alcohol from the diet; this is not difficult with B$_{15}$ for it also has the property of neutralising the addiction to alcohol). As an aid to the body's protein synthesis and by providing protection against modern pollution dangers, B$_{15}$ also contributes towards an increased life span. For many people, this is the main benefit of this vitamin, explaining why the Russian scientists have stated: "The time will come when there will be calcium pangamate on the table of every family with people past 40".

Food sources: Apricot kernels, rice bran (another reason why rice should never be dehusked), brewer's yeast, whole grains, all seeds, especially pumpkin seeds (pepitas) and most of the usual B-complex foods.

Dosages: Not only is there no RDA, but law-abiding citizens are urged by their governments to avoid this vitamin, although they refuse to thoroughly research it, for apparently no valid reasons. However, so much proof exists to establish the value of B_{15} in many overseas countries that wherever it has been made available for therapeutic use, some amazing results have been achieved. Daily therapeutic dosages have been known to vary from 50 mg to 500 mg, although care has to be taken with the larger doses as nausea has been known to develop. This might suggest that when RDAs are established (and they must eventually, for people will not permit governments to keep them in ignorance), they will be in the order of 10 mg.

VITAMIN B_{17} — LAETRILE ($C_{14}H_{15}NO_7$)

Characteristics: This is one of the most controversial nutrients of all time. Most researchers regard it as a poison for its cyanide content. But those who have used it with success as an anti-cancer nutrient forcefully claim it to be a vitamin. It was discovered by Krebs and Krebs in California and patented in Britain in 1958. (Many valuable books have been written about it, one of the best being *World Without Cancer*, by G. Edward Griffin; American Media, California, 1974, reprinted nine times to 1978.) Chemically, laetrile is a compound of two saccharine molecules, benzaldehyde and cyanide. This is known as an amygdaline — as nitriloside when used therapeutically.

Benefits: Governments rejecting laetrile do so on the grounds that it is a poison. If this criterion applied to all drugs used in medicine today, it would convert all medicos into nutritionists and herbalists, for they would have little to prescribe other than foods and herbs. It is quite possible that, for a healthy person, laetrile in extremely high doses could be slightly poisonous. But in small doses it is believed to provide increased resistance to cancer. Some practitioners consider that in large doses, it can greatly assist a cancer sufferer to remit the disease, so long as he undertakes a raw foods vegetarian diet. This treatment can only be prescribed by a medical practitioner who is acquainted with laetrile and who can obtain sources of it. In the USA, it is banned by the FDA in all except fifteen states, where its use has been legalised. In Australia, it is virtually banned, although in Western Australia some practitioners are using it with medical support. Some states, especially NSW, have outlawed a non-medical practitioner making any claims for or treating cancer, yet conventional medicine has not yet found a reliable cure from its vast annals of available drugs, so many of which confer iatrogenic illnesses upon the patients; chemotherapy and radiation treatment are particularly severe in this area.

Food sources: The most reliable source of information on B_{17} foods comes from Dr Abram Hoffer, the famed orthomolecular psychiatrist, in his latest book, *Nutrients to Age Without Senility* (Keats Publishing, Connecticut, 1980). Those foods with more than 500 mg laetrile per 100 g edible portion he lists as: wild blackberry, elderberry, seeds of deciduous fruit trees, mung beans, bitter almonds, macadamia nuts, bamboo and alfalfa sprouts. Foods with between 100 mg and 500 mg per 100 g are: other berry fruits, including currants, also quince, buckwheat, linseed, millet, kidney beans, lentils and lima beans. It is the only B-vitamin not found in brewer's yeast.

Dosages: Obviously, no RDA has been set. There are also some wide variations of opinion about its therapeutic dosages. Up to 1000 mg taken thrice daily is considered a safe but maximum dosage, although no levels of toxicity have been established. Dosages between this level and 250 mg daily are the usual prescribed in conjunction with diet changes, as mentioned earlier.

BIOTIN — CO-ENZYME R ($C_{10}H_{16}N_2O_3S$)

Characteristics: Sometimes known as vitamin H, biotin is actually a part of the B-complex family, having similar characteristics to most other members, especially its water solubility and its synergistic activity with vitamins B_2, B_3 and B_6. It is essential for the normal metabolism of protein and fat, for it generally occurs bound to protein. It is a very important growth-promoting factor in humans and in animals and works towards the conversion of some essential amino acids to those not obtained from foods. It is found in every living cell in minute amounts and is metabolically related to pantothenic acid and folic acid.

Absorption: Its extensive presence in foods generally ensures that adequate biotin is absorbed in metabolism. Rarely does absorption become a problem, except in the presence of raw egg white, where the proteinaceous compound, avidin, bonds with biotin to form a nonabsorbable complex. Biotin aids the synthesising of ascorbic acid in the body.

Loss factors: The major loss factor is avidin, as described above, implying that if eggs are to be eaten raw, such as in an egg-flip, the yolks must be separated from the whites and the whites avoided. Other loss factors for biotin are the same as for other B-vitamins.

Deficiency symptoms: Extreme exhaustion, drowsiness, muscle pains and anorexia (loss of appetite) are some of the symptoms expected from lack of adequate biotin. Others are eczema of the face and body, when insufficient vitamin A is present in the diet also.

Benefits: As biotin can be synthesised by intestinal bacteria, it should always be present to afford benefits to the body. These include assisting to maintain the hair in its natural colour, rather than greying; helping to avoid baldness, one of the causes being a deficiency of nourishment to the scalp, facilitated by adequate nutrients and massage; and alleviating dermatitis, eczema and loss of body weight.

Food sources: In the natural food range, brewer's yeast, soya beans and their products (such as TVP, soya flour, soya grits and soya milk), rice bran and brown rice, egg yolk, nuts, whole grains, peas, cauliflower, mushrooms, wheat bran and lentils. In the animal food category are livers, fish and chicken. All these items possess at least 10 µg per 100 g edible portion.

Dosages: RDA is given as 150 µg to 200 µg daily, with 50 µg for infants. Therapeutic doses are rarely needed as isolated nutrients, for biotin is usually included as a component of a B-complex formulation, as well as in most multiple-vitamin tablets. Toxicity is not a potential problem with biotin.

CHOLINE — ($C_5H_{15}NO_2$)

Characteristics: A member of the B-complex and a vital constituent of lecithin, choline is classed also as a lipotropic — a fat emulsifier. It was discovered in 1950 and is important in the natural human diet, but essential in the modern diet due to its higher fat content. It is also essential in the diets of non-vegetarian animals. Choline is one of the very few substances able to penetrate the brain-blood barrier (protector of the brain against variations in the daily diet), passing directly to the brain's memory cells where it produces a chemical compound for aiding the memory.

Absorption: Choline can be synthesised in the human gastrointestinal tract if not attendant in foods. It requires methionine (an amino acid), folic acid and B_{12}, plus a number of other minor ingredients to be internally synthesised, but this is rarely necessary since it is one of the most abundant vitamins in natural foods. It has an interesting alternative role where, as part of lecithin, it can temporarily replace methionine if it is deficient in the diet.

Loss factors: Choline has the same inhibitors as all other B-vitamins listed earlier, but as its daily requirements are very flexible and easily provided from any reasonable diet, loss is rarely a problem.

Deficiency symptoms: Loss of memory, leading to possible senility or Alzheimer's disease (in older people), is often a symptom of deficiency of choline. Arteriosclerosis is another condition which might occur from a deficiency of choline, especially on the modern diet. However, these symptoms can also occur for other reasons, even when choline is adequately present.

Benefits: As a component of lecithin, with inositol, it works to utilise fats and cholesterol, so that the fat can provide energy and the cholesterol can be kept from settling against the arterial wall or in the gall bladder. By nourishing the liver, it aids in the elimination of poisons and drugs from human bodies and in overcoming the risk of cirrhosis, especially in heavy drinkers. Many cases of nervousness and nervous twitching or fidgeting have been overcome by choline increase. Vitiligo, the skin disease where photosensitivity creates white patches in the skin and premature greying of the hair, can be remedied by daily doses of choline in more than 50 per cent of the sufferers.

Food sources: Availability of choline from the diet is both extensive and abundant, with many foods providing more than 100 mg per 100 g edible portion. These include lecithin, egg yolk, wheat germ, soya beans, blackeye peas, brewer's yeast, chickpeas, lentils, split peas, brown rice and other whole grains, plus peanuts. Only liver, ham and veal, amongst the meats, come within the high-choline group, although they are not recommended as part of the optimum diet. Vegetables are also very valuable sources of choline.

Dosages: RDA has not yet been established, but intakes of around 250 mg for children and 400 mg to 800 mg for adults are considered reasonable each day. Therapeutic doses vary considerably — lecithin can provide the most suitable intake, for then it is in balance with inositol. Well balanced B-complex formulations can also be highly suitable in providing up to a few hundred milligrams daily. But for conditions such as vitiligo, where around 2000 mg are required daily, choline bitartrate tablets should be taken — they are often formulated to 250 mg choline and the same of inositol. If taking lecithin for its choline content, one should also increase the intake of calcium to maintain the calcium–phosphorus balance, for lecithin tends to increase the body's phosphorus.

FOLIC ACID — ($C_{19}H_{19}N_7O_6$)

Characteristics: Another of the many members of the B-complex vitamin group, folic acid derives primarily from foliage, as its name implies. This explains why its highest concentration is found in animal livers. The first monograph on it appeared in the Journal of the American Chemistry Society in 1941, since when much important research has been undertaken into its nutritional properties. It is water soluble and vital to the body's utilisation of amino acids and sugars. It is also important in the body's production of the nucleic acids RNA and DNA.

Absorption: The body will easily absorb folic acid so long as it is not afflicted with too many medicinal or addictive drugs, especially alcohol. Otherwise, the absorption of folic acid from the diet is relatively uninhibited. Its importance should cause one to ensure adequate greens are consumed each day, for folic acid is essential to the body's cellular mitosis (division and replacement).

Loss factors: Folic acid can be destroyed by being stored, or those foods containing it being stored, in open, unprotected conditions for extended periods, even at room temperature. It is also destroyed by boiling foods containing it, and by sunlight. As with all B-vitamins, folic acid is destroyed by alcohol, inducing its deficiency in alcoholics, often manifesting in anaemia and bone marrow deficiencies. If a high intake of vitamin C is being undertaken, folic acid should similarly be increased since high levels of vitamin C tend to increase the excretion of folic acid. Many drugs create a loss of folic acid from the body, especially oestrogens, aspirin and sulphur drugs, so this loss should be compensated by an increase in folic acid intake.

Deficiency symptoms: Anaemia is one of the common deficiency symptoms of folic acid — important to detect because it is often masked by what appears to be a deficiency of iron. With folic acid so vital to the formation of red blood cells, a condition of nutritional anaemia can occur if too little folic acid is appropriated by the body. As well, such a deficiency can be created by too little green vegetable intake, or by overcooking them. Such anaemic conditions can be indicated by lethargy and muscle weakness, lack of energy, loss of appetite and digestive disturbances indicated by gas formation, abdominal distension and/or diarrhoea, plus sleeplessness, forgetfulness and irritability. Not only do women on the oral contraceptive pill need increased folic acid, but so do pregnant women. The unborn child demands a high quantity of folic acid, often more than the mother can provide — unless she has been on a natural foods diet. More than 50 per cent of pregnant women have inadequate folic acid and this deficiency can be responsible for spontaneous abortions and miscarriages.

Benefits: Abundant folic acid will never be a load to carry. It will promote healthy skin and hair, maintain a good appetite and guard against intestinal parasites and food poisoning. In therapeutic quantities, it can act as an analgesic and will heal canker sores in the mouth. For nursing mothers, it can improve the milk flow, especially in conjunction with alfalfa tablets and sprouts.

Food sources: Brewer's yeast is again the number one source, then torula yeast. Other important vegetarian sources are blackeye peas, wheat germ and bran, all legumes, green vegetables and nuts. Liver is the only significant meat source, although it is quite unnecessary to partake of second-hand folic acid when so much is available from natural sources.

Dosages: RDA for adults is 500 μg to 600 μg, increasing to 800 μg for pregnant or lactating women. Infants and children can need as much as adults — premature babies can need up to eight times as much, due to their anaemia potential. In fact, the tendency towards infantile anaemia is best offset by increased folic acid availability by either lightly steamed and strained green vegetables or, under professional guidance, therapeutic doses.

INOSITOL — ($C_6H_{12}O_6$)

Characteristics: Part of the B-complex group and, with choline, part of lecithin. As such, inositol is also a lipotropic — a fat emulsifier. It is curious that inositol has the identical formula to fructose, fruit sugar, although it does possess a different molecular structure in that it is a single molecule, rather than the double molecule of fructose. Its characteristic sweetness has caused inositol to be sometimes called "meat sugar" and is responsible for the semi-sweet taste of lecithin.

Absorption: The body's ability to metabolise fats and fatty substances is largely dependent on inositol, choline and biotin, adequate intakes of which contribute towards avoiding cholesterol build up. It is very easily absorbed from the gastrointestinal tract. As a component of lecithin, it mixes in most liquids especially well, particularly in fruit juices. Lecithin is also an excellent way to maximise the effectiveness of vitamin E.

Loss factors: Dietary items which destroy other B-vitamins also affect inositol. But two additional factors are disruptive here — coffee and lindane. Coffee has been tested in conjunction with inositol when it was discovered that the caffeine in coffee caused normal amounts of inositol to be rendered ineffective — large quantities of inositol were therapeutically required to overcome the effects of the drug. Lindane is a chemical pesticide of the chlorinated hydrocarbon family which includes DDT. As Rachel Carson reported in her book *Silent Spring*, lindane is effective as an insecticide by its power to destroy inositol in its quarries. This has the potential of rebounding on its users and anyone coming within its sphere of influence, including consumers. The consequential deprivation of inositol soon becomes apparent in many of the deficiency symptoms.

Deficiency symptoms: The most noticeable symptom of inositol deficiency is hair loss. This can also be accompanied by eczema and, sometimes, by digestive problems, especially with fats. Premature hair loss is a key indicator that the diet is deficient in inositol and should be treated immediately it is recognised by supplementary lecithin.

Benefits: Nourishment of the skin, especially at the highest part of the body, where the heart has to pump the hardest for the blood to transmit its nourishment, is an important benefit for one's scalp protection. The scalp reacts to a deficiency of inositol by shedding its covering in the same way that it reacts to a deficiency of biotin by the appearance of dandruff and to a deficiency of choline by loss of the hair's colour. This proves how closely these three vitamins work in maintaining the body's optimum health. Inositol also maintains the body's efficient distribution of fat and cholesterol.

Food sources: Inositol is found in the same foods and similar concentrations as is choline, but now some fruits are being included in the list of abundant sources. These include oranges, grapefruit, raisins, cantaloupes and peaches.

Dosages: No RDA has yet been established, which appears strange since inositol is no less important than choline, also remaining largely unrecognised by government scientific circles. As inositol is used a little more by the body, its average daily requirements should be a little more than choline's — around 800 mg to 1000 mg for adults, 400 mg for children. Daily therapeutic dosages can vary up to 500 mg if the diet includes some of the food sources in which inositol is found; if totally deficient in these, up to 1000 mg should be taken, together with up to 500 mg of calcium (preferably in chelated form) to balance the phosphorus increase caused by inositol.

PABA — PARA-AMINOBENZOIC ACID ($C_7H_7NO_2$)

Characteristics: This water-soluble vitamin is one of the newest members of the B-complex family. Although it has been occasionally known for nearly fifty years, it was not until the early 1950s that intensive research established its primary uses. Even today, although we know of its relationship to hair and skin, as well as its effect on sulphur drugs, we do not know the reasons for these factors.

Absorption: Although PABA can be synthesised in the body, dietary and/or therapeutic dosages are necessary for it to have its most beneficial effects. PABA is probably a component of folic acid, which it helps to form in the body, in turn aiding the utilisation of protein.

Loss factors: Again we find that the factors of handling, preparation and diet that affect B-vitamins in general, also affect PABA. Sulphur drugs have been shown to inhibit B-vitamin utilisation, but now the table is turned — PABA was found to have a similar formula to "sulfanilimide" when it first came into use during World War II. Fortunately, PABA was able to protect most bodies from the toxicity of this drug by rendering it largely inactive. In cases of severe depletion of PABA, eczema and hair loss have been noted, as with inositol. A milder deficiency of PABA is manifested by loss of hair colour, turning it either grey or white. The skin can also show white blotches under such conditions.

Benefits: Its ability to aid in the natural recolouring of faded hair, in conjunction with choline and B_5, is a recently proven property of PABA. But perhaps its most important modern application is its effectiveness as a sun-screen for protecting the skin against serious sunburn, both from direct rays of the sun and from ultraviolet sunlamps. This property was not recognised until the late 1960s, but is now so widely known as to form an essential ingredient in every effective suntan lotion or cream. Every sunbather should check its inclusion in the list of ingredients before buying a suntanning aid — and should never consider lying in the sun without applying such a lotion or cream. Such application will not only afford protection, but also nourish the skin and contribute to its smoothness and healthful appearance.

Food sources: To date, very little research has been completed on defining food sources of PABA. In general terms, however, those foods found to be abundant sources of other B-vitamins are certain to be valuable sources of PABA.

Dosages: Again, no RDA has been established by government scientists, nor have therapeutic dosages been established for varying conditions. Until such guidelines do emerge, reasonable care should be exercised in the potency and duration of therapeutic applications for PABA. It should be quite safe to consider taking up to 100 mg thrice daily for the remedying of any of the above deficiency conditions. For general therapeutic support, the usual 30 mg of PABA found in well-formulated B-complex tablets should be considered a useful minimum.

VITAMIN C — ASCORBIC ACID ($C_6H_8O_6$)

Characteristics: Pure vitamin C is in the form of a white powder, soluble in water and stable to air when dry. In liquid form, as a component of a food, it is readily oxidised and should not be exposed to the air for more than a minute or two to avoid any significant loss. It cannot be stored in the human body, so should be made available daily — most other animal bodies can synthesise vitamin C in their livers or kidneys, but a mutation occurring some millions of years ago ceased this function in the human body.

Absorption: The human body absorbs vitamin C with ease. It rapidly puts into use those quantities required, excreting through the urine any unwanted amounts. Many healing practitioners and researchers, unsupported by research grants from drug producers, have independently attested to the vital need of vitamin C for a huge diversity of conditions from lengthy observations. None has ever reported toxicity, even with massive doses administered by injection or orally.

Loss factors: Other than those loss factors mentioned above, probably the greatest depletion of the body's absorption and utilisation of vitamin C is caused by stress. This habit, for it is a habit in that it can only occur if a person allows it into his or her lifestyle, is known to precipitate emotional disharmonies, then depression, leading to any of the many mental illnesses coming within the term "schizophrenia". These conditions of illness are traceable to lack of vitamin C, although this lack rarely precipitates the symptom. Therefore, treating the symptom with vitamin C must be accompanied by constructive counselling for a more complete remission. Other forms of vitamin C loss are caused by poisonous chemicals destroying it soon after it enters the body. Of these, perhaps the most pernicious is tobacco and other smoked drugs. When we consider that one cigarette destroys 25 mg of vitamin C, imagine how much is destroyed by a pipe, a cigar, or worse, "grass". Cooking in copper pots also causes loss of vitamin C even before the foods reach the body — vitamin E is also lost this way. Modern food processing and refining also precipitate losses.

Deficiency symptoms: The only people who refuse to accept the research findings of dual Nobel Prize winner, Dr Linus Pauling, are those who allow their prejudices, for any number of selfish or ignorant reasons, to occlude their rational faculty. Here is a brilliant research scientist who has stated that a deficiency of vitamin C can be a cause of cancer in many of the body's organs. It is not the only cause, he states, but a very significant one — let those who refuse to accept, prove otherwise. (He also proves it to be an excellent controller of colds — his own daily dose is 13 000 mg.) Vitamin C is missing from so many processed foods, as is bran and many other nutrients, that all can be regarded as attributable to cancer formation — but Dr Pauling says that lack of C is a major factor. Likewise, Australia's Dr Archie Kalokerinos has proved that a vitamin C deficiency is primarily responsible for the syndrome now known as "sudden infant death syndrome" or "cot deaths". His astounding reduction in the death rate of Australian Aboriginal children is proof of his correctness (see *Every Second Child*, Keats Publishing, Connecticut, 1981). Last on our list of proved deficiency symptoms is the condition with which vitamin C was originally associated — scurvy. This "cure" was one of the earliest for which a vitamin was recognised.

Benefits: When Captain Cook fed his sailors fresh limes and became one of the first to prevent death from scurvy among his crew, little did he realise that such a small quantity of vitamin C could mean the difference between life and death. For this he became almost as famous as for his discovery of so much new land for the British Crown. But the benefits of vitamin C have since far exceeded the control of scurvy. Its important role in the formation, maintenance and health of collagen in every body cell, from the smallest of capillaries to the connective tissues, teeth and bones, gives vitamin C a most exhaustive role in the body's manifold functions. These include healing wounds and burns, broken bones and bleeding gums, the maintenance of the white blood corpuscles (which surround damaged or infected tissue to isolate the condition) and of the adrenal glands (which aid the balancing of our emotions). Healing after surgery (with vitamin E) and strengthening the infant after childbirth, if the mother's health is at all below par, are further benefits of vitamin C. So too is the detoxification of poisons (even at the expense of destroying the vitamin C used), the decreasing of serum cholesterol and the lowering of blood clot incidence in the veins and varicose veins. In short, adequate vitamin C can be of material assistance to protein in preserving life and allowing it to be extended to its pristine span of six times its maturing (see Stage 1).

Food sources: Not even a meat-eating person can contest the vital role of fresh fruits and vegetables in providing essential sources of vitamin C. In fact, meat, nuts, seeds, grains, seafoods and eggs are devoid of any vitamin C. Milk possesses only minimal amounts of vitamin C. The richest sources are, in order of descent: guavas, capsicums, blackcurrants, parsley, Brussels sprouts, broccoli, watercress, pawpaw, red cabbage and kohlrabi, all of which possess above 60 mg per 100 g edible portion. Then follow other fruits and vegetables. Freshly sprouted legumes, seeds, etc. are also very rich sources of vitamin C, offering the most reliably fresh source available.

Dosages: RDA for adults is currently regarded as being 45 mg, with higher doses recommended for pregnant or lactating women. This figure is an increase on that recommended a decade ago, and on that recommended in the previous decade. Gradually, government scientists are accepting that vitamin C should be increased in recommended dietary intakes as modern living becomes more demanding, more polluted and more deficient in natural foods. It is now suggested that a minimum daily recommended allowance of vitamin C be as follows: infants, 40 mg; children, 50 mg to 80 mg; adults 100 mg; sports people, pregnant and lactating women, 150 mg. A wide variety of vitamin C in supplement form is available, including the usual tablet, powder (as ascorbic acid, calcium ascorbate and sodium ascorbate, or combinations of these), as syrups, as flavoured chewable tablets, as time-release tablets and now, the latest form, as effervescent tablets. The range of potencies is no less variable, some being as low as 100 mg, but most now commence at 250 mg and range up to 1000 mg, with some tablets containing 1200 mg or even 1500 mg. These extremely high potencies should always be protein-coated, time-release varieties, otherwise one's urine takes on a new, expensive quality. Probably the best supplement form is a C-complex which includes rutin and the "citrus salts" bioflavonoids and hesperidin; another includes rose hips and/or acerola, cherry extract (the two richest, natural forms of vitamin C). Supplemental dosage varies from 250 mg to over 5000 mg daily.

VITAMIN D — "THE SUNSHINE VITAMIN" ($C_{56}H_{88}O_2$)

Characteristics: This complex and lengthy formula is actually a combination of two compounds, each with the same formula: vitamin D_1 (lumisterol) and D_2 (calciferol or, as it is sometimes known, ergosterol). They vary only in the physical arrangements of their molecules, the former being the most widely spaced. Each has the formula $C_{28}H_{44}O$, but the total compound is that obtained by the body from sunlight and/or fish liver oils. Vitamin D_2 (calciferol) is the synthesised form prepared from ergosterol by ultraviolet radiation. It is interesting to note that, although the synthetic form is chemically identical, its molecular arrangement is different to the natural form — being a tighter molecule, it is not quite so easily assimilated into the body. Vitamin D is insoluble in water — it is a fat-soluble vitamin, similar to vitamins A and E in this regard. Thus, it can be stored in the body and is not required on a daily basis.

Absorption: As its primary source for the body is from sunlight, nature has been most thoughtful in programming it for body storage, since some climates experience weeks or months without sunshine (in the latter category, supplementation is often needed as people turn to more processed foods). A prime reason for tropic-dwelling people to be dark-skinned is for protection from intense sunlight. This heavy pigment protected them, yet allowed adequate absorption of vitamin D from the sun's rays. As people moved away from the tropics, their skins gradually became lighter to allow increased absorption during the shorter durations of sunshine and the lower intensity of ultraviolet light. To a large extent, the body became adjusted to receiving less light from being more heavily clothed. This encouraged food supplements of vitamin D, these being grown in temperate climates, or extracted from cold-water fish or milk products. We have learned that sunshine and natural foods are vital ingredients to human health, but when these are not occurring in adequate proportion to human needs, a disease such as rickets will manifest. With plenty of exercise, the body will be kept warmer in winter and will not need so many clothes; for the abundance of clothes and the lack of exposure to the sun do not permit the skin to synthesise adequate vitamin D. Dietary supplements of vitamin D are taken orally and absorbed through the walls of the small intestine with dietary fats.

Loss factors: Factors which destroy vitamin D are fewer than for most other vitamins. Smog is one, and so is glass. Both reduce the amount of ultraviolet light available directly to the body. Sitting in a room into which sunlight filters through a closed window will do nothing for the body's vitamin D intake — one must be out in the direct sunlight, for glass considerably filters out ultraviolet rays, as does smog. So even if one sunbathes in the proximity of an industrial or heavy traffic area, ultraviolet rays will not be absorbed, because of the smog. Mineral oil as a laxative is the other major loss factor. Not as many people use it today as they did decades ago when it was heavily promoted, and millions of people, especially Americans, were hoodwinked into believing that this load of toxic chemicals helped to regulate the bowels.

Deficiency symptoms: Hypovitaminosis D is the deficiency syndrome through which rickets develops. Symptoms are initially recognisable by continuous bowel trouble, excessive perspiration during sleep and distension of the abdomen. Further symptoms develop as the disease grows — the ribcage becomes compressed, wrists and ankles appear swollen, arms and legs become bowed. Rickets has been known for more than a century, but it was only at the beginning of this century that it was recognised as a nutritional deficiency disease, although no one knew which nutrient was deficient. Codliver oil was found to be beneficial in correcting the disease, so it was assumed that fat was the cause. Ultimately, it was found to be vitamin D deficiency. Now that sunlight and certain foods have been found to remedy the deficiency, rickets rarely occurs — if it does, it is due either to ignorance or sheer neglect on the part of the parents. An adult form of rickets, osteomalacia, is occasionally evidenced by some of the above symptoms, together with spinal curvature. This occurs more with older people. Other, less frequent, symptoms are severe tooth decay and osteoporosis (bone calcium deficiency caused by inadequate utilisation of calcium from the diet due to a lack of vitamin D).

Benefits: If any vitamin ever undertook a major single function in life, it is vitamin D. So important is its ability to assist the body's utilisation of calcium and phosphorus that any other benefit pales by comparison. Thanks to the recognition of the essential nutritional role of vitamin D, rickets is a disease rarely encountered in the Western world today. Vitamin D also benefits in the treatment of conjunctivitis and aids the body in the assimilation of vitamin A.

Food sources: Seafoods, butter, sunflower seed kernels, liver, eggs, mushrooms and natural cheeses are best food sources of vitamin D. Fortified milk is next, although this is a poor source for youths or adults — milk being so unsuitable to them in many other ways. But no food source can compare with the sun's rays.

Dosages: RDA is universally accepted as being 400 international units (i.u.) daily for all ages. Supplementary intakes vary from 400 to 1200 i.u., although some patients with severe deficiency symptoms can require up to 4000 i.u. daily at the commencement of their treatment, reducing gradually after the first few days. Careful observation is necessary on such high dosages, due to possible toxicity. Symptoms of such toxicity can include excessive thirst, irritable eyes and skin, vomiting, persistent diarrhoea; internally, there will be high deposits of calcium inside the walls of blood vessels, kidneys, lungs and/or stomach.

VITAMIN E — ALPHA TOCOPHEROL ($C_{29}H_{50}O$)

Characteristics: The name tocopherol is a general description of the family of chemicals classified as vitamin E. There are eight in the group, but it is usual for only the first of them, alpha, to be therapeutically prepared for human need since it is the most effective. In nature, the tocopherols are usually found together and they possess slightly differing formulae. There are two forms of alpha tocopherol available for therapeutic application. That known as "natural" is d-alpha tocopherol acetate, derived from natural sources; the other is known as dl-alpha tocopherol acetate, regarded as being "synthetic". To the consumer, the difference is that the natural variety is about 36 per cent more potent than the synthetic and is derived from natural food oils, usually soya and/or wheat germ. The acetate form of vitamin E is that which is prepared for therapeutic use for greater stability and has the formula $C_{31}H_{52}O_3$. Vitamin E is insoluble in water, soluble in fat. It is stored in the liver, fatty tissues, heart, muscles, blood, and many of the body's glands, but for a short time only.

Absorption: As it can be stored for later use in the body, daily intakes of vitamin E are not always essential, but they are desirable. The internal loss factor of vitamin E is in the order of 65 per cent being excreted via the faeces. This can be too large a loss for some people whose vitamin E intake is barely adequate or their absorption ability diminished. Therefore, daily intake is recommended by many practitioners. If fats in the gastrointestinal tract are in any way spoilt or rancid, vitamin E absorption will be severely limited. Likewise, where foods containing vitamin E have become rancid, they will not be of any value so far as vitamin E absorption is concerned. One of the important functions of vitamin E is to prevent fats becoming rancid and this can only occur if the E is assimilable. Then it can do its work in protecting vitamins A and C from oxidation loss and the unsaturated oils from rancidity. Vitamin E has been known for over half a century, having been discovered in 1922 and studied in depth since 1936. Although thousands of research papers have been written on it, much of its character, its absorption into the body and its healing benefits remain undisclosed.

Loss factors: Heat and oxygen are two of the major causes of rancidity and loss of vitamin E. Special care should be exercised in choosing for consumption such foods as are highly susceptible to loss in these ways, especially wheat germ and unrefined oils. Other loss factors include inorganic iron in the form of ferrous sulphate, usually used in therapeutic dosages — vitamin E should not be therapeutically consumed within eight hours (either way) of this enemy. Chlorine in drinking water is also a loss-causing influence, again emphasising the importance of consuming distilled or filtered water. Mineral oil should also be avoided, for the same reasons as apply to vitamin D. Long storage in freezers and modern processing techniques also induce loss of vitamin E. Women need to take special care to avoid losses caused by oral contraceptives, or any other hormone intake, by the changes taking place in their body while going through the menopause, or when pregnant or nursing.

Deficiency symptoms: Lack of vitality is one of the major deficiency symptoms, indicating that either overwork or undernourishment, or both, are prevailing. Actually, people rarely overwork, they simply fail to handle their affairs in a balanced manner. This also indicates lack of certain nutritional factors. In most of these conditions, vitamin E will be found to be lacking. With insufficient available to the body, red blood cells will be destroyed above the normal level, the muscles will register degeneration due to sluggishness, and reproductive systems will become disordered. There exists little doubt that many more deficiency symptoms will be discovered as research continues. A significant amount of this research is being undertaken by Dr Wilfred Shute at the Shute Foundation Research Laboratories in London, Ontario, Canada. This organisation was originally partnered by the two Shute brothers, but Dr Evan Shute died a few years ago, leaving Wilfred to continue the pioneering work about which he lectured during his Australian visit in 1980. At these lectures, he projected graphic photographs of many skin conditions before and after, as well as during, treatment with improved diet, general vitamin therapy and massive doses of vitamin E. These skin problems ranged from ulcers and open sores to severe burns and gangrene, all of which responded significantly, usually with total healing, to vitamin E as the major form of treatment.

Benefits: The human heart is an amazing organ in its ability to work unceasingly from birth until death. But often it is overtaxed by unbalanced emotions and unsuitable nutrition. Vitamin E can certainly benefit the latter condition, and in so doing will indirectly help to overcome the former. Businesspeople, sports people and the elderly will be especially benefited by vitamin E. In its manner of nourishing the muscles to overcome lethargy, vitamin E mildly stimulates the heart muscles by enabling us to exist on that reduced oxygen level which so many people find now prevails in their environment and lifestyle. Smoking is one of those critical oxygen users, pollution minimises its availability and confined atmospheres increase the carbon dioxide ratio to oxygen. This benefit of vitamin E works to nourish the red blood cells so that their loss rate does not exceed their regeneration. Also, by detoxifying many of the poisons which find their way into the body, vitamin E aids the reproductive systems of both sexes by improving virility and the condition of the sperm, as well as strengthening the female abdominal membranes to avert a spontaneous abortion or miscarriage. Other benefits of vitamin E include its ability to help arteries expand, thereby stimulating the circulation to avert strokes, carrying the improved blood circulation right to the surface of the skin where its healing will become speedier. It will help overcome varicose veins, cystic mastitis and will even delay ageing.

Food sources: Since there are so few foods abundant in vitamin E, their therapeutic support is rather important. The list commences with wheat germ oil (containing up to 300 mg per 100 g); then sunflower seeds, sunflower oil, safflower oil, almonds, other vegetable oils, wheat germ and peanuts.

Dosages: RDA has been increased in the past decade and even now remains too low. Recommended minimum daily requirements now appear to be 20 mg to 40 mg for adults, proportionately less for children and infants; 50 mg for pregnant or lactating women. Therapeutic dosages vary from 100 mg to 1000 mg daily, even higher for severe symptoms. Doses are increased in potency if 25 μg selenium is added to tablet or capsule.

VITAMIN K — PHYTONADIONE ($C_{31}H_{46}O_2$)

Characteristics: The somewhat little-known vitamin K which occurs naturally in many green vegetables is closely related to two other vitamins called "K". Some writers and practitioners consider vitamin K, the dietary supplement and nutrient, to be a trio, numbered 1, 2 and 3. But, strictly speaking, this is not the case. Vitamin K_1, phytonadione, is the naturally occurring extract from alfalfa, isolated by the Germans in the 1920s and called "Koagulationsvitamin" — the blood-coagulating vitamin. Vitamins K_2 and K_3 are the synthesised counterparts and are known to have toxic effects on the body. Vitamin K is fat-soluble, insoluble in water and exists so extensively in higher green plants as to be considered unnecessary, in general, as a therapeutic nutrient. But there are exceptions.

Absorption: Easily assimilated through the intestine by normal digestion, vitamin K is found in many foods in adequate quantity. It can also be synthesised by the intestinal flora should the human diet be considered by the body's innate intelligence to be deficient in vitamin K.

Loss factors: Many of the common enemies of modern living are inhibitors to the body's absorption of vitamin K. Such loss factors include general radiation and X-rays, air pollution, oral antibiotics, aspirin and rancidity. Mineral oil laxatives are also inhibitors, as found with other fat-soluble vitamins.

Deficiency symptoms: The anaemia and chronic diarrhoea condition known as sprue is often a symptom of vitamin K deficiency. Excessive bleeding due to inefficient blood clotting, leading to haemophilia (which is often inherited, but sometimes found to be congenital) is also occasionally a nutritional-deficiency condition in which vitamin K plays a leading role. Colitis, related to inadequate bowel bacteria, resulting in malodorous stools, can also indicate lack of adequate vitamin K in the body (as well as incorrect food and/or indigestion). Coeliac disease is considered by some people to be caused by gluten in the diet, but this is not the full story (see Stage 13); however, it does respond to increased vitamin K by consuming far more green vegetables, especially alfalfa.

Benefits: Primary role in human health for vitamin K is to ensure the formation of the blood-clotting chemical, prothrombin. This ensures a person will not bleed to death from a tiny scratch to the skin. It also prevents internal haemorrhaging. Vitamin K as an aid to regulating menstrual flow is obviously also important. Sufferers from irregular nosebleeding will benefit from more vitamin K-rich foods.

Food sources: Leading food sources are all green vegetables and alfalfa sprouts, followed by liver, cheese, butter and whole grains. Yogurt, vegetable oils and egg yolks come next.

Dosages: No RDA has been established, but a daily intake of 300 µg is usually considered adequate — equivalent to 150 g of broccoli lightly steamed. Newborn infants require more than this adult need. The best therapeutic sources are alfalfa tablets and liquid chlorophyll (which is prepared from concentrated alfalfa leaves). Suggested maximum dosage is 600 µg daily.

VITAMIN P — BIOFLAVONOIDS

Characteristics: This group of compounds is closely related to vitamin C and necessary to its proper functioning and absorption. The group comprises rutin and hesperidin, as well as flavones and flavals. The flavonoids are the compounds found in the piths of citrus fruits and their role in maintaining capillary permeability gives this group the name of vitamin P.

Absorption: The ease with which vitamin P is absorbed is similar to vitamin C, with which it works synergistically. It plays the important role of preventing oxidation destroying vitamin C.

Deficiency symptoms: As this group rarely works on its own in human nutrition, it is difficult to isolate specific deficiency symptoms, other than the tendency to bruise easily (indicating capillaries are too fragile) and frequently bleeding gums, noticeable after cleaning teeth. If you find you are susceptible to many infectious conditions even though you consider you are taking adequate vitamin C, chances are you are deficient in the bioflavonoids.

Benefits: In strengthening and regulating the absorption of the capillaries, vitamin P works to maintain a more robust skin and a greater effectiveness of vitamins C and E. Vitamin P conjoins with its "big brother", vitamin C, to be of relief assistance to women in their menopause, especially in regard to the balancing of physical and emotional discomforts.

Food sources: By far the best natural source of vitamin P is the under-skin, the white pith of citrus fruits. For this important reason, only the outer, coloured skin should be removed, leaving plenty of pith around the inside flesh.

Dosages: No RDA has been established; however it has been found that vitamin P works best with vitamin C in the ratio of 1 : 5. Thus, average daily requirement should be in the range of 20 mg to 30 mg. Therapeutically, it is usually found that vitamin P complex is a part of a vitamin C complex tablet. It is possible to obtain tablets of vitamin P only, in which case the bioflavonoids are usually in the order of 500 mg in total, with 50 mg each of rutin and hesperidin.

It must be recognised that much has yet to be uncovered in the complex realm of vitamins. What is presented here is intended to be a valuable general guide for the everyday use of people who eat and for those who guide people in what they should eat. But it must always be remembered that vitamins plus minerals plus fats plus carbohydrates plus proteins, when totalled and added to water, still do not equal the total of man's ideal diet. The major missing factor is life force. No reliable analyses are yet available for this nebulous component, but it will always be greatest when food is eaten fresh and grown organically (see Stage 14).

For greater detail on the nutrient content of foods, researched tables of average values for Australian foods (200 of them) are provided, together with graduated lists of each nutrient, in my book *Guidebook to Nutritional Factors in Edible Foods*, Pythagorean Press, Sydney, 1977 and Woodbridge Press, California, USA, 1979.

STAGE NINE

Secrets of Food Combining

Custom may lead a man into many errors, but it justifies none.

Henry Fielding (1707-1754)

In terms of his dietary habits, man has certainly been led into many errors. Could English novelist Henry Fielding have been referring to that infamous English habit of the customary three-course meal and a cup (or two) of tea, when he wrote of errors?

It appears that wherever the English have settled throughout the world — which is almost everywhere — habits of overeating have followed. So long as the stomach is filled, little regard is placed on the nature of the filling. This appears to be the custom.

Habit seems to have decreed that every meal should include every nutrient in huge, concentrated portions. No regard appears to be given to the fact that it is impossible for several different chemical reactions to ensue simultaneously in the same receptacle without conflict. Does man think his stomach can be the exception?

It is basic scientific knowledge that diverse chemical reactions, requiring different concentrations of acidity or alkalinity, cannot occupy the same receptacle at the same time. If they did, the risk of an explosion from the volatile gases emitted would be very high. This is just what occurs in the human stomach after a large, complex meal, as we all well know.

The history of human indigestion is as long as that of overeating. Yet a study of the chemistry of the stomach reveals that most digestive problems arise there, being caused by man's naivety in expecting a chemical impossibility. The human stomach is only one receptacle, therefore it can effectively support only one chemical reaction at a time. With its basic purpose of initiating the breakdown of proteins, the stomach must be allowed the freedom of fulfilling its object without the interference caused when different types of protein, together with fats and carbohydrate concentrates, are imposed at the same time and in similar proportions. This implies that meals should not comprise a conglomeration of many different concentrated foods. It further implies the need to practise the science of proper food combining as a vital, yet much neglected aspect of human nutritional science, to discover this last science of good digestion.

From Table to Stomach

Inasmuch as we have found it advantageous to acquire a working knowledge of items such as our car, lawn mower, and sewing machine, it is so much more important to understand the hidden activities which take place within us when food disappears into the mouth at mealtimes.

The practice of rules of food combining is neither faddist nor restrictive. It is a simple, scientifically based system of choosing foods which are compatible. Rather than restrict, it more correctly channels our choices into particular directions. When we realise that we have at our disposal at any one time of the year a selection of many different types of foods from which to choose, it becomes apparent that we need some principles of guidance in selecting those foods which will combine well and best facilitate digestion and after-meal comfort.

Preparatory to understanding the rules of food combining, we must check that we are thoroughly conversant with the basic digestive processes. For this reason we need to know the major functions of that 9 metre long cavern (in the average adult), called the human gastrointestinal tract.

The Mouth

Its first receptacle is the mouth, in which the food intake is prepared for despatch to the stomach. Food spends less time here than in any other part of the gastrointestinal tract — often far too little time. The two primary functions of the mouth are taste and chewing. Taste is intended to convey the suitability, or otherwise, of the food through the sensual reaction of pleasure or displeasure. The teeth then act upon the mouth's contents to render the food into smaller pieces, to pulverise and reduce it all to a creamy substance. This is facilitated by the intermixing with saliva, requiring the food to be retained in the mouth until it has been thus properly prepared for acceptance by the stomach.

Human saliva contains the important enzyme ptyalin. Its purpose is to initiate the catabolism of carbohydrates by converting starches into sugars. (Catabolism is the breakdown of foods into component nutrients; the second part of the metabolic process is anabolism, which is the building-up of cellular structure by absorption and transfer of the nutrients.)

This action of ptyalin in saliva greatly improves the later work of the duodenum and the small intestine, as they take over carbohydrate breakdown when the food has left the stomach.

Saliva also performs the important role of adequately moistening the food. This facilitates chewing and allows the tongue to finally roll the food into a ball for its passage from the mouth into the oesophagus, the narrow tube which carries food into the stomach.

It is important to note that ptyalin is not present in the saliva of an infant. It requires about twenty-four months for ptyalin to commence to become a part of the saliva in sufficient quantity to regulate the digestion of starches. This implies the dangers associated with the feeding of starchy foods to infants and children under the age of two. Ignorance of this factor can result in the development of a starch intolerance and can contribute to such problems as coeliac disease.

Story of the Stomach

Immediately after food enters the human stomach, it is churned and impregnated with gastric juice. The primary agent of activity in gastric juice is hydrochloric acid (HCl), the concentration of which is determined by the nature of protein concentration in the meal received. Accompanying HCl is the enzyme pepsin, the purpose of which is to hasten the action of HCl upon the protein without actually taking part in the reaction. Mucus is also present in gastric juice to act as a lubricant.

An additional enzyme, rennin, plays an important role in the stomach of the infant. Its purpose is to coagulate milk to enable its protein (caseinogen) to be catabolised. However, substantial proof exists to testify that rennin begins to diminish in the infant as its teeth commence to form. By the time the child has a full set of first teeth and is able to thoroughly chew solid foods, around the age of seven or eight years, the gastric juice no longer contains rennin. Without this enzyme of infant need, milk is no longer an acceptable food in its liquid state. Its continued consumption, therefore, is considered by some to result in probable indigestion and possible allergies.

The purpose of the stomach, then, is to receive and hold food to enable the reduction of its protein components into simpler chemical forms. Complex food proteins are thereby broken down into amino acid chains, called polypeptides. During this process, starch catabolism is suspended, drawing to a close the work of ptyalin from the saliva (ptyalin acts only in a neutral or alkaline medium and is rendered ineffective by the stomach's essential acidity).

Some nutritionists seem to believe that the stomach also contains a "gastric lipase" for the preliminary breakdown of fats. No evidence supports this claim. Catabolism of lipids (food fats and oils) cannot take place until emulsification has occurred and this depends upon the next stage of digestion, in the duodenum.

With food in the stomach, the lower escape valve, the pylorus, remains closed until adequate gastric action has taken place. If proper digestion is allowed, the opening of the pylorus will be delayed until all proteins are converted to their simplified polypeptide chains, preparing them perfectly for their next stage of breakdown. Alternatively, if food is taken into the stomach before adequate breakdown of the previous meal's proteins, the pylorus may be forced to allow the premature evacuation of some or all of the inadequately prepared food, thereby placing undue burden on the facilities of the lower gastrointestinal tract.

Duration of a meal in the stomach will primarily depend on the quantity and type of protein contained therein. There are definite limits to the amount of gastric juice available to the stomach and if this has to be shared with a huge quantity of protein, gastric catabolism will be delayed. Also, certain protein types of foods contain more complex molecules of protein than others — animal meats being at the head of the list, requiring the highest concentration of HCl. Fresh vegetables possess the most easily digested protein, followed by seeds and nuts. Food will also be unduly delayed in the stomach if the meal contains concentrations of fats or sugars, as will be discussed in relation to food combining.

Duties of the Duodenum

When food leaves the stomach, its passage through the pylorus takes it directly into the duodenum, which is the beginning of the small intestine. No absorption of food has taken place from the stomach, for digestion has not reached a sufficient stage of completion at that point. Alcohol is, fortunately, the only exception. Its absorption through the gastric mucosa protects the intestines from its harsh effects, but the brain must suffer because alcohol seems to find its way there from the bloodstream, almost as a direct warning against its use.

When first entering the duodenum, food is greeted by bile, composed of salts, acids, water and mucus. Bile is stored in the gall bladder, fed from the liver. It is secreted to act upon lipids (fats) by emulsifying them in preparation for subsequent enzyme action. A little further along the duodenum, pancreatic juice enters. Now commences the major activity in the food's general catabolism.

While food is moving along the duodenum, its condition of general acidity, created in the stomach, diminishes until alkalinity prevails. This is hastened by the entrance of pancreatic juice which comprises three important enzymes — trypsin, lipase and amylase. The purpose of trypsin is to act upon proteins, now in their state of partial breakdown; of lipase to act upon fats, now emulsified by the bile; of amylase to act upon carbohydrates, taking up where ptyalin left off.

It is interesting to note the relative quantities of digestive juices available in the average-sized person of good health. The maximum gastric juice available is around 2 litres (nearly 5 pints). But the stomach will also contain some saliva, of which approximately 1 litre (1¾ pints) is available for the digestion to draw upon. Of maximum availability to the duodenum are 0.75 litre (just over 1¼ pints) of bile and a little over 0.5 litre (1 pint) of pancreatic juice. In the small intestine, another 0.25 litre (almost ½ pint) of intestinal juice is available, essentially in the form of mucus.

Small and Large Intestines

Through the duodenum, the food passes along the small intestine, slowly increasing its alkalinity as the intestinal enzymes complete their catabolic actions. Gradually, all nutrients are separated as much as possible from each other and from cellulose and other residues.

Proteins have now been split into their component amino acids. As such, they are absorbed through the intestinal wall and transported to the liver for detoxification. From the liver, amino acids are taken to various parts of the body for suitable combination and build-up into body proteins. As the body cannot store amino acids, any excess must be converted into carbohydrates and fats by the liver, releasing nitrogen.

Carbohydrates are now reduced to the simple sugars and are absorbed at various stages along the intestinal wall, almost entirely from the small intestine. The bloodstream transports carbohydrates to the liver, where some are stored as glycogen for supplying muscle energy as subsequently required. Excess sugars flow over into the bloodstream, where the floating balance should be maintained in proportion to the body's energy needs by the regulator, insulin. Insulin is manufactured in the pancreas (in the Islets of Langerhans) for secretion into the bloodstream as required, the pancreas acting as the reservoir.

All lipids have been broken down into component fatty acids in the small intestine. When ready for absorption, they are taken up by the lymph-stream and transported to the various bodily locations having greatest need for them. They, alone, bypass the liver.

The small intestine is, paradoxically, the longest component of the gastrointestinal tract. At an average length of some seven metres, it is also the longest organ in the body. Because its diameter is smaller than that of the colon, it is referred to as the "small" intestine; in contrast the colon is called the "large" intestine, although its length is only an average of 1.5 metres.

Residues of food components, remaining after the absorption of needed nutrients, continue to pass along the small intestine until they enter the large intestine, or colon, at the ileocaecal junction. Unlike the small intestine which hangs in coiled loops from attachments along the posterior abdominal wall, the colon is in a relatively fixed position and tends to provide a frame within which the small intestine nestles.

From the ileocaecal valve, the large intestine rises along the inside of the lower trunk's right side. At the waistline, the ascending colon turns left to form the transverse colon. This slightly dips as it travels towards the left side of the trunk where it moves to the rear and turns down to form the descending colon and finally the sigmoid colon which feeds the faeces into the rectum for eventual evacuation through the anus.

Just two or three centimetres up from the beginning of the ascending colon lies the base of the vermiform appendix. This curious little narrow tube, closed at its other end, varies in length from 2 cm to 20 cm, averaging 9 cm. It is longer in children than in adults, appearing to shrink with progressive ageing. Its function is largely unknown, although popular opinion tends to attribute to it an ability to provide the colon and small intestine with disease-resistant properties, especially against cancer.

But our primary concern here is with the body's handling of the residues of digestion. The accumulation of food residues into "stools" in the colon takes place in an alkaline medium, creating a favourable environment for the survival and activity of intestinal bacteria. These work to decompose the residues and render them ready for final evacuation through the anus. Prior to this, water and a few trace mineral salts are absorbed through the colon walls, but sufficient moisture should be retained for the smooth movement of faeces along the colon. If transit time is too short (as in cases of diarrhoea), too much water will create liquid faeces instead of semi-solid stools. If transit time is too long (as in cases of constipation, generally when insufficient fibre is included in the diet), stools become hard and compacted, for too much water has been absorbed during the abnormally long transit time.

Intestinal bacteria are vital to the final breakdown of previously incomplete digestion. The resultant putrefaction is normal; however, its excess will probably cause flatulence and an unpleasant odour. This often occurs when food has been too hastily evacuated from the stomach to make way for an additional intake. Other likely causes include insufficient chewing, emotional upsets at or close to mealtime and unsuitable food combinations. Drugs and chemicals are other frequent causes of improper functioning of the colon, resulting in its evacuating as infrequently as once a day or once each second day, instead of the normal twice each day regularity.

Many modern drugs act to kill the colon's normal bacteria because they have not been tested adequately prior to prescription. But this is not only limited to the colon. As we now recognise the fact that human digestion is primarily a chemical function, we are better able to understand how much damage can be done to the body's delicate chemical balance by the introduction of foreign chemicals. Such impaired digestion can often be traced to strong prescription drugs, as well as to food-preparation chemicals.

Processed foods imply a further digestion problem. They are generally seriously deficient in bulk (vital dietary fibre found in all natural foods), resulting either from milling or slaughtering. The removal of fibre-rich bran from wheat and rice grains by stripping the outer layer to make white flour and polished rice has been the greatest single cause of colonic malfunction in the world.

A close second is the huge amount of animal meat, dairy produce, eggs, poultry and fish consumed in modern society — far too much for the human gastrointestinal tract to handle, especially as these items are often consumed with little or no fibre-rich natural foods, such as vegetables and fruits. The human colon was not designed to handle this imbalance and be flooded with fibreless animal foods.*

Another factor which interferes with the normal balance of digestion is the modern habit of including in a meal a huge variety of rich foods, many of which will have been heavily processed. This overload will interfere with the proper functioning of the stomach, the intestines and the body's general health pattern and will give rise to a variety of pathological problems.

---

* For comparative nutritional factors in foods, refer to my food analysis book: *Guidebook to Nutritional Factors in Edible Foods*, Pythagorean Press, Sydney, 1977 and Woodbridge Press, California, 1979.

Food Classifications

For the reader to gain a reliable understanding of the science of food combining, it is first necessary to recognise the different food groups and the foods classified within each group. Such classification is based on the nutrient content of each food so far as the three major nutrient groups are concerned, viz. proteins, fats and carbohydrates.

By virtue of the special properties of certain types of foods, various subdivisions are made. This is not done to create complications, but to afford the most complete classifications for those who wish to adopt food combining for maximum benefits. To this extent, there are nine classifications, as follows:

1. Primary Proteins

Protein is the most important nutrient, therefore any concentrated food will come within its classification when it contains at least 15 per cent protein by volume. Primary proteins are those which comprise the simplest molecular structure for protein-rich foods, being therefore easiest to digest. They are all plant proteins, principally raw nuts and seeds, as under:

Pumpkin, sunflower, safflower and sesame seed kernels;
Pignolia and pine-nut kernels;
Almond, Brazil and cashew nut kernels;
Walnut, hazelnut and pistachio nut kernels;
Soya beans — best when sprouted then lightly cooked;
Lecithin, the nutrient-rich supplement extracted from soya beans;
Wheat germ — fresh, raw and unstabilised (processing will inhibit rancidity but will destroy some protein and cause saturation of the essential fatty acids present).

Wheat germ and lecithin are not whole foods, as are the other items included in this list, but their value as food supplements is attested by the fact that they possess the majority of the nutrients found in the original whole food from which they are extracted.

2. Secondary Proteins

These comprise other edible concentrated protein-rich foods, most of which are of animal origin. The exception is the peanut, not included in the previous list because of its digestive difficulty when eaten as a protein-rich food in quantity of around one hundred grams, its high concentration of saturated and mono-unsaturated fatty acids, together with its anti-digestive enzymes. These are characteristic of many types of legume, peanuts belonging to the legume family, for it is botanically not a nut. The list, therefore, comprises:

Eggs — preferably free-range;
Cheese and yogurt;
Peanut kernels — raw and unsalted;
Animal meats, poultry, fish.

Some qualifying notes on these foods will assist in their best utilisation: Eggs are always more nutritious when eaten raw, after separating yolks and discarding whites. Yolks contain abundant lecithin which coagulates and becomes useless when cooked, yet when raw is a most effective negator to the heavy concentration of cholesterol in the yolks. Egg whites are almost pure albumin and difficult for the digestion to handle unless coagulated in cooking, but cooking would reduce nutritional properties of yolks.

Cheese comes in many shapes and recipes, but the most nutritionally desirable are those without salt, made from raw milk and with no chemical additives. In Australia, it is almost impossible to achieve this ideal, so we must settle for the best compromises. Natural Swiss Emmentaler cheese is almost ideal. It is made from raw milk, with minimal salt and no chemical additives. It therefore has a low shelf life compared with other block cheeses, but its nut-sweet flavour makes it a most desirable and characteristically different cheese. Ricotta cheese is also low in salt, but is even lower in fat, making it very desirable for people seeking a low-fat diet. Both it and cottage cheese are regarded as "soft" cheeses and are very easily digested when properly combined. Other cheeses are less nutritionally desirable, unless they are home made without additives.

Yogurt is also preferred to raw milk, especially if made from goat's milk. But take care not to overeat this item, for it does introduce foreign bacteria into the colon which, if in large quantities, would tend to clash with the bowel's normal flora. Thus, a reasonable daily maximum would be 100 g. Again, the best yogurt is that made in one's home from raw goat's milk — it has a far richer flavour than anything available commercially and is much more nutritious.

The inclusion of animal meats, etc., is solely for those people who are not yet ready to become vegetarian. But care should be taken to exclude processed meats (such as sausage), pork, salted meats (such as ham and bacon) and battery-bred poultry. Free-range poultry is acceptable in this category.

3. *Fats*

Included in this group are those foods, other than protein-concentrates, known to contain fatty acids in excess of 10 per cent by volume. Although not long, it is nonetheless an important list, comprising:

Macadamia nuts, pecan nuts, chestnuts, beechnuts;
Coconut flesh and milk;
Avocados and olives;
Vegetable oils.

Nuts included in this list possess up to ten times as much dietary fat as protein. In fact, macadamias and pecans are the richest sources of fats of any natural whole food. Vegetable oils are top of the fat scale with almost 100 per cent content, implying virtually no other nutrient of any significant value. These oils are best used from cold-pressed sources and purposely exclude animal fats, for they are too highly saturated and contain cholesterol. Vegetable oils contain no cholesterol and are far more poly-unsaturated fats than oils derived from animal sources, such as cod liver oil, butter, margarine from whale blubber, etc.

Coconut flesh and milk provides a very rich food, known to have sustained tropical natives when other foods were not available. However, it is not the whole food many people assume, for it lacks vitamins A and C, as well as being low in B-complex vitamins, calcium and magnesium. Whole coconut does provide a reasonably fat-concentrated meal in itself and is best eaten on its own or with other fruits.

Avocados and olives are unusual fruits in that they possess such high concentrations of fat (up to 21 per cent). They will combine well with most vegetables and afford a fair combination with most fruits. Avocado offers the very best spread for bread, being especially nutritious on a whole-grain bread, taking the place of both butter and the spread. (The only other highly nutritious spreads for bread are raw nut butters — cashew, almond and, to a lesser extent, peanut butter.)

4. Starches

Carbohydrate-rich foods are divided into starches and sugars because of the varying reaction to each in the gastrointestinal tract. Starches include a few fruits and vegetables, together with grains and pulses, all of which possess at least 15 per cent starch content by volume and have not been included in protein or fat classifications. These foods are:

Fruits — breadfruit and jackfruit (both tropical products);
Vegetables — potatoes, sweet potatoes, pumpkins, squash, yams, taro and Jerusalem artichokes;
Grains — rice, wheat, corn, rye, millet, buckwheat, oats, triticale and sorghum;
Pulses — all beans, dried peas and lentils.

5. Fresh Vegetables

These include all non-starch plant products not included in the foregoing lists or in the following fruit lists. They encompass every other type of salad and garden vegetable including starch-type dry foods which have been sprouted into fresh foods, such as alfalfa, lentil, mung bean, wheat and any other sprouts.

6. Sweet Fruits

This classification includes fresh and dried fruits possessing a high fructose concentration, causing them to come within the broad classification of carbohydrate-rich foods. However, because the carbohydrate is primarily sugar, rather than starch, digestion does not depend so much on ptyalin in the saliva as with starch-concentrated foods. This group does not include melons, but does include:

Bananas, figs, persimmons, custard apples and monstera deliciosa;
All dried fruits — sun-dried and chemical-free are always preferred to chemically-assisted dried fruits.

7. Melons

By virtue of their unusually high water content, high sugar concentration and low percentages of other nutrients, melons often create digestive problems for many people. Another reason for this is the tendency many people have to overeat melons. For these reasons, melons are classified separately to include:

Cantaloupes, watermelons, honeydew melons and casaba melons.

8. Sub-acid Fruits

Some nutritionists prefer to call this grouping "neutral fruits". Either term is acceptable, for both describe the nature of this group of fresh fruits; they are mid-way between the group of sweet fruits and acid fruits. Comprised are primarily fruits of deciduous trees and vines, with a few sub-tropical fruits included:

Mulberries, blackberries, raspberries, blueberries and loganberries;
Pears, apples, apricots, peaches, nectarines, plums and cherries;
Paw paws, mangoes, guavas, grapes and lychees — these sub-tropical fruits are higher in fructose than the others and almost border onto the "sweet fruit" classification, so care should be taken not to eat too much of them if proteins are being consumed at the same meal.

9. Acid Fruits

This final grouping comprises all those fresh fruits possessing a distinctly acid taste, even though some are also quite sweet to the taste buds. They include:

Citrus fruits — oranges, lemons, limes, mandarins and grapefruit;
Pineapples, strawberries, gooseberries, kiwi fruit and passionfruit.

How to Use the Food Combining Rules and Tables

Food combining is designed to facilitate easier digestion. Its emphasis is on the reaction of different foods to each other in the stomach. The chart on page 149 diagrammatically presents the full set of food combining rules in an easy-to-refer-to form. Accompanying this chart are the lists of foods in their correct classifications.

To use the food combining chart, simply select the food you wish to eat as the main part of your meal. Find where it appears in the classification lists. Then locate that classification in the left-hand column under Food Groups. By looking along the horizontal line, you will come to "good" in a few places. This means that the food groups heading the vertical column above "good" are the best combinations to eat with your main choice for the best and easiest digestion to take place. Then you refer back to the foods listed under that or those food classification headings and select from that or those lists, the food or foods you wish to eat with your main choice.

For example, if your main choice is cashew nuts, referring to the classification lists, you find cashews are Primary Proteins. On your Food Combining Chart, Primary Proteins occupy the first horizontal line. Then as you look along that line, you will find "good" appearing three times. At the head of these three lists, you will see that primary proteins, vegetables and acid fruits are shown to be compatible with your main choice of cashew nuts. Returning to the food classification lists, you will find that you have a vast range of food from which to choose to eat with your cashews. You will soon read in the explanation of the food combining rules that you do not mix too many different proteins together and that you do not mix too many fruits and vegetables together. But you still have a vast range from which to choose to make a delicious vegetable or fruit salad, or a steamed vegetable casserole to accompany your cashew nuts.

The qualification "fair" on the horizontal line of your main choice implies that such a combination would not provide the best digestive partner. But if you wish to go ahead with that choice, so long as the quantities were very modest, you should have no digestive problems, unless you are already suffering from indigestion (in which case you should stay strictly with only the "good" combinations).

Where the qualification "poor" appears, avoid this combination wherever possible. Failure to do so might not appear to induce indigestion or apparent food combining problems, but you are not always conscious of what is going on inside. In my practice, I have found many instances of patients suffering from repeated headaches which have been attributed to tension or nervous problems, when they can be simply traced to suppressed indigestion, palliated with antacid tablets or the like.

To the person who has not previously considered the scientific combining of his foods, who has eaten anything and everything placed in front of him, food combining could appear too much trouble and fuss! Certainly it is almost like learning to eat all over again, for it makes you think before you choose what to eat with what. And because you have rarely thought of this before, except insofar as mere taste is concerned, you might be initially reluctant to undertake this "new" concept.

But food combining is not new. It has been practised by many religious groups for centuries, although their purpose was more for spiritual than scientific reasons. Learning to correctly combine foods is much easier than learning to drive a car or to type; indeed thousands of people have learned these rules without much effort and very little complaint. But learning to drive or to type cannot compare to learning correct food combining rules insofar as your total health is concerned. So why hesitate?

After a week or two of practice, most of the food combining rules will be easily remembered and applied. After a month, you will not even need to make more than the occasional reference to the rules. In fact, after a few months, you will possibly modify some of the rules to suit your particular digestive requirements. By this time, food combining will have become second nature and you will wonder why you uttered those words of protest in the beginning.

Here are the seven food combining rules, broken into two groups — four primary and three secondary rules. Remember that these rules are scientifically propounded for the average human gastrointestinal tract to facilitate the easiest and most efficient digestion. As people's digestive systems are marginally different, you might find, as already mentioned, that some of these rules can be modified for your particular needs. Do not rush into doing this: stay with the basic rules for some weeks until you are familiar with them and their effects on your body, for it is not always possible to know from the outside what is going on inside.

Primary Food Combining Rules

Rule 1: Avoid Mixing Protein and Carbohydrate Concentrated Foods in the Same Meal

Although every food contains some protein, those regarded as protein-concentrated foods demand the longest digestion times. They are held in the stomach for some hours until the gastric juice has performed its task. This can vary from two and a half to six hours, depending upon the complexity of the protein in the food. But if properly combined and in moderate quantities, no protein-concentrated food should require more than four and a half hours in the stomach.

If a protein food is accompanied by starch-concentrated or sugar-concentrated foods, fermentation will usually result. This is sure to create some degree of indigestion and probable gas in the stomach. In turn, this will reduce the efficiency of protein digestion in the stomach and might even give rise to food allergy conditions.

Animal-food proteins (meats, fish, cheese, etc.) demand very high concentrations of hydrochloric acid (HCl), as previously explained. Thus, if their gastric digestion is inhibited, as it can be by carbohydrate fermentation in the stomach, increased discomfort will be caused by some putrefaction of the meat, etc. This will create more gas and discomfort. Eating meat with potatoes and/or bread and/or sweets should especially be avoided.

Concentrated protein foods are always best digested when eaten with a fresh vegetable salad. Primary protein foods also combine very well with acid fruits and, to a slightly lesser extent, with sub-acid fruits, especially paw paw. These fruits and vegetables are valuable natural sources of vitamin C, which greatly aids protein digestion.

Rule 2: Avoid Mixing Proteins and Fats at the Same Meal

Fat in foods will inhibit the secretion of gastric juice through the stomach wall. Thus, when most fat-concentrated foods are consumed at the same time as protein-concentrated food, gastric catabolism is decreased by the degree of lipid concentration in the stomach. As with carbohydrates, fats will undergo no digestion in the stomach, taking a vacation while gastric juice goes to work on the complex protein molecules.

Even though all primary protein foods possess high concentrations of fat, such lipids will be held in suspension, awaiting catabolism in the lower intestine, without impeding gastric action. Free fats, such as oils, butter, margarine and milk fats, tend to coat the gastric mucosa, thereby inhibiting its effort to secrete gastric juice. This can become quite a problem if heavy concentrations of HCl are required to act on high concentrations of protein, particularly animal proteins.

Drinking milk at or just prior to a meal has precisely this effect. But the fat content of milk is not the only problem. If it were, skim milk with meals would be acceptable. Milk creates two other problems in the stomach — with its alkalinity and its protein digestion. The alkaline nature of milk will tend to reduce the effectiveness of HCl, especially when the heavy acid concentration is required to catabolise animal protein foods in the stomach. Effective digestion of the protein in milk demands that its gastric catabolism begins only when it has been coagulated into a more solid form with the aid of the enzyme rennin, yet this no longer exists in the human stomach once the child's first set of teeth have been fully formed. This creates a need for large quantities of mucus as the stomach attempts to compensate for the lack of rennin. That mucus secretion is delayed for a time by the fat coating the gastric mucosa. Eventually it will fight its way through; meanwhile the milk will have become somewhat soured in the heat of the stomach and in the delay before catabolism commences.

Fat surrounding fried foods is also regarded as free fat, tending to interfere with gastric catabolism. The intense heat of frying lipids is bad enough, altering, as it does, the molecular structure of the fat or oil used. As previously explained, this creates a tendency for grave carcinogenic risks, completely out of proportion to whatever pleasure the fried food might temporarily provide. If food is to be cooked, it should be lightly steamed in "waterless" cookware or supported by a flexible stainless steel steamer stand inside a saucepan. This will retain maximum nourishment. If meat must be consumed, it should be lightly grilled, never fried. It should also be fresh meat — remember, on the infrequent occasions when natural man did eat meat, it was raw and freshly killed. It was also very lean meat, being wild and extremely muscular.

Rule 3: Avoid Combining Totally Different Proteins in the Same Meal

Any variety of nuts or any variety of seeds will usually combine quite satisfactorily with each other in the same meal. Any variety of cheeses will usually combine with each other; as will any variety of fresh meats on their own. This is not to endorse variety, rather to indicate its acceptability within each group so long as small quantities are consumed. But it is important to recognise that the different protein groups do not combine well in the same meal, due to their varying requirements of concentration of HCl.

To comprehend acid concentration levels, we must refer to the chemical scale by which hydrogen ion concentrations are measured. This is called the pH scale; the concentration of an acid (or alkali) being measured by its pH number. Mid-way on the scale of 1-14 is the number 7, representing a neutral solution, such as pure water. As the concentration of acid in a solution increases, the pH number reduces — a pH of 6 is a weak acid, whereas a pH of 1 is extremely strong. As the concentration of an alkali increases, its pH rises from 8 to 14.

When the stomach is given the task of digesting protein in foods, it amasses a concentration of HCl appropriate to the nature of the protein's chemical composition.

For plant proteins, such as nuts and seeds, HCl concentration is rather low during the early stages of catabolism, at a pH of between 5 and 5.5. As catabolism develops in the stomach, the concentration of HCl increases until its pH reaches a figure of around 4.

In contrast, the concentration of HCl for cheese catabolism in the stomach will commence around 3.5. This will reduce to just under 3 as HCl concentration is called upon to increase during the course of cheese digestion in the stomach. For eggs, the pH concentration also commences around 3.5, but it increases far more than for cheese, rising to 2 on the pH scale towards the end of gastric digestion.

Meats demand the highest concentrations of HCl of all protein foods. This is recognised by tests of the carnivore stomach where a pH of 1 can be developed to facilitate the rapid catabolism of meat protein. This is ten times the highest level of HCl concentration in the human stomach, where the highest pH concentration usually possible is 2. Thus, when meat is ingested by man, his stomach seeks to secrete its most concentrated level of HCl from the outset and to hold this throughout the period meat is in the stomach. This intensely high acid strength, maintained for so many hours, can induce burning of the sensitive gastric mucosa and lead to gastric ulcers.

What all this implies is the difficulty of imposing upon the stomach the task of supplying gastric juice with two different concentrations of HCl at the same time. For instance, if nuts and meats are consumed in the same meal (as so often occurs when eating in a Chinese restaurant), how can the stomach supply the correct concentrations of HCl for both when meat demands up to thirty times the concentration of nuts at the commencement of their gastric digestion?

This is impossible since man has only one stomach. Therefore, some considerable degree of indigestion must occur, for the protein of greatest quantity will usually come nearer to winning the battle. This will be to the detriment of both protein foods, especially that requiring the greater HCl level, for it will inevitably pass into the duodenum improperly prepared. Sometimes the lower intestines can handle this extra catabolic burden, but invariably some of the meat or dairy proteins will pass into the bloodstream a little short of being properly prepared. Body cells often find these unsuitable, seeking to throw them out, occasionally giving rise to differing forms of food allergies.

Rule 4: Avoid Mixing Carbohydrates and Acid Fruits in the Same Meal

Remember that the starch-splitting enzyme ptyalin has an important job to perform as the food is chewed. This is why ptyalin is included in the saliva. Its role in initiating the reduction of complex starch molecules towards simpler sugars is second only in importance to chewing. How beneficial, then, that both can take place simultaneously. So why spoil this clever plan of nature?

Ptyalin demands a neutral or slightly alkaline medium for proper functioning and this is the normal condition of the saliva in the mouth. However, when acid foods are eaten, the action of ptyalin is halted. It is, therefore, most advisable to avoid including acid fruits in the same meal as sweet fruits or starches. So tomatoes should not be eaten with starches, especially potatoes or bread (no more tomato sandwiches!).

Refined sugar products are also acidic, both in the mouth and in the bloodstream. The acidifying of the saliva by sucrose is widely recognised as one of the principal factors in the formation of tooth decay, but few people realise how damaging this can also be to the digestion by its destruction of ptyalin. With the annual average consumption of refined sugar running at over 50 kg per person in Australia (equivalent to a cupful per person per day), it is no wonder that we find sugar in virtually all packaged foods. This induces quite a pernicious problem to the health — especially to the digestion, when sugar is consumed in the same meal as protein or starch foods. Packaged breakfast cereals are some of the worst offenders of this repelling digestive combination, imposing an overwhelming burden upon the digestive system when the metabolic rate (indicating the ease by which the body can digest foods) is at its lowest for the day. Many graduate nutritionists no doubt were told during their training, as I was, that the contents of most packages of breakfast cereals contain less nourishment than is found in the cardboard comprising the package!

Secondary Combining Rules

Once the primary rules have become a matter of general habit by their daily application to one's choice of meal components, it will be time to take notice of a further set of combining rules. These should be used in conjunction with those already established, for they complement the primary rules to provide a full set of guidelines for greatly improved digestion.

Rule 5: Melons Should Be Eaten Alone

Because of the unique properties of melons, as already mentioned, their digestion is best facilitated when no other food is eaten at the same meal. Melons can provide a very satisfying meal on their own for either breakfast or lunch — it is wise not to have them for the evening meal because their very high water content could result in undue disturbance to your night's rest!

Experience has proved that in cases where eating melons has caused indigestion, they have always been consumed as part of a complex or multi-course meal. Melons are the easiest of foods to digest, proved by the short time they require to pass from the stomach. However, when eaten with other foods, melons are retained in the stomach until protein in the other meal components has been suitably broken down. By that time, fermentation of the melon's sugars has commenced, creating its characteristic gas problem.

Many people have found that melons can combine with sweet fruits or sub-acid fruits in a fruit salad without creating any problems in their digestion. There is no scientific objection to this, provided that quantities of all ingredients are reasonably moderate. However, with such a mixture it is wise to avoid dried fruits, since they have a high fibre and protein content compared with other fruits.

Rule 6: Many Fruits and Vegetables Do Not Mix Well in the Same Meal

Compared with vegetables, fruits possess a higher natural sugar content (fruit sugar — fructose) and a lower starch content; their protein content is also lower than that of vegetables. Fruits, therefore, require less chewing and ensalivation, less catabolism in the stomach and, in general, prefer a speedier digestive process than vegetables. If slowed down too much in the stomach by the presence of fibrous vegetables and/or complex protein foods, the fermentation of fructose could commence, especially with sweet fruits. This can create stomach distension and severe discomfort.

Certain acid fruits provide exceptions to this rule. Citrus fruits in small quantities can be eaten with a fresh vegetable salad or with primary proteins. In fact, many people have found that citrus fruits and nuts make an excellent combination, offering the easiest means for the digestion of nuts as a primary protein source. But in general, nuts will be found to combine best with fresh vegetable salad.

Food Combining Chart

Food Groups	Primary Proteins	Secondary Proteins	Fats	Starches	Melons	Vegetables	Sweet Fruits	Sub-acid Fruits	Acid Fruits
Primary Proteins	Good	Poor	Poor	Poor	Poor	Good	Poor	Fair	Good
Secondary Proteins	Poor	Fair	Poor	Poor	Poor	Good	Poor	Poor	Fair
Fats	Poor	Poor	Good	Fair	Poor	Good	Fair	Fair	Fair
Starches	Poor	Poor	Fair	Good	Poor	Good	Fair	Fair	Poor
Melons	Poor	Poor	Poor	Poor	Good	Poor	Fair	Fair	Poor
Vegetables	Good	Good	Good	Good	Poor	Good	Poor	Poor	Poor
Sweet Fruits	Poor	Poor	Fair	Fair	Fair	Poor	Good	Good	Poor
Sub-acid Fruits	Fair	Poor	Fair	Fair	Fair	Poor	Good	Good	Good
Acid Fruits	Good	Fair	Fair	Poor	Poor	Poor	Poor	Good	Good

PROTEINS
Primary
Almonds
Brazil Nuts
Cashew Nuts
Hazel Nuts
Pine Nuts
Pistachios
Walnuts
Pepitas
Sunflower Seeds
Wheat germ
Sesame Seeds
Lecithin
Soya beans
Secondary
Peanuts
Cheese
Eggs
Yogurt
Poultry*
Meat*
Fish*
*Not recommended for good nutrition

STARCHES
Rice
Wheat
Corn
Rye
Millet
Buckwheat
Lima Beans
Red Beans
Pinto Beans
Navy Beans
Mung Beans
Broad Beans
Garbanzos
Lentils
Chestnuts
Breadfruit
Jackfruit
Potato
Sweet Potato
Jerusalem Artichokes
Pumpkin
Taro
Yams

FATS
Avocados
Oils
Macadamia Nuts
Pecan Nuts
Coconut
Olives
Butter, Margarine

MELONS
Cantaloupes
Watermelon
Honeydew

VEGETABLES
Globe Artichokes
Beetroot
Carrots
Capsicums
Cucumbers
Swedes
Parsley
Brussels Sprouts
Cauliflower
Cabbage
Celery
Lettuce
Turnips
Fresh Beans
Fresh Sprouts
Fresh Peas
Zucchini
Chokoes
Squash
Broccoli
Asparagus
Eggplant
Silverbeet
New Zealand Spinach
Tomatoes
 (not with starches)
Onions
 (best cooked)

SWEET FRUITS
Bananas
Figs
Custard Apples
Monstera Deliciosa
Persimmons
All dried fruits

SUB-ACID FRUITS
Mulberries
Raspberries
Blackberries
Blueberries
Grapes
Pears
Apples
Cherries
Apricots
Peaches
Plums
Nectarines
Paw paws
Mangoes
Guavas

ACID FRUITS
Grapefruit
Lemons
Oranges
Limes
Mandarins
Pineapples
Strawberries
Passionfruit

Because of their high mineral and vitamin contents, fresh vegetables combine well with all proteins, fats and starch foods. In particular, no protein-concentrate meal should ever be eaten without the accompaniment of a fresh salad for maximum digestive benefits and total enjoyment, both in the eating and absence of unpleasant after-affects.

Of all vegetables, those that should be carefully avoided or, if demanded, eaten sparingly, include: onions, radish, garlic, horseradish, chili peppers, scallions (shallots), etc. All of them possess digestive irritants. Although not strictly members of the same botanical family, each of these vegetables contains mild poisons, such as mustard oil, which are dangerous to the sensitive mucus lining of the intestines.

Rule 7: Milk Does Not Mix with Any Other Food

We have established that milk is only suitable for the natural feeding of infants. Even then, it should only be mother's milk (refer Stage 6, page 78). Milk is a singular type of food which is best digested on its own, for it is known to impede the gastric catabolism of any other foods which might be simultaneously in the stomach.

Fortunately, milk requires only a moderate concentration of HCl to break down its protein. This can only be facilitated in the presence of the enzyme rennin, which, in humans, is found only in the stomachs of infants and young children. For its best digestion to be facilitated, milk should be able to pass through the stomach in well under an hour, otherwise gastric fermentation of its lactose milk sugar and resultant indigestion can occur. Mother's milk and, to a lesser extent, goat's milk on their own qualify in this respect. But cow's milk, even on its own, is more complex and concentrated in its protein structure, requiring from one to two hours to pass through the stomach. But if any other food proteins are simultaneously in the stomach, gastric digestion time will be extended by far too long, creating indigestion.

It is important to realise that quite a serious indigestion problem can arise when milk is consumed with a meal containing protein-rich foods. Whether the milk is drunk just before, during or just after the meal, its fat content will act as a coating to the gastric mucosa. This will impede the secretion of gastric juice, especially HCl, into the stomach, thereby delaying protein catabolism. The degree of impediment will, of course, depend on the quantity of milk consumed and the concentration of fat in the milk.

This rule is of utmost importance in the correct feeding of infants when supplementary food is given, just as it is important to young children when milk becomes the supplementary food after weaning. Parents should exclude any other food, especially one that is protein-rich, when milk is in the stomach. This will mean a half-hour's wait when mother's milk or goat's milk is given; at least an hour when cow's milk is given.

From this it is easy to recognise the low desirability of cow's milk for infants and, in fact, for all humans. As stated previously, older children and adults should avoid milk at all times in any quantity. If nature intended them to drink milk, they would not have needed teeth!

Acid and Alkaline Foods

Many people become confused with the classifying of foods in the two chemical categories, acid and alkaline. These are not classifications we have thus far considered in our food combining rules. Indeed, they do not enter our consideration of food combinations, for these, as previously explained, pertain to gastric digestion.

The digestive activities within the mouth and the stomach command the initial major scenes in the food digestion drama. Thus, these must be considered in terms of the acid concentration and requirements of the gastric juice and the alkaline requirements of the saliva to avoid the drama becoming a tragedy. And that is the constant mealtime play known as Food Combining.

In the small intestine, another theatrical performance takes place. The atmosphere is an alkaline medium where all classifications of foods come together with no notable star performer, as protein is in the stomach. As the final scenes of digestion take place, nutrients are absorbed into the body's systems by gliding off stage into the wings as they disappear from the gastrointestinal tract. It is then up to the liver and kidneys to handle food nutrients and residues in accordance with their acid or alkaline natures. This is where the importance of considering the acidity or alkalinity of a food comes into play.

"Acid" or "alkaline" foods are classed as those which have an acidic or alkaline reaction in the body after digestion. It refers to the chemical nature of their ash residues, determined by whichever minerals assert their presence in the blood after catabolism; and the presence or absence of acid residues in the blood is the further factor in the determination. The taste of the food itself does not determine its acidity or alkalinity from a nutritional standpoint, contrary to opinions expressed by many untrained "nutritionists".

Alkali-producing foods are, in general, all fresh fruits and vegetables, as well as sprouted foods. Exceptions are blueberries and globe artichokes. Many fruits taste acid, but this is physiological, not chemical. This acidity is due to the presence of a variety of organic acids in the fruits — citric acid, malic acid and tartaric acid in different fruits. All of these are oxidised in catabolism, converting the fruit to alkaline in the process. The only acid not thus handled is oxalic acid, for the body finds this very difficult to absorb and seeks to neutralise it in the kidneys with the vital alkalising minerals calcium and magnesium. It is these two minerals, plus sodium, potassium and iron which are the major factors in determining whether a food is alkaline.

Acid-producing foods are generally concentrated sources of protein and starch. They are foods whose residues contain more of the acid-producing minerals sulphur, phosphorus and chlorine than the alkalising minerals listed in the previous paragraph. Other chemical producers of acidity are the organic acids such as oxalic and tannic. Beverages such as tea, coffee and cocoa are extremely acid-forming, due to their high concentration of oxalic acid and, in tea, tannic acid. Other highly acid-forming foods are animal meats, refined sugar products and grains.

This indicates the need for the human diet to adhere to the 75 per cent-25 per cent rule (fresh foods to concentrates) to maintain the correct balance between alkaline and acid foods. More about this in Stage 10. Meanwhile, here is a list of acid-forming foods as a guide for health-conscious people to minimise their intake, in the interests of improved health:

Grains — rye, wheat and rice are the most acidic;

Animal foods — meat, poultry and fish, with eggs only slightly;

Beans and lentils — unless they are sprouted;

Nuts — especially peanuts and walnuts; to a lesser extent, Brazil nuts and hazelnuts (note that almonds are very alkalising);

As mentioned previously, olives and blueberries are slightly acidic, but sugar and the products in which it is included (which are most baked and processed foods) all come under the category of being particularly acidic. This is another reason for avoiding them in your regular diet — a small quantity very occasionally should not cause any problem to a healthy person, but it certainly could to anyone suffering from allergy conditions.

Temptations of Intemperance

Probably deriving from some primitive instinct of eating as much as could be stuffed into the stomach whenever possible, modern humans appear to have forgotten that they now have storage facilities outside the stomach which are eminently capable of catering for tomorrow's needs. No longer must we inflict our bodies with unneeded fatty tissue to avert hunger during lean times. There are no more lean times in the Western world.

Intellectually, we have no problem in recognising that the refrigerator and the corner store have replaced the need for excess adipose tissue. But old habits, stimulated by appetite seducers, die hard. Chemicals, sugar and spices, compounded by gimmicky advertising, have ensnared humans to eat, eat, eat. Motives of profit from increased manufacture and sales far outweigh nutritional values of promoted products. In fact, if advertisers were compelled to state the nutritional factors and harmful properties in their products, intelligent people would avoid them (as they do cigarettes and tobacco since compelled to carry the health hazard warning on their packages).

Westerners need no longer maintain gastronomic indulgence, for many could live very comfortably on half their present food intake. The other half usually feeds their doctor! All they need to do is to ensure that their intake is more nutritious and less processed.

Residents of many "underdeveloped" countries are in a somewhat different situation, for their country is usually over-populated and under-productive in terms of suitable food crops. This is often the result of thoughtless habit and gross mismanagement. If only the huge areas of cultivated tea in India, poppies in Indochina, coffee in South and Central America, wine in Iberia were to be partly converted to food cropping suited to their climates, we would not be hearing about "world food shortages".

Another prime cause for overindulgence in the Western world is the stress and tension, worry and anxiety we create in our own lives. No one inflicts these upon us; we do it all ourselves by failing to exercise adequate command of our emotions. We find repeatedly that people turn to overeating when they allow themselves to become emotionally disturbed. And the junk they invariably eat actually exacerbates the problem by nutritionally and emotionally unbalancing them further. Much of the sadness and crime in the world today can be traced to improper nutrition and inadequate emotional control.

Whatever the reason for overindulgence, we must recognise the fact that if we want to eat more, we must eat less — that way we will live longer and ultimately be able to eat more! This is especially evident when we consider the most suitable combining of foods for best digestion, for without indigestion, we can certainly enjoy our food more. Whenever a large variety of foods comprise a meal, we risk conflict within our gastrointestinal tract and, by such discomfort, conflict between ourselves and other people. Is it worth the few minutes of taste pleasure when the consequences are so distasteful? Just as much taste pleasure can be derived from more suitable food combinations, given the time to consider them. And if there is no time to think about what one is intending to eat (as I have so often heard people say), perhaps there is insufficient time to have the meal. To digest food properly, one must be relaxed and not rushing from crisis to crisis.

"Variety is the spice of gluttony", says Dr Herbert M. Shelton* in his book, *Superior Nutrition*. Indeed, variety so often induces people to overeat by exciting their taste buds into a frenzy of demands. But the few seconds on the tongue are not worth the extra kilograms on the waist or possible hours of internal discomfort.

Perhaps the argument is that, with modern chemical agricultural techniques, quality is sacrificed for quantity so that food no longer offers the extensive nutrient value once expected of it. To some extent, this is correct. So perhaps we do need more than one food per meal to obtain our balance of nutrients. We also know that concentrated protein foods are easier to digest when suitably combined with a vegetable salad or, in the case of nuts, with citrus fruit. Thus, the ideal appears to lie between the two extremes. Monotrophism, however, is less dangerous than gluttony, by far. It is better to be a little underweight than grossly overfed.

The happy medium is the intelligent choice of meals to comprise suitably combined ingredients in moderate proportions. The best guide to quantity is to finish eating when you still feel you could eat a little more, remembering it is better to throw food away before eating it than to waste it through incomplete digestion with the accompanying burden of excessive food in your gastrointestinal tract. However, fresh food can often be kept in the refrigerator until the next day — only cooked food should be discarded. (Even so, when thrown out, it is not really wasted so long as you have wisely built a compost heap!)

Cooking food produces the most serious temptation to overeating. The smell of food being "spoiled" in a frypan seems to stimulate the appetite, yet food which is cooked or processed in any way must sacrifice much of its optimum nutrient content (the degree of loss depending on the method and duration of cooking or processing). It also softens the food fibres so that less chewing is required; thus less ensalivation takes place. Both factors lead to overeating.

It is time to realise that a full stomach is no guarantee of nutritional satisfaction. To compile a meal with the intent that "it must be nutritious because it stays with you so long" is to be ignorant of the role of the stomach in nutrition. That desire for fullness is really no more than a nonrational craving based on a primitive fear of hunger, perhaps encouraged by overindulgent parents. It has no substance in reality, but rather indicates that one's digestion is at fault if such fullness persists for an overlong period.

One of the important aspects of food combining is the recognition that its rules are designed for the average digestion. Many people are already suffering from digestive impediments, suggesting the employment of some slight modifications to the basic combining rules to allow for their particular problems. This is impossible to develop through the pages of a book, for so many variables are involved. Thus, it is suggested that in such a condition, one should seek a consultation with a health practitioner whose training has embraced the full scope of nutritional science, especially in the fields of natural hygiene and wholistic health.

In any case, one's own powers of observation will always be a reasonable guide to the modifications which might be necessary for the preparation of a suitable diet. Based upon the foregoing basic rules, such observations should take into account the facts of nutrition, guided by indications from within. Care should be taken to disregard any emotional desires, such as might be based on habit, fear or conformity.

---

* Dr Herbert M. Shelton, following the lead of Dr William Howard Hay, has undertaken more research and provided more testimony supporting the value of proper food combining than any other nutritionalist we could name, past or present.

To be of some guidance in this regard, the foregoing food combining chart shows many combinations as "fair". These can be good combinations for some people, or poor for others. Personal experience will be the real guide.

It is important to remember that one's needs must always take precedence over one's desires. Needs are permanent, so far as the present is concerned; desires are the demands of transient emotions which, to the person in command of his feelings, can be easily phased into harmony with his needs. Thus guided, the changes which will be introduced into one's dietary habits will be gratefully accepted by the gastrointestinal tract and, ultimately, every organ of the body, even if they do create some minor emotional objections. But these are only products of old habit, touched with a bit of laziness!

STAGE TEN

Man's Ideal Diet

Always rise from the table with an appetite and you will never sit down without one.

William Penn (1644-1718)

Man has two vastly different diets. The first is his mental diet — sense experiences and thoughts which are fed to his consciousness. The second is his material diet — products from the surface of his planet which are fed to his mouth. Yet it is the first which always determines the second.

In his early years of earthly experience, infant man is conditioned first by parents, then by school and beyond-family associations. These experiences comprise the foundations for his mental diet. They form impressions which condition the emerging consciousness, building the framework for those habits by which he will be identified as he reaches physical maturity. But because these habits all too often become welded into an inviolable web of conformity, mental maturity rarely accompanies physical maturity.

From his open-minded wonder at the world, which characterises infant experience, the human child grows into the pattern set by his elder influences in much the same manner as in most families of two- and four-legged animals. But human mentality has far greater potential. It is not intended to blindly conform — creating a basis for frustration when it does.

The child is taught to become the reflection of the parents, conditioning which is nowhere more poignantly expressed than in his eating habits. Parents who rarely possess suitable qualifications for dietary training inflict their habits upon innocent offspring — habits which coalesce into such a solid foundation that with them the child becomes firmly identified. Thus, rarely are such habits brought into question unless exceptional circumstances prevail.

The Dietary Revolution

Exceptional circumstances certainly do prevail today. As the new age of enlightenment draws nearer, we are witnessing many severances of old habits, the most important of which is the revolt against the revolting diet!

That man is learning to think independently, to emancipate himself from infant influences and evaluate his life in terms of its total purpose is a major step forward. As he opens his mind to a redeveloping consciousness, man is reforming his mental diet by questioning, investigating and, where necessary, changing. And he is discovering that one of the most vital areas for change lies in the realm of his material diet. Man is at last recognising that the only way by which he can achieve his purpose on earth is to assume total command of his physical charge — his body. He is learning that unless the body is able to give perfect expression to the psyche, his growth will be hampered by limitations which will frustrate his fulfilment of purpose.

The most uncomfortable and restrictive of all such limitations is illness. Any condition of ill health in the body is more than a discomfort, it is a testimony of unsuitable diet — both mental and physical. And it is only by correction of such unsuitability that total comfort may be restored and restrictiveness dispelled.

It should, therefore, create no great surprise that the young men and women of today are rebelling against unsuitable conditions of blind conformity. They recognise the need to depart from habits which have been deteriorating at a more rapid pace with man's increasing research into specialised, often quite unrelated, facets of life. The growing awareness is inspiring a return to the natural, simple system of living and the dietary revolution is its obvious expression.

Abandoning Pernicious Habits

The tendency to veer away from natural living has led man into one poisonous habit after another. Each was, at first, seemingly unrelated and apparently quite safe. But this was more the impression created by the promoters of the products, rather than the actual effects of each upon the human organism or the interactions which resulted when two or more poisonous habits were adopted simultaneously. This is more the rule than the exception.

1. *Chemicals*

As people are tempted away from natural foods to "convenience foods", their intake of man-made chemcials is greatly increased. More than 3000 different chemicals are now employed in what is termed "food manufacturing". None of these chemicals is tested in relationship with the others as to their combined effects in the human gastrointestinal tract; nor is it known what kind of cellular or psychic effects may result from various combinations of the artificial chemicals.

Chemicals are employed to create artificial flavours, perfumes, colourings, textures and appetite stimulation to induce greater consumption of products. They suggest that the foods with which they are associated are fresh, wholesome and nourishing. They represent, and this is the primary reason for their growing use, a huge industrial investment with an exceptionally high profit.

But the concern of thinking people evidences a trend back to natural foods. And as this is seen to develop, the consequential improvement in health is probably the greatest testimony in support of man's ideal diet, and the greatest condemnation of the artificial.

The only chemicals man needs are those in the natural, ionised state, forming an inherent part of the products of our earth. Every nutrient, flavour, texture and colour which will satisfy man's health and aesthetic needs is to be found in his ideal diet of natural foods.

2. *Appetite Stimulants*

Probably the most subtle and pernicious role of chemicals in the diet is their employment to stimulate overeating. To overeat on even a diet of fresh, natural foods is to create discomfort and waste. But when processed foods are involved, the intake of many different chemicals will introduce definite inhibitions in all the body's systems, with an overflow into the psychic.

Spices, strong herbs, common salt and condiments are commonly employed as artificial appetite stimulants, which induce a greater consumption of processed products. Their effects upon the body's delicate chemical balance, the sensitive lining of the gastrointestinal tract and the body's growth pattern are disastrous. The low nutritive value, high calorie content and general addictive nature of processed foods are creating many a sick, overweight body and a sluggish, uncreative brain.

Human taste buds are intended to indicate the suitability, or otherwise, of the food with which they are in contact. They are highly sensitive cells which rapidly lose their acute abilities when subjected to violent shocks, such as those caused by the use of the appetite stimulants mentioned above. We thus soon lose the pleasures of delicate taste treats as our tongue loses its ability to discriminate between the real and the artificial, between the suitable and the poisonous.

The general penalty for overeating is overweight, but when overeating involves an addiction to chemicals, it also creates a foundation for chronic illness. This situation is compounded if the diet contains chemicals or influences with inherent psychic dangers, such as accompany the consumption of animal meats and organs (see below).

Obviously it is better in every way to eat only as much as we need, for only in that manner can our total health be ensured. And if there is no natural appetite at mealtime, then miss the meal, for the body is obviously not then in need of food. Do not eat by the clock, for your needs vary each day.

3. Meat Eating

Over 2500 years ago, Pythagoras warned judges that they should avoid the consumption of animal meats for at least twelve hours prior to adjudicating at a trial. Meat eating clouded the reasoning powers, he asserted. And those of us who have been meat eaters in the past and have since converted to a non-meat diet can personally witness that such advice is assuredly no less valid.

Animals are under severe emotional stress prior to and at time of death. Their flesh is fed by a bloodstream which is loaded with stress hormones, lactic acid and other toxic waste products, most of which constitute the "delicious flavours" associated with cooked animal flesh. All those free chemicals are ingested without realisation that they are materially contributing towards modern man's mental unbalance.

Is it not apparent that the pressure of modern living becomes too much for man when his natural psychic balance is disturbed by foreign chemicals? Especially so, when these are chemicals from disturbed animals in fear of their lives.

Research carried out at certain independent (this word has a vital import)* academic centres, such as Loma Linda University in Riverside, California, and Walla Walla College in Washington State, has shown that meat eating, especially in the quantities consumed by today's eaters, is a contributor to mental unbalance.

Dr Joseph Barnes, as Professor of Biology at Walla Walla College in the 1960s, devised a long series of experiments with monkeys, then with willing students, proving some of the mental and emotional dangers associated with meat consumption. These experiments showed that so much of the insensitivity, instability, nerviness and aggressiveness of meat-eating humans was a schizophrenic reaction in both human and monkey that directly related to their consumption of animal flesh.

These psychotic illnesses are becoming more and more apparent in this century, almost in direct proportion to increasing meat consumption. This hitherto unsuspected relationship was found to be substantially attributable to the transmitting of stress hormone, adrenalin, from the blood of the fear-ridden, slaughter-sensing animal into that of the consuming human.

---

* Many other academic and research institutions are endowed with funds from industrial enterprises with vested interests in perpetuating many of man's modern habits.

In recent years, many people have come to realise the cholesterol and saturated fatty acid problems associated with their consumption of pigs, cattle, sheep and other animals. Turning to seafood for their major protein intake has slightly overcome these health inhibitors; a far greater improvement being accorded those who have turned to plant protein sources — nuts, seeds, legumes and sprouts.

Unfortunately, many people turn from meat to chicken under the erroneous impression that "white meat" provides a better protein source. Little do they realise the vast difference in quality between today's battery-bred, commercial birds and those of yesteryear which were healthy, contented farm-yard fossickers. With so much demand, stimulated by skilful advertising, poultry producers have become large corporate managers controlling enormous flocks of "clockwork chicks". A chicken's birth is today usually artificially stimulated, it lives its short life in pigeon-holed space confinement so that it even finds difficulty in spreading its wings. It is fed processed and chemicalised mush designed to fatten it rapidly; it is injected with other chemicals to suppress its many illnesses and is finally slaughtered, frozen and sold before it has time to die from one of the many illnesses of devitalisation which would otherwise finally overtake the poor bird.

A similar problem besets four-legged meat. The quality of modern beasts has declined considerably in the clutches of a greedy pastoral industry which now resorts to the use of artificial feeding to "prepare" animals for sale by fattening them in the most economical manner to bring the highest prices, regardless of the quality of the meat about to be inflicted upon an unsuspecting and trusting public. Minced newsprint, textile wastes, sawdust and even polyethylene plastic pellets are among the tasteless morsels mixed into the animal's usual feed. Little wonder animal fat is today so poorly constituted and animal protein so deficient when compared with its quality of half a century ago.

Such departures from man's natural diet can only shorten his life by inflicting upon him symptoms of ill health in a chain reaction of intensifying morbidity.

4. *"Pure, White and Deadly"* — *Refined Sugar*

This appropriate description of refined sugar was used by Professor John Yudkin of London University in his exposé* of one of modern man's debilitating habits. With the per capita consumption of processed cane sugar currently running at around 50 kg per annum in Australia (and most Western countries), it is saddening that so many millions of hectares of fertile land are deprived from food crops to produce this "foodless" enemy of tooth enamel. And a further sad fact is that once land has been continually monocropped with sugar, it is extremely difficult to restore it to optimum fertility for cultivating food crops. But all this is not surprising when we realise how many millions of dollars in export income are derived from sugar, how many large corporations depend on it for profit and how much government prestige and voting power is related to sugar production.

It is as though human health were relegated to an inferior position of concern when government involvement is considered. Some years ago, a leading Labor politician in Canberra (and a doctor of medicine in private life), stated in Parliament that sugar "is a third-rate poison". Whereupon those members of Parliament whose electorates and/or financial interests would be threatened by such a revelation, indignantly denied such a charge as grossly misleading. The matter was never again raised!

---

* *Pure, White and Deadly*, by John Yudkin, published by Davis-Poynter, London, 1972.

Honest researchers and many consumers realise that refined sugar contains no nourishment, only empty calories. This also applies to raw and coloured sugars — although they offer a few milligrams of alkalising minerals from their molasses contents, these are insufficient to counteract the 94 per cent or more of sucrose which is their major constituent. But resulting from the empty calories is the serious problem of mineral-leaching created by sugar consumption.

The digestion of refined sugar is only possible with the aid of alkalising minerals. As sugar does not possess such properties, they must be withdrawn from the body's storehouse. Thus, stored calcium and magnesium are utilised, thereby depriving the body, particularly the bones, of these vital growth and repair minerals. This is one of the factors contributing to osteoporosis (chronic porousness of the bones, causing easy fractures, especially in older people).

In the mouth, sugar has the pernicious habit of sticking to the teeth where its extreme acidity attacks the enamel, initiating dental caries (decay). In the gastrointestinal tract, sugar rapidly ferments in the stomach when protein foods are simultaneously present and delays the desired rapid departure of sugar. This gives rise to the formation of stomach gas and belching, for sugar does not undergo any catabolism in the stomach — that takes place in the duodenum once the pylorus opens and sugar is released from the stomach.

Sugar is not only one of those foodless waste crops (in the same category as tea, coffee, cocoa and hops), but its use in the modern diet to sweeten substances which might be otherwise rejected by the palate makes it an accessary to fraud. By masking the real taste of otherwise unpalatable "foods", sugar provides a means of disguise by which such substances as unripe fruits, packaged breakfast cereals, chocolate, candies, cookies, cordials and carbonated drinks are consumed in the belief that "if they taste okay, they must be okay". In this way many unhealthy addictions are formed.

There is little doubt that, if packaged breakfast cereals were not well sugared, their normally bland taste would see them rejected for the foodlessness they offer. Likewise would chocolate be rejected without the heavy sweetening (sometimes over 50 per cent) of sugar. It would be so bitter that it, too, would be left on the shelf, thereby saving many kidneys from the oxalic bombardment caused by cocoa.

To replace sugar with sorbitol, saccharine or any other chemical sweetener is almost as dangerous, nutritionally, but potentially far more dangerous chemically (far too little research has been undertaken to ascertain how much interacting takes place between chemicals in the body). One of the worst features of sugar and the artificial sweeteners is their tendency to create inducements to snacking of unhealthy and foodless "foods" between meals. Many a parent has complained that their child has come to the dinner table without an appetite for a nourishing meal, due solely to its addiction to snacking on junk "foods". This is not only constipating, emotionally destabilising and generally unhealthy, but it is potentially weight-producing, laying a foundation for obesity and many future illnesses.

It is important to note the difference between refined cane sugar or beet sugar (sucrose) and natural fruit sugar (fructose) as found in natural foods. Each has a different chemical formula and vastly different origin. Sucrose ($C_{12}H_{22}O_{11}$) is taken out of its natural context and combined with many other chemicals in its processing into an almost 100 per cent pure, nutrient-devoid food additive. It is certainly not a food in any manner of consideration. Fructose ($C_6H_{12}O_6$) is, by contrast, a naturally occurring substance found in fresh fruits, vegetables, etc., physically and chemically associated with other nutrients and nutritional factors and providing the consumer with a rapid source of nourishing energy. Fructose is a simple sugar, classed as a monosaccharide —

sucrose is a more complex sugar, classed as a disaccharide of fructose plus glucose which have to be split by hydrolysis in the process of heat or digestion (in which considerable insulin, plus calcium and magnesium are robbed from the body). Fructose does not require insulin and, in its natural state, brings its associated minerals and vitamins into the digestion process.

Honey and maple syrup are two other sources of concentrated sugars. They are progressively better than sugar and their virtues and vices will be discussed in Stage 11.

The very best sweetener is to be found in the form of dried fruits. These will also be discussed in Stage 11, for they are valuable sources of many nutrients, not only fructose.

5. Snacking — One Meal A Day

With so much advertising directed at inducing human indulgence in an all-day-long eating escapade, it is difficult for people to understand that they can really overeat. Many people believe that so long as they eat "good food", such as potato chips, chocolate bars, thick shakes, etc., they are looking after their bodies. To them, obesity or illnesses of overeating are unrelated to their commercially promoted appetites.

But these people are not entirely to blame for their addiction to eating. This pattern was probably set before they could know anything about it, set by their unknowing parents who, in an effort to avoid malnutrition, created an over-correction. The delight they derive from cuddling a chubby little baby is not in the long-term interests of the emerging child.

Once the stomach has learned to accommodate excessive amounts of food, the body will develop excessive fat cells to store the unused intake of nutrients. This will set a pattern for the body from which future deviation presents a very difficult task for most. It will demand considerable strength of will in later life when the person is sometimes shunned for his fatness, rather than cuddled; when he realises how ugly such excesses actually appear, how much more difficult it is for him to move with ease and agility, and without perspiring all over those in his immediate vicinity.

Indeed, overindulgence by parents is a serious disservice, rarely recognised until its effect is too entrenched to easily alter. Most people eat only one meal a day — it commences within minutes of their waking in the morning and concludes with their going to bed at night. Their eating habits are so consistent that they rarely like to let an hour pass without putting something into their mouths. This incessant snacking does not allow time for the previous intake to be properly catabolised in the stomach before it is forced through the pylorus to enter the duodenum, inadequately prepared for proper digestion. The overworking this demands of all the body's digestive, eliminating and storage facilities is reflected in so many instances of early degenerative disease.

Compounding the felony, snacking is almost invariably not upon whole, natural foods, but on processed confections and the like, contributing little more than abundant carbohydrates and calories to the body. Far in excess of their needs, these factors induce the production of fat cells which first flatter, then, as they accumulate, coarsen the body's appearance.

6. Drugs

The ingestion of drugs, irrespective of what form or for what reason, predisposes towards an almost limitless variety of physical and psychic illnesses. With so many writers offering so much information on the dangers of drug ingestion, it is amazing to realise that the consumption of drugs continues to accelerate. Is it that the drugs impair one's reading ability, or one's mental faculties?

Apart from widely recognised dangers associated with the voluntary drugs, how many people recognise their commitment to the involuntary ones? Well known to the former category are the medical and hallucinatory drugs of addiction (including tranquillisers, stimulants, etc.), plus alcohol, tobacco and the like. But in the latter category are those dangerous drugs which, by their general nonrecognition, can inflict serious damage upon the organism without any suspicion to provide protection. Classic examples are (1) systemic agricultural poisons, (2) oxalic acid "cocktails" and (3) carbonated beverages.

1) In Stage 14, we take an in-depth look at the natural alternative to modern agricultural techniques. Now, let us briefly look at those highly toxic organic phosphate chemical sprays (e.g., malathion and parathion) used on many fruit trees to kill alighting insects. Known as systemic poisons, they not only effectively poison insects, but also act on the sensitive nervous system of man, should he unwittingly consume the products of such trees. We know that their effects are not so noticeable on man from single contact; but being cumulative, these poisons can muster a dangerous long-term toxicity. The effects of other agricultural chemicals on the environment are becoming well known, but action to avoid the use of any of them requires considerable persuasion at the teaching level, so committed are educationalists to the chemical theory of food production. Aerial spraying spreads the poisons over vast areas, well beyond those originally intended. Aided by prevailing winds, these poisonous chemicals are carried onto pastures grazed by meat-producing herds, some members of which are often close to death by slaughter time.

2) Is it any great surprise that kidney failure is on the increase throughout the world? Wherever tea, coffee, cocoa and meat are consumed in quantity, the accumulation of oxalic acid, inherent in each of these, will actively degenerate the kidneys, developing into "gravel" crystals and kidney stones. It will also seriously deplete the body's reserves of calcium and magnesium in heroic efforts at neutralising this dangerous acid. Thus, it is not uncommon to find that people who evidence kidney disorders also suffer from osteomalacia (softening of the bones), although this might not become apparent until they suffer a fracture and discover its knitting to be an unduly lengthy process. The caffeine, theobromine and tannic acid present in the beverages mentioned should be sufficient to warn people of their dangers; but the compounding danger of oxalic acid induces so serious a condition as to warrant the withdrawal of these substances from the market for human consumption.

Herb teas and coffee substitutes, such as dandelion or barley-based beverages which are sold in health food stores, are generally quite harmless to the body and can often provide healing benefits. Most gastric upsets will respond to a drink of warm water, but if a mild alfalfa or comfrey tea is taken instead, the added alkalising influence will help neutralise the condition of hyperacidity caused by fermentation in the stomach. More details of herb tea benefits are in Stage 13.

3) An episode in my youth created a lasting impression on my mind — perhaps because of its unexpected outcome. A group of lads decided to have a "water fight" after a hot morning of tennis. Instead of water, carbonated cola beverages were fizzed and sprayed over each other, some of us taking cover behind a new car belonging to one of the group. The battle lasted about a quarter of an hour before all contestants adjourned for lunch, intending to return later to wash the car.

The need to wash the car did not eventuate. By the time we returned, it had lost most of its paintwork. Such is the abrasive action of cola-type drinks — imagine what they can do to one's stomach!

On a hot day, the most refreshing drink is cool, pure water; the most nourishing is cool, fresh fruit juice. These are non-addictive, non-sweetened by any additive and totally natural. They are truly thirst quenchers and so simple for the gastrointestinal tract to handle. So-called "soft drinks" have quite the opposite effect on the gastrointestinal tract. They are acid-forming in the lower digestive system; the same acid effect is extremely drying in the mouth and upper digestive tract. This creates the addictive need for the person to take another drink a little later, under the misconception that the earlier drink "quenched" their thirst. Sugar or artificial sweetening contained in all these drinks also causes a residual thirst by lingering in the saliva.

In this manner, the majority of people remain uninformed and addicted to carbonated beverages. They are intentionally misled by the promoters whose greedy attempts to increase consumption of these unhealthy "refreshers" drugs the body with unwanted acids, undesirable stimulants and unhealthy sweetening as it sticks to the teeth and precipitates decay.

Thus a gloomy picture is painted when man departs from a natural diet pattern and becomes addicted to processed, "foodless" foods and drinks. Those with an understanding of the relationship between food and health can always be of assistance to the non-thinkers whose addictions exceed their knowledge. Their deep fear that they will be robbed of "all their pleasures" by abandoning unhealthy habits can be negated by we who have learned that nature has tastier and healthier products to offer man than ever the devising mind of the chemist could conceive.

The Seven Basic Rules

We now realise that eating should be much more than a blind indulgence. Eating has to be enjoyable, but its primary purpose is to nourish. The ideal diet combines the requirements of both these in offering seven basic rules for best digestion:

1. *Ensure you are relaxed before and during the meal and, at least for a short period, following its completion.* This enables maximum enjoyment of flavours being eaten and of company with whom the meal is being shared. Suitable music or prior meditation are the best aids to good digestion.

2. *Every meal should consist of either fresh, ripe fruits or vegetables as its basis.* If they can be obtained organically grown, so much the better in terms of flavour, texture and nutrient value. Any protein concentrates (seeds, nuts, pulses, grains, etc.) should be eaten raw (or sprouted) and unsalted. Dried fruits should be sun-dried. All should be guaranteed chemical-free. This may demand some searching, but every Western country has such sources available — they are quite abundant in the United States, England, Canada, Australia, etc.

3. *Simplest meal composition is generally easiest on the digestive system.* The more varieties within the meal, the greater demand on the gastric juice. An ideal meal will be limited to no more than five varieties, although a breakfast of fresh fruit is even better when comprising only two or three varieties. Observe proper food-combining rules for easiest digestion and most efficient intake of nutrients. Always choose fresh, natural foods in preference to those canned or processed in any way. Always avoid soups and sweets — when they surround a meal, they significantly impair digestive efficiency and guarantee some measure of indigestion.

4. *Drinking does not mix with eating.* Fluids, taken in any significant quantity either just before, during or after the meal while it is still in the stomach, will impede gastric digestion. This applies to water, soft drinks, alcohol, tea, coffee or cocoa. Certain herb

teas can actually aid the digestion, as will be discussed in the next Stage. A small quantity of water or suitable fruit or vegetable juice during a meal is generally satisfactory, but each person needs to check his or her individual gastric reaction — if any gas or other form of indigestion should become apparent after such a combination, it is best avoided. The creation of a thirst during or after eating usually implies unsuitable seasonings or spices used in the meal. The most natural way to eradicate the thirst is to thoroughly chew an apple or a portion of cucumber after the meal, then brush the teeth. This will remove the thirst-inducing items from around the teeth, but if they persist in the tongue or throat, a cup of warm alfalfa-mint herb tea will do the trick. When fresh fruits or vegetables are the major components of the meal, rarely will an unnatural thirst develop.

5. *Choose the type of meal to suit your intended activities following its completion.* The digestion of food demands energy — the more complex and concentrated the meal, the greater the demand. It is unwise to consume a heavy meal if hard work is intended following its completion; under such circumstances, it is best to consume a meal of fruit, maybe with dried fruits, but no concentrated protein foods.

6. *Eat only one meal at a time.* Do not eat when food from the previous meal remains in the stomach. Eat only on an empty stomach to ensure proper digestion.

7. *When food is not desired, do not force it to be eaten.* It is better to miss a meal than to eat when no appetite exists. A short fast is the best remedy for a lost appetite and a very positive way to keep weight under control.

A Balanced Diet

The oft-expressed concept of the balanced diet is one of the least understood aspects of human nutrition. Certainly a dietary balance is essential for the provision of vital nutrients, but this does not imply that every nutrient must be ingested every day.

If the diet comprises 75 per cent fresh fruits and vegetables, with 25 per cent concentrates of protein, carbohydrate and fat sources, it will provide the necessary balance over a period when adequate varieties are consumed during that period (for example, a week). It is impossible to ingest all the known amino acids, vitamins, minerals, fatty acids and carbohydrates each and every day. But over a few consecutive days of wise eating, this balance will be obtained and maintained.

With a view to such practical guidance, let us look at each of the three daily meals, then develop a basic chart of menus for a week to include a balanced eating programme.

Breakfast

Whether it is eaten in the early or midmorning, or at midday, the first meal of the day is breakfast. So named because it is the meal which breaks the short fast following the departure of the previous night's meal from the stomach during sleep, breakfast has a special importance in man's eating programme.

When the stomach is emptied during sleep, the feeling of emptiness ("hunger") which would accompany such emptying during the day is avoided. During the night's unconsciousness, the stomach is allowed to relax and contract slightly — a highly desirable respite from its unending daytime activity. Awakening from sleep, the body's functions are slow to get going; especially so is the metabolic rate. Thus, it is quite natural that little appetite for food will develop for some hours after rising.

If the appetite has not developed before departing for work, then miss breakfast and take along some fruit to relish during the morning when the natural development of the appetite makes the meal enjoyable. To artificially stimulate the appetite or to habitually force down a breakfast because it is the "done thing" is to afflict the gastrointestinal tract with an undesirable load.

Some people awaken feeling eager to eat, but usually it is at least an hour after rising before a genuine appetite develops. Still other people do not feel an appetite until nearer the middle of the day and for them, two meals a day are usually quite adequate.

Some food writers are in the habit of expressing the opinion that breakfast is the main meal of the day and should be the largest meal. No evidence exists in nutritional science for such an assertion. Instead, it will be found that such people are merely expressing their own preferences, invariably the consequence of personal predilections from years of habit. It is no more sensible to get into your car in the morning and race away at top speed before the engine has time to warm up, than it is to inflict a heavy breakfast on the unprepared gastrointestinal tract.

The very best breakfast is fresh fruit. It has numerous advantages — it is easiest to digest, offers a valuable source of ready energy and is quickest to prepare. Fruits are the most convenient food God ever gave to man — they come in skins which retain nourishment, indicate the state of ripeness and can often themselves be eaten for added nutrients. Fruits are available throughout the year, with a vast variety of flavours and textures; and they can, if necessary, be kept for surprisingly long periods without deterioration, if stored properly. Added advantages are their juiciness, delicious flavours and readily metabolised nutrients.

For breakfast, fruits should be chosen which combine best for easiest digestion (as discussed in Stage 9). They should be served whole to avoid the oxidation which would otherwise somewhat diminish their optimum nutritional value and flavour. They should be organically grown, where possible, and should always be mature and as ripe as is practical.

For both nutritional and psychic reasons, it is most beneficial to choose those fruits (and vegetables) which are produced in the most peaceful surroundings. Admittedly it is not always possible to know this, but every endeavour should be made to ascertain the source of one's food. Some people maintain that food grown in their immediate neighbourhood has definite advantages, but this is only true if the environment is a peaceful one. That fruit might have to be transported hundreds of kilometres is, of itself, no derogatory factor. It is the nature of the environment, rather than its distance, which implies greater influence.

Depending upon appetite, age and body proportions, the quantity of fruit to be eaten for breakfast can vary from 450 to 900 grams. If the appetite is especially ravenous, the addition of sun-dried fruits to the breakfast is recommended, provided acid fruits are not eaten at that meal. If acid fruits are preferred, a few nuts or seeds can be added for extra nourishment. But these added concentrated foods should not be eaten unless one is engaged in much mental or physical work and has a hearty appetite.

Other people with a hearty appetite at breakfast prefer yogurt with their fruit. It is best to limit the quantity of yogurt to half a carton (around 125 g) and no more often than each second day. The best yogurt is that made from raw milk, goat's milk being far superior to cow's milk; ideal if you can make it yourself to avoid the uncertainty of undesirable settling agents or other additives, as are often found in commercial yogurts. Too much yogurt can interfere with one's natural colon bacteria activity, possibly resulting in unnatural bowel movements.

Lunch

For those people who eat only two meals a day, their lunch is their breakfast. However, to provide adequate nourishment, its size would need to be somewhat larger than a normal early breakfast, especially when working. Lunch can be a medium-sized meal, but not as large as the evening meal. If not working, lunch should be the main meal of the day and the evening meal somewhat smaller. It should be remembered that man's metabolic rate, indicating the efficiency of his digestion, is generally at its height around 1 pm (its lowest rate is around 2 am, indicating the error of late-late suppers and party snacking).

It is best to have the protein-concentrated meal at lunch-time — but only if one can relax afterwards. Otherwise, choose the evening meal for the largest of the day, as most people do. Night-workers, retired people and Latins (those smart people who invented the siesta), and any others who can take at least an hour to relax after a meal, are ideally suited to having their lunch as the principal meal of the day.

For the working person, for whom lunch is smaller than dinner, two basic types of meal can be successfully planned. One is primarily a fruit meal, the other a vegetable meal. If the period during which lunch can be eaten is relatively short, the fruit meal will be the wiser choice, being easier to digest. The addition of a little concentrated food, such as dried fruits, nuts, seeds or avocado (depending on the choice of fruits) will make this meal larger than breakfast and more sustaining during the afternoon. The alternative style of lunch, centred around a salad, also allows for the inclusion of suitable concentrated foods to make for a sustaining meal which is relatively easily digested. Many people prefer sandwiches for lunch because they are easy to handle — this is satisfactory provided the bread is totally whole grain and suitable salad fillings are chosen, with either a nut butter or avocado as the spread.

Sandwiches are especially important for school children, for they prefer to conform rather than be different — their comfort and feelings, their acceptance by fellow pupils, all must be considered. Parents who have achieved sufficient maturity to dare to be different and choose only natural foods for themselves will often find it difficult to understand how their child can be so responsive to the opinions of their peers. Perhaps they should cast their memories back to their own school days to recall how important it was to be "one of the mob".

The school sandwich does not have to be the non-nutritive white apology for food known to most children, nor any of the "junk foods" sometimes proffered by school canteens. The thoughtful, nutritionally aware mother can have her children conform very closely to the accepted daily habits by baking her own bread and making sandwiches which contain suitably combined, nutritious vegetables. She can use steamed and mashed potatoes with green peas or grated carrot or similar vegetables, avocado with sliced and quartered cucumber and lettuce, raw nut butter and finely chopped celery, steamed lentils mashed with grated beets with a sprinkling of alfalfa sprouts. So many variations are available that room does not permit their listing here, but at least the foregoing guide will set one's mind working along this theme, with ingenious results.

If a protein-concentrated lunch has been eaten, the dinner should comprise starch concentrates with vegetables. If starches or sweet fruits were eaten at lunch, proteins should be considered for the dinner concentrates.

Dinner

For people who enjoy cooked foods, dinner is usually the best meal for such foods.

Many people avoid cooked food at any meal, even at dinner, for they realise that raw foods are not only more nutritious, but also possess more natural flavour. And these people will be healthier for the choice, so long as they do not hanker after the occasional cooked meal, for this will create emotional discontent, negating much of the nutritional good they would otherwise achieve. It would be far better for them to include the occasional cooked meal in their weekly diet — and dinner is the best time for this if they are working people.

The cooked evening meal has hitherto been one of those unquestioned rituals in most households, even in the tropics. This can be readily understood on a cold winter's night, but it has no intelligent foundation in the heat of summer. It would be better if the dinner were to comprise an ample salad, when both improved nourishment and improved refreshment would be enjoyed.

Another cogent reason for cooked dinners being popular in most households is that the family can all get together for at least this one important meal of the day. It is also usually the meal at which friends are entertained and the housewife seeks to express her catering talents. Even greater versatility would be expressed if she were to serve a meal combining raw and cooked foods in a nutritional and artistic presentation. Remember that the company of your friends is just as important as their health and the health of your family — so do not serve junk "food" and poorly combined items that will lead to intestinal distress.

Whether the meal is intended only for the family, or for a huge gathering of friends, it should be not only nutritionally sound but also attractively presented. Many people eat with their eyes. Their saliva run is initiated by what they see, just as much as by what they smell or think about. There is a lot of satisfying artistic ability to be expressed in the attractive preparation of the evening meal. And natural foods lend themselves so well to such a display. Many mothers have complained to me that their children do not take easily to natural foods, after years of "anything goes". Invariably, the mother has no concept of how to make these foods look attractive — she merely plonks them on the plate, the kids take one look and run!

Dinner is that important meal of the day when the family gets together, so make it an occasion for a mini-celebration by combining all the foregoing advice — and listen to the appreciation it attracts. Always serve a tempting salad, either as the main course with a suitably combined protein food, or as the accompanying course of a cooked dish or two. Ensure that the salad includes abundant sprouts, for the essential nourishment of the meal will be provided by the salad.

Cooking Methods

There are many different ways of cooking foods. The concept came into being to soften certain harder foods (such as the potato family, beetroot, pumpkin, etc.) in order to render them more edible and more enjoyable. But, as with many original concepts, centuries of habit have produced a mushy consequence.

To boil foods until they are soft enough to be eaten without teeth has become the standard which many home cooks and restaurant chefs have set themselves. All are apparently oblivious of the nutritional damage they sustain both to the food and the people they seek to satisfy.

What boiling does to foods can be compared with the action of an agitator in a clothes washing machine, whereby dirt is aggressively removed from the clothes and dissolved in the washing water. By boiling foods much of their nutrient properties are similarly lost in the boiling water — soluble minerals and natural sugars, as well as most of the water-soluble vitamins are removed from the food sources and permanently destroyed. With these nutrients goes much of the flavour, inducing many people to add table salt and other condiments (generally to the detriment of their health) in an attempt to gain some taste satisfaction from their cooked food.

A far better method of cooking is to steam the food. Only stainless steel cookware should be used, thereby avoiding the possible poisonous effect of aluminium oxidation, the result of food acids reacting with the metal during cooking. It is known that some of the released metal is ingested with foods served from an aluminium saucepan or frypan. By far the best cooking utensils are those made from heavy gauge stainless steel — ideal if they possess an external copper base (for fast and even heat distribution) and a heavily machined lid (for retaining a partial vacuum and permitting low-temperature cooking). Do not use utensils with an inner coating of copper, enamel, "teflon" or the like, for these have many recognised disadvantages, as any nutritionally oriented chef is aware.

Steaming at less than the normal boiling point of water is made possible only under conditions of partial vacuum. Simply place the vegetables on a perforated steamer stand (the flexible type which snugly fits into any size saucepan, but ensure it is entirely stainless steel and not aluminium; add a little water (0.5–1 cm); and bring to the boil. As soon as boiling commences, reduce heat to lowest level, ensuring the lid is squarely in position. With the reduction in temperature, water will cease boiling and steam within the saucepan will condense, forming a slight pressure reduction and partial vacuum. This will hold the lid tightly in position.

Remember how, at school, we learned in physics that temperature and pressure are directly proportional? This applies equally in cooking. With the slight reduction in pressure to a partial vacuum within the saucepan, water will boil at a lower temperature. This creates more steam to facilitate the cooking, but at many degrees below the normal boiling point of water. It also reduces loss of the water-soluble vitamins C and B-complex.

If vegetables are to be cooked, their nutritional loss can be further reduced by not peeling or cutting them. This considerably reduces oxidation, sugar loss and flavour loss. Fruit should never be cooked, for it so rapidly loses its natural sugars that very little flavour remains, indicating a catastrophic reduction in nourishment.

Other forms of cooking should be assiduously avoided. Baking in a dry-heat oven is the least pernicious of these, but the higher temperatures and prolonged cooking at these temperatures will materially diminish the food's potential nourishment far more than steaming. Frying in cold-pressed vegetable oil is preferred to the use of solid fats, but either implies excessive temperatures and the risks of molecular restructuring of the fatty acids with their attendant carcinogenic risks (especially prevalent when animal fats are used). If the fats are re-used, the cancer risk is considerably amplified and becomes a potentially serious health hazard. This is an unnecessary risk attending those who frequent many commercial eating houses. The worst offenders are sleek take-aways featuring "fast foods" — the "eat-it-and-beat-it" "joints". Their specialties are the fried and greasy mass-produced missiles which originated in America and which have since conquered almost the entire world's casual eating habits.

Many of the ethnic eating houses also use the "re-fried" process. Perhaps that is why, in their own countries, where so much of their food is re-fried, such high levels of gastrointestinal illness prevail. When these groups introduce their food styles on a commercial basis in Western countries, they combine the worst of both worlds by adding such chemical flavourings as MSG (monosodium glutamate). This "flavour enhancer" is a suspected carcinogen which is used with liberal quantities of common salt to stimulate the jaded taste buds of the average smoking/drinking unnatural food eater. Such meals are invariably prepared by the Asian cooks; Latin cooks use more of the heavy spices (such as cayenne) — not so much carcinogenic as ulcer-inducing.

An Ideal General Menu

By way of guidance to the selection of a healthy and delicious menu for day-to-day use, the following should serve to illustrate just how much variety is possible, while retaining relative simplicity in meal formation. Remember, this is only a guide. It should be altered to suit the season, food availability and needs of each person.

We should remember that these suggested menus are intended for everyday use. When we eat out or entertain at home, it is obvious that such meals will be beyond the basic plan of good nutrition, as these occasions are beyond the scope of a basic, simple menu pattern. Even so, we generally are offered a choice of foods and can always express our preferences for those closest to our understanding of sound nutrition.

In preparing this guide to an ideal menu, care has been taken to cater to the most general requirements. Thus, for those preferring only two meals a day, or for school children, workers involved in the expenditure of considerable energy, or sports-people, this menu will need modification to suit individual needs.

An Ideal General Menu for One Week
For the Average Healthy Adult

Breakfast	*Lunch*	*Dinner*
MONDAY		
1 cantaloupe or ½ honeydew melon or ¼ watermelon.	Potato salad — with 2 steamed potatoes, grated carrot and beetroot, cucumber, capsicum, lettuce and celery. Avocado can be included.	Vegetable salad — with finely shredded cabbage, parsley, small mushrooms, tomato, alfalfa sprouts, lettuce — 60 g sunflower kernels.
TUESDAY		
up to 400 g cherries and 2 nectarines or 2 red apples and 2 oranges.	½ paw paw, 1 banana and 60-100 g raisins or sun-dried dates.	Soya bean or lentil casserole — with sautéed onion, celery and capsicum — and steamed broccoli, zucchini and cauliflower, and a side salad of tomato, sprouts, cucumber, lettuce.
WEDNESDAY		
up to 700 g stone-fruit incl. apricots, plums, peaches, nectarines.	3-4 slices whole-grain bread spread with avocado, sliced cucumber and fresh sprouts.	Vegetable salad — with tomato, capsicum, lettuce, celery, parsley, small mushrooms — and up to 125 g almonds (skinned).

Man's Ideal Diet

Breakfast	*Lunch*	*Dinner*
	THURSDAY	
up to 500 g grapes and 1 pear or peach or ½ paw paw and 2 passionfruit.	Vegetable salad — with fresh sprouts, tomato, cucumber, carrot, celery — and up to 150 g fresh ricotta or cottage cheese.	Potatoes, steamed or baked and sprinkled with oil, and steamed green peas, beetroot, artichokes (either type) and steamed or baked pumpkin.
	FRIDAY	
½ pineapple, 1 pear, 1 apple or ½ punnet strawberries, 1 kiwifruit, 1 apple.	½ paw paw, 1 banana and either 2 fresh figs or up to 100 g sun-dried fruits.	Sprout salad — with 2 or 3 varieties fresh sprouts — and tomato, small zucchini, grated beetroot, and 100 g Brazil or hazel nuts.
	SATURDAY	
2 persimmons and 250 g berry fruits or grapes or 1 mango and up to 300 g stone-fruit.	Vegetable salad — with capsicum, tomato, parsley, cucumber, lettuce, celery — and up to 60 g pumpkin kernels.	Steamed buckwheat or rice casserole with sautéed onions and steamed Brussels sprouts, egg plant, green beans, turnip or carrots.
	SUNDAY	
Fresh fruit (any choice) or muesli (recipe follows)	2 oranges and 1 apple or 1 grapefruit and 2 mandarins, and up to 125 g cashew nuts.	Steamed sweet corn and sweet potato and small vegetable salad with celery, carrot, lettuce and fresh sprouts.

This menu is designed to give those who hunger for variety the spice they seek, yet offer maximum nourishment. For those not so insistent upon variety, easy modification of the menu is possible.

When choosing fruits, it is important to select those in season and avoid, wherever possible, those that have been in cold storage. If in doubt, call your local marketing authority to learn which fruits are available and when — there is considerable variation from state to state and country to country. For example, cherries, grapes, apricots and other deciduous fruits are usually only available during summer and early autumn. It is wise, therefore, to enjoy their nutritional, flavoursome offerings while they are in season. Some people prefer to eat the same seasonal fruit for breakfast for many consecutive days and there is nothing wrong with this so long as there is a balanced nutritional intake over the entire day.

In compiling this menu, account has been taken of the fact that most people are a little heavier than they would prefer to be. Thus they will find that by adhering to the Ideal Menu concept of fruit and vegetables, with nothing to eat between meals, their body weight will gradually normalise and be maintained.

A modified version of this menu should be used by those who would like to gain weight, those expending above-average calories at work or play, or by young people still growing. Some major modifications can be made at breakfast by adding a little yogurt with the fruit or by replacing the fruit some mornings with a suitable muesli (recipe to follow). Their weekday dinners or weekend lunches could be increased in size and include an occasional omelette or cheese or added wholegrain bread. They could also include a little health-food dressing, such as made by Norganic or Hain, over their salads. (For others, who seek to avoid salad dressing, a little freshly squeezed lemon juice is most suitable.)

For a breakfast muesli, one of the health food varieties is suitable so long as the person can digest such a vast combination of nutrients. Otherwise, to make one's own presents no problem. Always choose raw ingredients, rather than toasted, and do not add salt or sugar. The most desirable recipe, in my opinion, is based on wheat germ, rolled oats and soya flakes. Bran can also be added if a history of constipation prevails. If extra "chewiness" and sweetness are required, dried fruits can also be included, the best being sun-dried (natural) sultanas. Prepared rolled oats and soya flakes will have been steam-cooked prior to being rolled at the mill, so they do not need cooking again. This muesli only needs to be allowed to stand for 10 or 15 minutes in its liquid to be ready for eating.

Muesli should not be moistened with milk. Most people think this is the only way to eat muesli but the two most suitable moisteners are either pure apple juice or soya milk. The advantage of soya milk is that it has better keeping qualities than apple juice, being available in powdered form with indefinite storage properties, and can be mixed when required. By far the best variety available in Australia and New Zealand is the "Soyvita" brand; in America, the best choice is "Soyagen" brand.

Preparing soya milk powder is extremely simple — it only needs the addition of water in proportions as recommended on the can. Additional benefits can be derived by adding a few supplements when mixing. The addition of brewer's or torula yeast will provide added protein, B-vitamins and minerals; maple syrup will provide added sweetness and calcium, and powdered lecithin will provide added protein, vitamins and minerals, as well as the anti-cholesterol factors needed by people not yet weaned off meat.

Muesli can thus provide a very filling and highly nutritious breakfast, but one which is extremely high in kilojoules. It should, therefore, be chosen only by people who need a high degree of morning sustenance to support heavy physical work, or by those who wish to gain weight. Sports-people and those who engage in a heavy physical training programme also find this a highly desirable breakfast. But be careful not to eat such a heavy breakfast soon after rising — one must have been out of bed for at least an hour and have completed a reasonable exercise programme to be able to digest a muesli breakfast with ease.

People should remember that it is not the ingredients of one or two meals that make for health, but what is chosen for the vast majority of meals — hence the guidance offered by the Ideal General Menu. Most people will want to eat out once or twice a week and will therefore depart somewhat from their Ideal Menu on those occasions. There should be no feeling of guilt in having done so, for one can still choose a very healthy meal when eating out, so long as the infamous "hasty-tasty joints" are avoided. We can enjoy the company of our friends without compromising our healthy eating habits.

STAGE ELEVEN

Uses of Health Foods and Herb Teas

A health food is a component of a person's diet which contributes to maintaining or improving their health. It possesses no magical or therapeutic properties in itself, but forms a part of a pattern of nourishment by which the person remains free from disease or disability.

There is no doubt, among thinking people, about the intimate relationship between diet and health. Those from an age when accepted habit formed the basis for nutritional knowledge are not so easily convinced. They stubbornly adhere to beliefs that are in opposition to scientific knowledge. For them, health foods are "all and any foods man chooses to eat", as was expressed in an interview in 1979 by one of Sydney's most outspoken dietitians. Of course, she was supporting her established viewpoint, simultaneously criticising health food stores as often compromising by stocking such unhealthy items as coffee, chocolate, home brewing kits, etc.

We often see these items in a health food store, but this does not imply that the store is not to be trusted to supply genuine health foods. Until more people become aware of the benefits of eating only health foods, the store owners will be obliged, for purely economic reasons, to stock these additional items.

Genuine Health Foods

Health food stores are the major source of top nourishment for the discriminating eater. Australia is most fortunate in this regard, having more health food stores, per capita, than any other country. With 950 health food stores throughout the country it represents a ratio of one store per 15,200 people — the United States, with its 6000 stores, represents a ratio of one store per 38,000 people. But, of course, the American stores are very much larger, with a greater turnover and range of foods. However, the rate of growth in size and number of Australian health food stores, together with their increasing range of local and imported health foods, implies that it is, indeed, the most favoured country in the world.

Most vitamins and food supplements are sold through health food stores, although supermarkets and pharmacies are endeavouring to rush into the field from a late start. In America, 56 per cent of the public in 1980 used one or more food supplements or vitamins on a regular basis. The figure for Australia is estimated at nearer 40 per cent. Nonetheless, with accelerating knowledge of the manifold virtues of health foods, more and more people are recognising that these represent a relief from medical drugs and most elective surgery which, hitherto, were offering the only hope (but which often fell short of providing the total remedy for the problem).

The modern, thinking person does not accept old habits and their poor track record. Information is being avidly sought on the dozens of health foods now available, on what they provide for the body and on how they are prepared or manufactured. In an endeavour to provide further knowledge of the subject, the following summaries of the most popular health foods now available is offered. The information is not intended to be exhaustive, but rather to provide basic guidance, first to the selection and nutritional uses of health foods (including those which are sometimes regarded as being healthy, but have proved to be otherwise); then to the selection and therapeutic usages of the most popular of the extensive herb tea range.

A Basic Guide

Alfalfa Widely cultivated, alfalfa is one of the most nutritionally versatile plants yet discovered. Its leaves and stems provide valuable properties for humans and grazing animals alike. Known to farmers as lucerne, alfalfa appears to have been named by the Arabs who have used it for centuries to feed their thoroughbred horses and who regard it as the "king of kings" of plants. This distinction derives from the plant's ability to penetrate as much as 12 metres into the subsoil so that its roots bring the nourishment of those elusive trace minerals from the depths into the plant's own chemical system. Manganese is the most important of these trace minerals, so vital to the human digestive system, especially in its manufacturing of insulin.

Alfalfa is a legume with rich, green leaves and purplish flowers appearing in summer. Its leaves are valuable sources of carotene (vitamin A), vitamins C, D, E and K_1, as well as calcium, potassium, iron, phosphorus and chlorophyll. These abundant nutrients have induced nutritional authorities to experiment with alfalfa as a ready form of easily digestible food for under-developed countries and as a protein concentrate (from leaf chlorophyll) for supplementing modern protein-deficient foods, such as breads, pastas, etc.

Currently, alfalfa is available in many different forms: as seeds for sprouting (delicious and nourishing in salads and on sandwiches); as tablets for therapeutic aid, especially for indigestion and hyperacidity, and for increasing the milk flow in nursing mothers; as flour, to enrich wheat flour and for therapeutic use; as chlorophyll for blood enrichment and skin improvement. Alfalfa is one of the highest sources of dietary fibre, containing up to 20 per cent by weight (twice as much as wheat bran). It is also used extensively in herb tea form, both singly and as part of many blends. Many natural healing ointments contain alfalfa for vital skin nourishment.

Bran Thanks to the valuable observational work of two British medical researchers, fewer people now suffer from constipation. Surgeon Dr T. L. Cleave, on duty aboard a British battleship during World War II, noted the high level of constipation among the crew, which he correctly attributed to lack of fresh fruits and vegetables. He found that by adding raw wheat bran to their diet, the problem was virtually eliminated! After the war, his researches were corroborated by the more eloquent Dr Denis Burkitt, whose extensive American tours commenced the new fashion — eating plenty of bran. Bowel problems were regarded as among the most pandemic in the Western world, varying from chronic constipation to acute diarrhoea, until bran became a favourite "medicine".

Many books have been written on the subject, the most erudite and therapeutically helpful being *The Saccharine Disease*, by Dr T. L. Cleave, Keats Publishing, Conn., USA, 1975, wherein the number of modern diseases traced to refined foods is exposed, directly incriminating lack of fibre and an excess of refined sugar. Refining wheat for bread, biscuit, cookie and cake baking has been the primary villain. Bran is removed from wheat grains early in the refining process. Bran is also removed from rice to make it white. Both types of bran are especially high in fibre (around 10 per cent) and both are being used effectively, not only to treat bowel problems, but also to supply important nutrients which have been separated from the grains in this thieving process called "refining". Brans contain very high concentrations of phosphorus, iron, potassium, magnesium and B-vitamins, especially niacin. Rice bran, in particular, is one of the highest sources of silicon known — the mineral so invaluable for the skin, connective tissues and cartilages.

Bran is found to normalise bowel movements by helping the bowel to form stools of correct size and softness for which the lower alimentary canal was designed. However, the natural foods diet of 75 per cent fresh fruits and vegetables would do this naturally, but so many people nowadays eat refined and animal-derived foods far in excess of their body's digestive ability. Worst offenders are meats, poultry, milk and its products, sugar, juices, margarine and fats, honey, chocolate, tea and coffee, soft and hard beverages. For many people, these constitute a major part of their food intake, yet not one of these items contains a milligram of fibre. Bread is the other offender — although it does possess about 1 per cent fibre (which is usually put back during mixing as "added fibre", as it is misleadingly advertised), it cannot possibly be regarded as a food offering adequate bulk. Rather than taking bran in its crude form, alter the diet to include fibre-rich natural foods. If this appears too radical, then buy bran and use it in breakfast muesli, pastry, muffins, etc. It is probably most effective when sprinkled over a fresh fruit salad.

Breakfast Cereals The "packet-to-plate" concept of breakfast cereals has become so popular with people who want to save time, that the question of nutritional desirability appears to have been completely overlooked, that is, until recently, when the popularity of muesli came into being. It was earlier this century, in Zurich, the largest city of Switzerland, that the Bircher-Benner Clinic developed the muesli concept, based on their research of under-nourished people who needed a complex, wholefood breakfast. Found to be nutritionally desirable for other people, especially those with heavy workloads and children at school, muesli has become known as the health food breakfast. It has become so popular that, in the past decade, even multinational food processors have joined the growing list of manufacturers. But true muesli requires very little manufacturing and is, therefore, a far cry from the usual highly processed flakes, bubbles and biscuits, hitherto considered the most desirable breakfasts.

One of the problems associated with "the cornflake era" is its inducement to sugar and milk consumption and the tendency towards the development of hypoglycaemia from the highly refined ingredients. Aware nutritionists have often spoken of the lack of nutrition in processed cereals, but the adding of "enrichment", by way of synthetic vitamins and minerals, made a little progress in overcoming the nutritional deficiency and a lot of progress in admitting the cereals to be nutritionally inadequate. Then the addition of fibre was seen as a further admission that processed foods induced constipation. Added sugar was an attempt to entice children to accept their breakfast of empty calories from the processors' packages, but ultimately muesli won the day in all households of thinking people.

The simplest and most easily digested muesli contains only a few ingredients. While this smaller mixture is a departure from the original muesli concept, it is more suited to our digestive processes. The two basic ingredients are raw wheat germ and rolled oats, to which can be added sultanas and/or soya flakes. (These additions are not strictly ideal food combinations, but most people can easily digest them if the quantities are moderate.) Other alternative ingredients are flaked barley, wheat, rice, rye or millet — flaked or rolled cereals are manufactured simply by steaming and hot-rolling the whole grains under pressure, thereby precooking them at the mill. The more expanded and complex health-food muesli usually comprises most of the above ingredients, together with bran, raisins, currants, cashews, sunflower seeds, cracked wheat berries, as porridge meal, and cracked buckwheat (or any combination of these). Some people can digest this mixture satisfactorily, others find it too complex. This is known as "raw" muesli, as opposed to "toasted" muesli, in which many of the ingredients have been pre-toasted for people addicted to a cooked (and nutritionally diminished) breakfast.

Both types of muesli will often be sweetened, usually with raw sugar. But this is totally unnecessary and undesirable, for dried fruits provide adequate natural sweetening (unless one is chronically addicted to sugar — and this is a good test). Some health food companies will also offer sugar-free muesli (even though sugar is one of the cheapest ingredients in the mixture); their concern for your health should justify your patronage if you seek muesli for breakfast.

None of the foregoing muesli combinations require further cooking, nor should they have a hot liquid added — this will destroy some of the optimum nourishment. Cool liquid added 10-15 minutes prior to eating will provide adequate soakage to all ingredients for comfortable chewing. Avoid the use of milk in your cereal. Many people have never considered another form of liquid, even though they might suffer from a milk intolerance. Some people prefer adding only water; for others who desire a liquid with more flavour and body, many healthy possibilities are available. Most enjoyable is fruit juice — apple is the usual choice, or apricot, grape, pineapple/coconut, etc. Another favourite is soya milk, to which lecithin powder and/or brewer's or torula yeast can be added for additional nutrients.

Bulghur Wheat ("Bourghal") Bulghur is the general name applying to grains which are prepared for imparting a special taste to some Middle Eastern dishes. It has been in use since biblical times, but in recent years has become more popular than ever before, probably with the ubiquitous migration of Middle-Eastern races throughout the modern world. The processes by which it is prepared vary little from old — the grain is steamed, dried, then cracked before a final drying.

Today, wheat is the most popular grain for such use and, in Australia, is generally found in health food stores under the name "bourghal"; it is also found as the primary ingredient in tabouly, a dried, savoury salad, also originating from the Middle East. Bulghur wheat has somewhat similar nutritional properties to whole wheat, but becomes far more palatable by its special method of preparation. It contains the bran and germ of the wheat, but because the grain has been cooked, it offers a far longer shelf life than the whole grain in its raw state. Many delicious recipes can be found for its dietary use, but it should be avoided by people who evidence a wheat intolerance.

Carob Many people who buy health foods are inclined to look upon carob as the alternative to chocolate. The truth is completely the reverse. Chocolate is not only the more modern alternative to carob, but if correctly classified by its contents, is a drug, whereas carob is a food. The cocoa bean has come into prominence within the last 200 years; carob was only introduced into the United States in 1860, by which time chocolate was already the snack food of the wealthier classes. So carob did not seem to offer any special advantage, even though it had been well known and in constant use in the Middle East and southern Europe for thousands of years — it was, in fact, mentioned a few times in the Bible, especially in relation to John the Baptist, from whom its alternative name, St John's Bread, originated. Carob tastes similar to chocolate, but is higher in natural sweetness, demanding less sweetening when prepared as a confection. Most brands of carob candies are sweetened with raw or white sugar (up to 35 per cent), rendering them unfit for healthy consumption, yet chocolate candies contain up to 60 per cent white sugar (or the equivalent in chemical sweetener), rendering them even more unworthy. Chocolate also contains caffeine, theobromine and oxalic acid, providing a horrifying assault upon the human organism. Carob contains none of these, instead it offers valuable nutrients, including all the alkalising minerals, fibre, B-vitamins, especially B_3, together with a reasonable quantity of protein (4.5 per cent).

Carob flour comes from the ground carob pods, the seeds enclosed by the pods being released for further tree propagation. The carob tree grows wild, lives 100 years or more and fruits with pods similar to other legumes (such as lima beans). Carob powder, used in cooking, is the pure flour ground from these pods. But when it is used in candy preparation, it should be used only with such added sweetening as dates, malted barley, etc., avoiding cane sugar product additives. These natural carob candies and confections are gradually becoming available in health food stores and, although more expensive, are amply rewarding to the taste buds and the health.

Chlorophyll The master action of nature — the complicated chemical process by which green plants store the sun's energy as food — is a vital function of chlorophyll. It acts to develop photosynthesis in plants in much the same way as haemoglobin acts in the blood of animals. Extracted from the green leaves of plants, chlorophyll is a valuable health food and is obtainable from most health food stores in liquid and tablet form. It is usually extracted from alfalfa leaves, although it can be obtained in the home from juicing green vegetables, especially the tops of root vegetables. A glass of "green drink" each day will provide a delightful energy renewal, as well as affording vital therapeutic properties for such conditions as anaemia, artery problems and bad breath (halitosis). The chemistry of chlorophyll is interesting, for it is quite a large molecule, centred around the important mineral, magnesium. The simple formula of plant chlorophyll is $C_{55}H_{72}MgN_4O_5$, and the vital life force of chlorophyll is of great benefit to people, especially those suffering from anorexia nervosa.

Cider Vinegar By the process of natural fermentation, apple cider vinegar is an ageing process which usually takes place in oak casks, in much the same way as wine production. When adequately aged, the best cider vinegar is promptly bottled ready for use, completely unfiltered. Its colour will vary in accordance with the variety of apples used, but always look for some sediment and cloudiness — these indicate the presence of "mother", natural apple residue, proving its unfiltered claim. Malt vinegar, by contrast, is rapidly distilled by chemicals and steam to provide a light-coloured, cheap product, quite adequate for those who only seek to add it to water for the effective cleaning of their windows. Malt vinegar possesses no enzymes and minimal nutrients, in poor comparison to cider vinegar with its potassium richness and enzyme benefits, as well as lesser quantities of phosphorus, chlorine, sodium, iron, copper, magnesium and silicon.

Paul Bragg, in his book *Apple Cider Vinegar* (Health Science, California), lists dozens of therapeutic and nutritional uses to which this product may be beneficially applied. These include overweight, detoxification, skin nourishment, combating headaches, corns, warts, sunburn, kidney and gall stones, arthritis and constipation.

Comfrey One of the oldest and most trusted herbs in use, comfrey is a perennial plant common to European meadows and Russia and Asia long before the USA "discovered" and brought it into popular health food use. England and Europe also did much to bring comfrey into practical use, both nutritionally and horticulturally (as an excellent soil nourisher). It is a plant which can be easily grown in most climates and soils — both leaves and roots having desirable properties for therapeutic use. Many people also find its leaves palatable in a salad or a drink, but others find them rather bitter. In dried form, as a herb tea, the leaves are universally popular; in tablet form, comfrey is used to aid the neutralising of hyperacidic conditions (such as in arthritis); in ointment form, it is used successfully to aid skin cellular regeneration and to reduce the formation of scar tissue. Occasionally the media makes havoc of some scientist's "discovery" that comfrey is "dangerous", after feeding rats huge quantities over a long period — lettuce would be just as dangerous, not to mention the sugar the scientist uses in his dangerous coffee!

Dolomite A naturally occurring mineral rock, dolomite is more valuable to human health and happiness than gold is to investors. It is a type of limestone in which the essential mineral, magnesium, is also present in the double compound of calcium carbonate and magnesium carbonate — $Ca(CO_3).Mg(CO_3)$. This compound is found extensively around the world as rock (the picturesque mountain range in northern Italy is named after it), from which it is powdered for both nutritional and horticultural use.

As will be discussed in Stage 14, dolomite is a valuable natural fertiliser, but now we will consider only its dietary applications. It can be taken directly in powder form, or in tablet form, either pure or combined with vitamins A and D for added skin and bone benefit, or with vitamin E for circulatory and internal tissue benefit. Dolomite is the safest and most economical form in which to obtain added magnesium for the body's mineral needs. (Magnesium oxide or magnesium orotate are the other forms, but these should only be taken under the direction of a competent practitioner.)

Some of the manifold therapeutic uses to which dolomite has been successfully applied in human health include relief from asthma; heart malfunction (with vitamin E); shrinking and healing of canker sores in the mouth, prostate and haemorrhoids (with vitamins A and D); relief of lower back pain and recurring headaches (in some cases, migraine). It is also an effective body deodoriser, especially for underarms and feet, as well as reducing intestinal odours from flatulence and in the stools — in this regard, it facilitates a more thorough digestive absorption, as well as improving the effectiveness of colonic flora in facilitating better bowel action.

Dried Fruits There are some fifteen different fruits available in health food stores in dried form. These provide concentrated sources of many important nutrients, far in excess of the same nutrient availability in the fresh state. But the primary purpose of drying fruits is to preserve them for long-term storage and availability throughout the year, long after the fresh fruit crop has expired. The natural method of drying fruits is to expose them to intense rays of the sun, thereby reducing their moisture content to around one-quarter of the original. This method applies effectively to virtually all fruits, with the exception of banana, the texture of which, being somewhat denser than other fruits, does not permit a totally effective penetration of solar rays, implying the need for dehydration in ovens at around 75°C for 24–48 hours. Commercial expediency now dictates that many other fruits are dehydrated at higher than solar ray temperatures, some even being further hastened by chemical use.

To provide simple classification of fruits suitable for drying, the fifteen varieties commonly recognised as suitable are divided into two basic groups — those which are primarily tropical and those from deciduous trees or vines. Of the tropical fruits, dates and figs are usually sun-dried. Both are essentially Mid-East fruits, although the finest crops are now produced in California — they are also the most expensive, especially the organically grown varieties, but their superior nutritional properties more than justify their cost. (Figs are unique in the fruit world because they are the only trees bearing two crops annually.)

Two other tropical fruits not so popular when sun-dried are pineapples and paw paws. Solar exposure tends to darken them quite severely, inducing most buyers to favour the dehydrated varieties produced in Taiwan, now the world's largest source of these, exporting to every continent. The unique texture of pineapples and paw paws has induced the Taiwanese to cook them before dehydration as a means of satisfying world demands for long shelf-life. The fruits are sliced, then boiled for twenty minutes to remove their acids and kill bacteria. This also dissolves their fructose. The missing sweetness is reintroduced by soaking the cooked fruit in a 5 per cent raw cane sugar solution for 24 hours before being dehydrated for another 48 hours. Another tropical fruit, mango, is as yet rare as a dried fruit, but its popularity is predicted to develop considerably during the 1980s, once a suitable dehydration technique has been developed and a market established.

Deciduous fruits form the larger percentage of dried fruits and can be divided into three sub-groups. Most popular are the berry fruits — currants, sultanas and raisins. Whereas sultanas and raisins are dried grapes, currants are small dried berries fruiting on a shrub which is native to northern European countries, imported to Australia and America from Britain. It is a favourite in cooking and in wine and brandy making. As a dried fruit, it is usually exposed to sun-drying initially, but the major moisture reduction occurs by dehydration in ovens. Sultanas and raisins are not generally dried this way, only the minority are prepared in this "natural" manner, as it is classified, for this is more time-consuming and costly. It also ensures that a higher level of nutrients remain, discernible by their darker appearance and sweeter taste.

The general method is to first dip the clusters of fruit into a caustic soda solution to split the skins to facilitate faster drying. This, unfortunately, also causes a loss of some of the fructose and soluble nutrients, plus an uptake of small amounts of caustic soda, further reducing natural sweetness. Sultanas are dried seedless sultana grapes (known in America as "thompson seedless grapes"); raisins are dried muscatel or waltham cross grapes — in Australia, it is generally the latter. Raisins, therefore, have seeds although most are now seeded prior to being sold; when sold unseeded, they are classed as "muscatels". A relatively new variety of raisin is becoming more generally available in natural seedless form. Called "manuka" raisins, they are grown on smaller acreages and are some 25 per cent more expensive to buy; but they are 95 per cent seedless, making them more desirable to many consumers, especially for feeding to children and for cooking. These must be naturally dried to retain their increased fructose level.

Apples, apricots, nectarines peaches, pears and prunes constitute the balance of those deciduous fruits suitable for drying. All of these undergo far more dehydration than sun-drying and, because all but prunes darken during natural drying, chemicals are usually applied to maintain their lighter appearance. Sulphur is used during dehydration, the yellow powder being burned in the ovens where it combines with atmospheric oxygen to form sulphur dioxide and precipitate onto the surface of fruits. This prevents darkening, caused by normal oxidation during dehydration, sun-drying and in storage. By far the most nutritious of these fruits are those exposed only to sun-drying — their darker surfaces indicate higher levels of vitamin and fructose than are found in the speedier, high temperature method of dehydration. Further, for many people, the combination of sulphur dioxide with body moisture during catabolism induces kidney problems from the resultant formation of sulphurous acid — a kidney irritant in moderate quantities. Prunes are also dehydrated but the chemical used is a mould inhibitor — potassium sorbate — it is popular in food and wine processing as a bacteriostat and antioxidant and is generally considered, on its own, to have no toxic effects in humans (no research has been done to ascertain its reactions, if any, with any of the other thousands of food chemicals in modern use).

Comparative nutritional values of the various dried fruits are being constantly sought by health-conscious people. Readers are referred to my popular food analysis book, *Guide Book to Nutritional Factors in Foods*, from which the following comparisons were extracted. Very similar kilojoule counts are common to all dried fruits — the average being 1100 per 100 grams (the 100 g quantity of edible portion is common to all food nutrient comparisons). When this is compared with lamb chops (1490 kilojoules, which is not regarded as a high-kilojoule food), it can be recognised that dried fruits are *not* high in kilojoules, especially when their general nutrient offerings are considered. General carbohydrate count is an average 73 per cent — this is high, but remember that most of it is in the form of easily metabolised fructose, an excellent energy source. Protein content is high for fruit, varying from apricots at 4.5 per cent, bananas 4.4 per cent, figs 3.8 per cent down to pears at 1.2 per cent. Fat is very low; pears being 1.8 per cent, apples 1.6 per cent, down to apricots 0.4 per cent. Fibre (part of the average 73 per cent carbohydrate) is importantly high in value, varying from 6.4 per cent in pears, 5.6 per cent in figs, 3.1 per cent in peaches and apples, down to 0.9 per cent in sultanas and raisins (yet this is the same as white bread). Calcium content of figs is exceptionally high at 240 mg — all other dried fruits possess reasonable calcium, varying from 90 mg in currants to 27 mg in apples. Iron is fairly high, with 6.0 mg in peaches, 4.3 mg in apricots, down to 1.1 mg in pears (average daily requirement being 11 mg). Potassium and magnesium are also abundant in dried fruits, especially in apricots, bananas, figs and peaches. All dried fruits possess reasonable amounts of B-complex vitamins, but are rather low in vitamin C. Vitamin A is also low in all except dried apricots where, at 0.88 mg (2.55 i.u.) half the body's average daily requirement is provided from 100 g.

Flour The cultivation of grains for human consumption was probably developed around 10 000 B.C.; and their grinding into meal to be made into a coarse bread evolved soon after. The modern-day use of steel mills has resulted in a very fine grade of flour, resulting in a considerable loss of nutrition. Flour, sugar and salt today constitute the "terrible trio" in human nutrition. Far too much emphasis is placed on the use of these products in modern dietary, to the exclusion of whole, natural foods. Flour should be used for the occasional baked product only, instead of its role having emerged as "essential" to human nutrition. In pre-historic days, flour was used when fresh food was scarce; even then it was only used immediately after being freshly ground, so that it did contain most of the original nourishment of the grain. With the abundance of fresh food available in most parts of the world today, flour should be far less used; and when it is, it should be freshly ground from the whole grain. Instead, the modern grain, although nutritionally richer than its original counterpart, loses so much nourishment when hulled, refined, ground, sterilised, bleached, etc., that the result is a grossly undernourished powder in which not even weevils can live. The "convenience" of buying ready-ground flour gave way to the further laziness of buying ready-made baked goods as the industrial revolution drew people away from their homes to spend more time making money with which to buy their bread, etc. These conditions do not apply today, with the enormous increase in free time won by assertive unions. But humans remain pampered, failing to realise how much nutritional loss they continue to suffer from sterile flour.

All grains can be ground into flour for baking nourishing breads, cookies and cakes, but the most popular varieties are wheat, rye, corn and buckwheat, as well as soya beans. When freshly ground at home (an easy operation with a small mill), the resulting flour is subjected to very little heat, oxidation or storage loss. To further minimise heat loss, the use of a stone mill, instead of steel grinding, generates less friction. The resulting flour will be slightly coarser, but will still be adequate for all forms of baking and will taste better in the finished product.

The foregoing nutritional logic will not impress everyone, for many will continue to buy prepared flour. While this is preferable to buying commercially baked products, it should be recognised that flour is best stored in a cool, dry place — the refrigerator is most suitable. Nutritionally, soya flour is by far the best. It exceeds all other flours in all major nutrients except niacin (in which wheat is superior), but soya flour cannot be so successfully used in cake or bread making, except in small quantities and in combination with rye or wheat; its major use is as a basis for soya milk powder, an ideal alternative to animal milk, especially for adults. For baking purposes, whole wheat, then buckwheat, flour lead the nutrient lists, followed by rye and cornmeal. Wheat is by far the most popular flour, but a significant difference prevails between wholemeal wheat and plain white wheat flours. When it is refined, wheat flour loses one-third of its protein, between half and three-quarters of all other nutrients, and a massive 87 per cent of its fibre. Certainly it has a longer shelf-life, but in terms of satisfying human nutritional needs, refined flour should never leave the store shelf!

Fructose The sweetest of all common sugars, fructose occurs naturally in all fruits and most vegetables, as well as in honey (in combination with other sugars). Being one of the easiest sugars to digest, it does not demand insulin through the pancreas, as does sucrose (cane sugar). It is therefore suitable for diabetics in modest quantities. Fructose is a ready source of energy for the body, indicating why fruits, whether fresh, dried or in juice form, are such valuable energy sources. It is now possible to buy fructose in pure powdered form from health food stores — it has been extracted from cornstarch, for corn is one exception to the general run of fruits and vegetables which, as they ripen, convert starches into sugar. Corn, by reverse, converts its sugar into starch as it matures.

Garlic With some health authorities declaring that garlic is poisonous to humans and others unable to find sufficient superlatives to describe its virtues, little wonder many people become confused. It is always important to experiment oneself, where practicable, or to research the experiments and results of practice of one who is uncommitted to a vested interest in commercial products. For this reason, no better informative source can be found than Dr Paavo Airola on the subject of garlic. He has used it in practice for many years with excellent therapeutic benefits for many people. Garlic juice has well-established antibacterial and antifungal properties, which have been demonstrated in every country, especially in Russia and Switzerland, and over many hundreds, sometimes thousands, of years. Hippocrates and Galen, considered pioneers in medical treatment, placed great store in garlic juice and raw garlic. Among the therapeutic benefits for which garlic is given credit are arthritis, cancer and other tumorous growths, hypertension and anaemia, intestinal putrefaction and colitis, hypoglycaemia and diabetes, whooping cough and colds, pneumonia and tuberculosis, many forms of allergies and, sometimes, asthma. Most people find that eating raw garlic is rather strong for the stomach and repulsive for their friends, especially for the quantity required if chronic symptoms prevail. Thus, odourless garlic extract in capsule form is wisest, for this also provides a greater concentration of the sulphur-containing acid allicin ($C_6H_{10}OS_2$), the most active therapeutic agent in garlic. If deciding to eat garlic cloves, be sure not to heat them in any way if remedial action of allicin is to be effective, for it is unstable and rapidly decomposes when heated.

Ginseng Probably the most famous and extensively used of all Chinese medicines, ginseng has more recently become a favourite in the West. Its use has been testified to over many thousands of years, not only in China, but also in Korea, Russia and even by the American Indians. To all, it has been considered a most remarkable panacea with a thousand uses, from stimulating the pituitary gland to improving one's sexual appetite. Korean ginseng extract is considered the most potent of all, attracting a price in the vicinity of gold. Slightly less expensive varieties are available from Manchuria and China; cheaper again from Siberia and from North America. And the effectiveness of each is generally considered to be in direct proportion to its cost. Where once ginseng grew wild in Asia and North America, over the past couple of decades its popularity has been so great that it has virtually been eliminated from its natural domain unless cultivated. These days, most of the ginseng used is from cultivated areas, where it requires four to six years to mature its desirable root system. Ginseng can be taken in liquid or powder form, as tablets or capsules, or as a herb tea. Its stimulating influence on the pituitary gland makes it somewhat unsuited to slim, highly active people, but for heavier, slower people, it is of utmost potential benefit. The range of therapeutic properties for ginseng covers hypoactivity, thyroid stimulation, fevers and inflammations, eases childbirth, helps menstrual problems, colds and respiratory problems and increases the body's natural fortitude against illness and inclement conditions. It is believed American Indians used ginseng chiefly as an emetic and to relieve nausea. Some care should be exercised in the administering of ginseng without understanding guidance, for many of its virtues could be in conflict with your own individual metabolic and emotional disposition. Exercise care as to how often and for how long you take it.

Glacé Fruits Many varieties of dried fruits are taken a step further by some processors to provide a higher level of sweetness and a shiny appearance to attract attention in display gift packs and atop glamorous cakes. The process is called "glacéing", implying a shiny, thin surface. However thin this surface was originally intended to be, its more recent development sees it growing slightly thicker each year, so that it is often found to exceed one millimetre all over. The process involves a sweetening agent (white sugar, raw sugar or honey) being held in position by a setting agent (gelatine or agar agar; sometimes pectin is used but this is usually too expensive). The result is an attractive display, but a piece of dried fruit with very diminished nutritional value in which the carbohydrate content has been greatly increased. So too is the risk of dental caries, due to the tendency of the setting material to hold the sucrose tightly to the teeth. Glacé fruits have become a traditional favourite as Christmas gifts. Wise advice would be to choose them only when prepared from sun-dried fruits, coated with agar agar or pectin and sweetened with honey. Even then, they should be consumed only occasionally, although they do make a very attractive gift and are far superior to chocolate or other sugar-based confectionery.

Grains Generally classified as the seeds of cereal plants, grains are characterised by their smallness, hardness and low water content. Barley, corn, millet, oats, rice, rye and wheat are the most commonly used grains for human consumption. Buckwheat is an American and European favourite, becoming more popular in Australia as its taste and nutritional virtues are recognised, especially as a replacement for rice and potatoes in main-course cooking, and to replace wheat in pancakes. Sorghum is a grain grown mainly for stock feed in the West, but long in use as a food in India and China (where it is also used for sweetening). It is slowly creeping into health food stores as a sweetener, somewhat like molasses. Newest grain to appear is triticale, a cross between wheat and rye, which was not fully developed until the 1960s. Careful selection and chemical treatment by an alkaloid are necessary to produce the final plant which is slowly gathering popularity both as a whole grain and a flour. And rightly so, for it is nutritionally far superior to both wheat and rye. Triticale is found to contain at least 2 per cent more protein than wheat, with a better amino acid balance as a bonus.

Certain general nutritional factors of grains are worthy of note. They are classified as carbohydrate-rich foods, for their average carbohydrate content is 75 per cent, whereas protein content varies from 14 per cent for wheat down to just under 7 per cent for rice. As the protein is usually not well balanced, being low in the essential amino acid lysine, diets based on grains for both protein and carbohydrate needs, such as in many less-developed countries, prove inadequate over the long-term. Many people turn to grains for their ease of growing, storage and preparing, but too much emphasis is given to their use in the diet. They do have an important role, but are no substitute for essential proteins. If sprouted, grains do provide an increase in protein balance, as well as in all other nutrients, especially vitamin C (with a slight reduction in carbohydrate and kilojoule values). Their complex form of carbohydrate, when in the whole state, is valuable for digestive needs, especially in providing excellent sources of vital fibre. Buckwheat is the richest source of dietary fibre of any whole food, being 9.9 per cent, with millet next at 3.2 per cent and wheat at 2.3 per cent. Buckwheat is also the richest grain in calcium and magnesium and second highest grain in potassium and vitamins B_1 and B_3. Millet is second highest in fibre and magnesium, but highest in iron and in vitamins B_1 and B_2. Direct comparison of all grains favours buckwheat as the most nutritious, followed by millet, oats, wheat, rye and rice. Barley and corn are near the end of the list, along with semolina, the wheat residue remaining after refining and milling. Triticale has not undergone sufficient analyses to provide an overall nutritional guide, although it does head the protein list for grains — and probably will be found rich in many other minerals and vitamins.

It is essential to realise that many of the valuable nutrients are lost when a grain is refined. People should demand all the nutrients produced by nature, instead of permitting robbery. The comparison between unpolished and polished rice says everything. When rice has its husk removed, the resultant white product has lost 6 per cent of its protein, one-third of its calcium and between 40 per cent and 75 per cent of all other nutrients; a disgraceful application of industrial interference. Finally, it is important to note that the kilojoule content of whole grains is very similar to that of meats — the average of 1400 is identical to lamb chops, so this does not justify the argument that whole grains are "too fattening".

Honey Those who regard honey as a sugar substitute have their chronology in disarray. Honey has been a favourite sweetener since long before human history was first recorded. It is referred to in many of the ancient texts, including the Bible, and has long been considered both a natural sweetener and an indication of a wealthy household, when honey was offered among members and guests. Today, honey is available in abundance, although its cost is far higher than refined sugar cane. Perhaps it is for this reason that honey is generally regarded as the alternative to sugar. Compared to sugar, honey is around one and a half times sweeter, for it comprises more than sucrose — as well, it is composed of fructose and dextrose, in varying proportions, depending upon the variety of pollen taken in by the bee. These sugars comprise 80 per cent of the weight of honey; of the remainder, 19 per cent is water and acids, 0.5 per cent protein and the balance is small quantities of vitamins and minerals. Honey would be an acid-forming substance in the gastrointestinal tract from its content of sugars alone, but is doubly so with its content of carbonic and formic acids. In fact, it is these acids which tend to induce gastric disturbances if too much honey is ingested. These acids are too strong for the small mineral content of honey to negate their presence, implying an important reason for honey to be used only in very small amounts.

Honey should not be regarded as a true health food, for it does not provide any significant nourishment for human beings. It is a far better sweetener than sugar, and a natural one at that. But because an item is natural, its health-giving properties should not be automatically imputed — hemlock is a natural plant, but Socrates did not take it for a health food (it was the poison by which he was sentenced to die). Of the minerals contained in honey, iron is regarded as the most abundant in terms of human needs, but an adult would require 1.25 kg of honey to obtain his recommended daily allowance of iron from honey alone. B-complex is the only vitamin present in any quantity in honey — even so, an adult would require 6 kg of honey for his RDA. In terms of honey's sweetness, the amount of vital nutrients present is minimal and totally inadequate for balancing the sugar and acid content. However, honey is far better than refined sugar, which is 99.9 per cent sucrose with virtually no minerals and absolutely no vitamin content. No grade of sucrose contains vitamins, which is one of its deficiency problems, but brown sugar, with its molasses addition, offers minerals in greater quantity than does honey — yet its lack of fructose makes any form of sugar cane difficult to digest. So the sweeteners which are superior to honey are molasses and maple syrup, both of which are yet to be discussed.

Naturopathic and storage properties of honey make it an important item to have in the home. It can be kept indefinitely in a cool, dry place because it does not spoil and is a natural preservative. It can be successfully used to preserve fruits due to its bactericidal properties. It can also be successfully used in cake and bread making; being hygroscopic it retains a certain amount of moisture to delay dehydration. Honey will only spoil if mixed with water and allowed to stand — it will ultimately ferment, but only after many days, sometimes weeks. Honey's formic acid also aids its preservative qualities. When buying honey, avoid impure offerings, such as mixtures of sugar, corn syrup and glucose, for this only dilutes honey's already meagre nutritional properties. Look for labels stating the honey is untreated, for this indicates it has not been heated during extraction from the comb. To avoid crystallisation, keep honey out of the refrigerator; stand the jar in warm water if honey does become candied.

Kefir The technique of curdling milk as the means of preserving it emerged in many countries from ancient times, giving rise to what we now know as yogurt, buttermilk and kefir. Many other varieties were developed and are still in use, but these three appear to have migrated to the West and are attracting increasing levels of popularity. Yogurt far outdistances all others, yet kefir appears to be rapidly gaining in popularity, especially in the USA. Kefir appears to have taken its origin from pre-Muslim times, for its popularity was already established in the days of Mohammed. The name "kefir" derived from the Arabic "keif" or "kief", translated as "well-being" or "good humoured", implying the general bodily feeling deriving from the consumption of kefir. Muslims thought so highly of this clabbered milk that they closely guarded the secret of its preparation, although it is alleged that Marco Polo penetrated this veil on one of his Eastern journeys at the end of the thirteenth century. At that time, the Western world was not interested and remained so until the early nineteenth century when kefir was recorded as having been prescribed for the treatment of tuberculosis. For many years kefir and yogurt were used for T.B. sufferers, the reasons being unknown today, although the disease usually afflicted undernourished people who must have decidedly benefited from the dietary modification.

Kefir is easily made from whole milk allowed to sour naturally in warm weather, or by being heated in cold weather. The souring is usually accelerated by the aid of "grains", the tiny solid particles which settle to the bottom of kefir and are strained out for subsequent use — they can be dried and stored indefinitely. This souring is a form of fermentation which produces a small quantity of alcohol from the lactobacilli (around 1 per cent), plus lactic and carbonic acids and peptones, enzymes by which human digestion is aided in the stomach. Being a semi-liquid, kefir is favoured by many people as a nourishing drink, a mini-meal in effect, but it should be drunk very slowly — each mouthful should actually be chewed before swallowing. General nutritional properties of kefir are similar to those of yogurt.

Kelp Kelp is a collective name for varieties of large seaweeds. They have been gathered, dried and powdered for their valuable mineral content since the early part of the last century, when it was realised that the mineral content of human blood is somewhat similar to that of sea water. Dried and weathered (to dissolve excess sea salt) kelp has been used in organic farming fertilising for many centuries, but only in the twentieth century has it occurred to health-conscious people that many of these valuable trace minerals can be ingested directly from powdered kelp. Thus kelp has become one of the most sought-after health foods and is now available in many forms — powder, granules, tablets, and as a drink. Even more recently, followers of the Japanese-originating macrobiotic regimen have popularised kelp in other forms, such as flakes, in soups, etc., and in different varieties of kelp for varying nutritional properties.

In general, kelp is highly advantageous for its iodine content, which, when taken in suitable quantities, averts goitre. Other minerals present in kelp include aluminium, iron, sulphur and silicon (around 1 per cent each), calcium nearly 3 per cent, potassium at 12½ per cent and sodium 15 per cent. Other minerals are in trace quantities, including iodine, manganese, magnesium, copper, phosphorus, zinc, cobalt, strontium, nickel, chromium, barium, titanium, bismuth, vanadium, silver and molybdenum. Kelp is largely harvested off the coasts of Norway, Japan and California, where it is commercially grown in huge beds. People with sodium problems should exercise care in the amounts taken — a small amount used as a seasoning should not create any difficulty.

Kitchen Appliances Many health foods can be made and prepared in the home with suitable appliances. Too often, people regard the oven, hot plates, refrigerator and cooking utensils as constituents of the complete kitchen and in so doing overlook half a dozen other important small items. The most important of these is the blender, for it can chop, whip, mix, grate, juice, purée and blend a vast variety of foods. It can speedily make salad dressings, nut creams, blended salads (ideal for people with dental and many gastrointestinal problems), soya and nut milks, liquefy fresh fruits into nectars and a whole host of gourmet delights for those special occasions. When choosing a blender, you should ensure that it is equipped with a sufficiently strong motor to handle all needs — its power rating should be at least 1.4 amps (336 watts).

Next in importance is the juicer. No health-conscious person can afford to be without a juicer, for freshly made fruit and vegetable juices are so far superior to commercially extracted juices that there is really no comparison in nutritional properties. Analyses of fresh juices compared with canned or bottled reveal that preserved juices indicated losses of up to 50 per cent of the original nutrient, due to the cooking and oxidation which usually accompanies large-scale extraction methods. Nutrients to suffer most are usually the vitamins, although in some cases minerals are also reduced — to a greater or lesser extent, depending on the variety. Due to the unstable nature of juices, they must be freshly extracted and immediately consumed for maximum nutritional advantages. Alternatively, one should (if unable to afford a juicer) buy only those juices whose labels guarantee freedom from preservatives or additives. Juicing is no substitute for the whole food, on a regular basis, but it does offer some very important advantages for certain therapeutic and maintenance needs. For slimming, hyperacidity, gastrointestinal and toxicity problems, juices are highly suited in lieu of solid meals; as a prelude to fasting and as a means of breaking the fast, juices are invaluable. Two basic types of juicers are available — the centrifugal and the "throw-out" models. The former holds fibrous residues in a spinning basket from which another 10 per cent of juice will be extracted after the cutter has done its job. This is the best style to buy, although it is more expensive. Price makes throw-out models more popular, but they have the added disadvantage that they do not last as long; so ultimately this style might not be the cheaper.

For people who drink quantities of citrus juice, especially large families, a citrus press is a very useful appliance. It enables many oranges, grapefruit and/or lemons to be juiced rapidly, thereby avoiding nutritional losses from oxidation when full tumblers are desired. Manually operated citrus presses are sometimes available, but they are rather bulky and difficult to install in the average kitchen. The electric models are best, for they also allow the separated flesh of the fruit to be included. There is, however, one distinct disadvantage in drinking orange juice, rather than eating the whole fruit — the loss of vitamin P (the bioflavonoids found in the pith, under the skin). Other than this, freshly squeezed orange juice is far superior to bottled.

The electric nut and seed grinder, for many families, is as important as their juicer. This appliance is not yet as readily available in stores as are blenders and juicers, but with a little searching you will find one marketed as a coffee mill. It is a small appliance, usually no more than 15 cm high, with an efficient little motor drawing around 130 watts. It will grind nuts, seeds, grains and beans at the touch of the button — the duration of the grinding action determines the degree of fineness attained. Nuts and beans can be partially broken for easier chewing or steaming, respectively. Nuts and seeds can be made into a coarse powder for sprinkling over a salad, especially for people with dentures, tender gums, etc. Grains can be readily reduced to a coarse or fine flour for baking breads or similar items on this very useful grinder. Although it only takes small quantities, around ⅓ cup at a time, its speed will allow 1 kg of flour to be produced in a little over one minute without clogging or generating heat.

For people who want to grind large quantities of flour, or who might like to bake a large quantity of bread at one time and freeze some loaves for future use, a small stone mill will be an advantage in the kitchen. These are often custom-made to order, although, with the accelerating price of bread, we expect to see a resourceful manufacturer introduce a variety of domestic flour mills on to the market soon. Stone mills are preferable to steel cutters to avoid generated heat destroying vitamins C and B-complex. This appliance has a more limited application than a blender, juicer or nut grinder and is more suited for the kitchen that "has everything". The only drawback is that it can lead to consuming too much bread, so be careful not to become addicted, for bread is really only a second-rate food (see Stage 7).

The final recommendation in small kitchen appliances is a set of reliable weighing scales. These are certainly not essential, but for those who enjoy specialised cooking or baking, accurate measuring is important, especially with metrics still rather new in concept. Scales which measure up to 500 g are too limited; those which register up to 1 kg are preferable.

Lecithin The complex compound, lecithin, is a phospholipid — or, to put it more simply, a combination of the mineral phosphorus and fats. It occurs in every cell of the body and is best known for its components from the B-complex group of vitamins, choline and inositol, two vital nutrients without which the body would not properly digest fats. Lecithin is the body's natural emulsifier of fats, for its function is to reduce large concentrations of fat molecules into smaller, digestible ones. This "emulsifying" effect allows the body to efficiently utilise fats, prohibiting their build-up and that of cholesterol, in the bloodstream. Lecithin, therefore, is valuable in a most extensive range of applications even beyond the health food area — it is used in making commercial ice cream, salad dressings, cookies and sweets, animal foods, cosmetics and soaps, for blending oils, as an antioxidant, etc.

The processing of foods removes lecithin, thereby depriving the body of that vital component it seeks from its food to assist in fat catabolism. Chemically extracted, refined oils used in domestic and commercial food preparation are among the worst offenders. Natural whole foods abundant in lecithin are listed under the section on choline in Stage 8. When insufficient amounts of these foods are found in the diet, supplementary lecithin is essential. This can always be obtained from the health food store in granular, powder, liquid or tablet form — the choice being up to the consumer's preference, for they are all similarly effective. This lecithin has usually been extracted from soya beans, for these provide the least expensive and most extensive source. Lecithin is also extracted from eggs, corn and most vegetable seeds, as well as from animal sources, although this last is the least desirable for human consumption.

With obesity existing as a symptom of modern dietary overbalance, many people are instructed to reduce their food intake, usually also excluding nuts, seeds, eggs and avocados, some of the best natural sources of lecithin. Consequently, their diet becomes deficient in lecithin, resulting in insufficient break-down of saturated fats derived from animal foods. Inadequacy of lecithin will so contribute to a build-up of cholesterol and fatty deposits in vital bodily organs that the heart is forced to work harder to effect desirable blood circulation and yet the person will generally find his or her energy potential under par. With the fat held in large globules and cholesterol clogged arteries, insufficient energy is available to muscle tissues. Hypertension is a frequent consequence, as are gallstones, due to those fatty deposits being located in the gall bladder.

Therapeutically, lecithin is invaluable as treatment in the correction of gallstones, hypertension, arteriosclerosis, various heart problems (often indicated by early chest pains), skin and nerve disorders, and R.D.S. This last-named condition is Respiratory Disease Syndrome, a fatal lung malfunction of some infants, where the normal expansion of these new lungs is inhibited by insufficient lecithin in the mother's body and thus deprived to the foetus, resulting in suffocation. There exists no RDA for lecithin; however, when it is established, 1000 mg is likely to be the figure, with half for children. When therapeutic dosages are required, these can vary with the severity of the need to possibly as high as 5 or 10 grams.

Legumes This name refers to the fruit (seed) of a leguminous plant, an annual from which the seeds are harvested in pods. A wide variety of human foods are classified as legumes, including peas, beans, lentils and peanuts (which are often mistakenly classified as a nut). Common to legumes are their hardness, ease of storage, low moisture content and rounded, smooth surface. Nutritional factors common to legumes are their high levels of protein, carbohydrate, fibre, iron and potassium. Care must be exercised when choosing legumes to supply the diet with essential protein, for legumes are traditionally low in methionine, therefore they are not ideal as a staple protein for daily human use. Legumes have a slightly acid metabolic residue which also tends to make them less favourable than nuts and seeds as everyday protein sources. Although their vitamin B content is above average, most legumes need prolonged cooking, thereby losing some of their B-vitamins. Where possible, legumes are best sprouted, mung beans and lentils being the most suited. Cooked legumes create digestion problems for many people, peanuts do so for others — if this applies to you, avoid cooked legumes, for heat in cooking will destroy many of the legume's natural enzymes, as well as bind together some of the nutrients. Many legumes have been known components of the human diet for over 5000 years, generally originating in Europe or Asia. They were used to advantage in the colder northern climates where they could be stored for long periods without spoiling. But in warmer climates where year-round growing seasons prevail, legumes are not regarded as a frequent or important component of the diet.

Licorice The characteristic sweetness and black appearance of licorice is quite different from the original substance from which this flavour is taken. It is the root of the licorice plant, a perennial shrub which is native to the warmer parts of Europe and Central Aisa. So popular has the licorice flavour become in modern times that it is now extensively cultivated, especially in the USA. Its dark brown roots have a yellowish pulp inside, from which the juice is extracted and concentrated for a wide variety of uses. Although this extract possesses a natural sweetness, demands of modern confectionery-eaters induced manufacturers to add refined sugar to the famous licorice stick and log, so that they now contain up to 28 per cent unnatural sweetening. Some health food manufacturers of licorice use raw sugar, but this minor improvement does not justify its consideration as a health food. As a herb tea, licorice offers a very pleasant and natural sweetness with a refreshing after-taste, but it should not be drunk too often, unless one suffers from constipation. Licorice is also used in powder and tablet form to relieve constipation, as well as in cough and anti-bronchial mixtures and as a sweetener for many medical preparations, and sometimes in beer and tobacco.

Liver The liver is the detoxifying and manufacturing organ of the human and animal body. No animal or human can live without it — but when animals are slaughtered, many humans seek to eat their livers as a vitally nourishing food. Since 1934, this habit has been developing, following the Nobel Prize for medicine being awarded to three American physicians for their discovery that the cure for pernicious anaemia was to take large quantities of liver and/or by the injection of liver extract. At that time, no one knew exactly what property in liver brought about the recovery from pernicious anaemia, just that many patients died from the dread disease without supplemental liver, but that none died after taking it — in fact, many lived to quite advanced ages.

The citation accompanying the Nobel Prize credited the three with discovering the "cause and cure of pernicious anaemia", yet the cause has largely remained unknown. The nutrient effecting the "cure" was thought to be folic acid, but in 1946 this was abandoned in favour of vitamin B_{12} (of which liver is the richest known source). Since then, brewer's yeast and whole grain cereal foods have been recognised as excellent sources of B_{12}, although they do not possess the potency of liver extract injections, which remain necessary for advanced cases of pernicious anaemia. But now, when we look to the cause, we find we can avert such treatment, for no healthy person should ever need to take medicine or meat in any form. The cause of anaemia is related to a lack of balanced calmness, as opposed to the tension so pandemic in modern living. Tension inhibits the proper functioning of the gastrointestinal tract, so that the more complex nutrients and large food molecules (such as iron and B_{12}) are often not catabolised from the food. With modern food processing, many foods do not even contain a fraction of their original iron or B_{12}, so the deficiency creates an additional handicap, inducing a disease which was virtually unknown before this century.

Macrobiotic Foods The famous Japanese medical scientist, Sakurazawa Nyoiti (whose Westernised name is Georges Ohsawa), researched for half a century to develop a health system based on the practices of Zen Buddhist monks whose ancient traditions were credited with bringing long life and virility to their followers. A prolific writer, Ohsawa has exercised enormous influence on Westerners, particularly young people, since the publication in 1965 of his best-selling book, *You Are All Sanpaku*. The essence of his "Unique Principle" is the marriage of philosophy with the science and art of food preparation. The foods are ostensibly selected and prepared to produce longevity and rejuvenation (being vegetarian in nature) based on the yin/yang (acid/alkaline) balance. But being primarily a grain diet, it tends to induce its own nutritional imbalance — fruits are generally avoided, salt is extensively used, as are fermented foods and seaweeds. The diet was intended to be an eliminating (toxicity-reducing) regimen, which can be beneficial to those addicted to the Western tendency to consume processed foods; but its duration was intended to be no more than ten days. Many people have adopted the strict macrobiotic diet as their regular regimen and many suffer from its limitations. Most competent nutritionists recognise the macrobiotic diet's limitations for Western application, while not denying that it might have been therapeutically suitable to ancient Easterners (fasting, a juice diet or a totally alkaline fresh fruit and vegetable diet are far superior for detoxification).

Some of the macrobiotic foods offer abundant nourishment, particularly tahini and rice cakes (prepared only from lightly cooked puffed brown rice and selected added grains, such as buckwheat and millet, with sesame). Some of the macrobiotic beverages have beneficial properties, such as mu tea (based on selected herbs, including ginseng), bancha tea, lotus, mint and thyme teas. Other macrobiotic foods are better avoided, due to their preparation techniques of fermentation, and to the liberal use of sea salt. These foods include tamari, miso, gomasio, sea vegetables (kombu and hiziki), mebosi and unrefined sea salt. Some of these, in very small quantities, can be used as seasonings, but the concentration of salt is counter-productive to good health — certainly the human body needs some salt in its system, but this should be obtained as natural sodium chloride direct from foods such as celery, beetroot, tomatoes, etc., otherwise it can poison the body and predispose towards arthritis, gout, arterio-sclerosis, and so on.

Maple Syrup One of the sweetest products of agriculture, maple syrup derives from the sap of one of the 75 different varieties of maple trees, the bird's-eye maple. It is collected by tapping the sap of the tree about 1.5 metres above the ground, from where the flow gathers in buckets or runs through plastic lines direct to the "sugar house". This is done in early spring before the deciduous maple trees begin to flower. At the sugar house, the sap is run into a huge heated tank where it is evaporated from a natural moisture content of 67 per cent down to 33 per cent. This concentrates the natural sugar, destroys any bacterial content and allows the syrup to be bottled for future use. Maple syrup was discovered by American Indians before white man settled the country; but it did not take the early settlers long to discover this sweet syrup. When refined sugar was introduced into North America, the demand for maple syrup diminished. Now, with our advanced knowledge of the dangers of refined sugar, demand for maple syrup continues to rise; more and more maple trees are being planted in north-eastern USA and bordering Canada, the homes of maple syrup.

Pure maple syrup is more than a sweetener: it is a food as well. As with any food, care must be taken not to overindulge. Fortunately, two factors avert this — normal appetites cannot handle high quantities of sweet foods and will "turn off" when sufficient has been eaten; the high cost of maple syrup will economically limit the amount people will buy. But for those who seek the best in their food choices, pure maple syrup will be included in their shopping list and used as a sweetener whenever one is required. As opposed to cane sugar, pure maple syrup contains natural minerals which aid its digestion — iron, calcium and potassium, in particular. It is lower in calories and in carbohydrates than both sugar and honey, although it has slightly lower B-vitamins than honey. The sugar content of maple syrup is 96 per cent sucrose — although this is the same as cane sugar, the accompanying minerals (plus many other trace minerals) vitally aid the body's breakdown of this disaccharide so that it is far more easily digested than cane or beet sugars. Although raw maple sap is clear and colourless, maple syrup takes on a brownish appearance, as does cane sugar when extracted and heated. The refining of cane sugar also bleaches it, whereas maple syrup is allowed to retain its colour. Maple syrup has the further advantage over cane sugar in its virtual lack of acidity in the human gastrointestinal tract (this is also an advantage over honey), for the pH range of maple syrup is from 6.8 to 7.3 — from close to neutral to slightly alkaline. Consequently, maple syrup presents no danger to tooth enamel.

Wherever the expression "maple syrup" has been used in the foregoing, it refers only to pure, condensed sap of the maple tree. Several brands of imitation maple syrup — "maple-like" or "maple-style" syrups, or those bold and immoral enough to not even indicate on the label that the contents are less than pure maple syrup — can be found in supermarkets (and occasionally even in health food stores which are not living up to their names). These products are either partially maple syrup with a majority of corn or cane sugar syrup added to lower the cost, or are totally devoid of pure maple syrup, using the imitation products with imitation maple colouring and flavouring, both of which are derivatives of coal tar, a possible carcinogen. Many restaurants engage in this fraud, compromising their conscience with an exaggerated cost consciousness. So much manual work is involved in the collecting, bottling and packaging of maple syrup, plus the costs of storing it for most of the year, of transporting it over long distances, that its comparatively high cost can be readily understood. We must also recognise that it does not attract any government subsidies, as does sugar cane — instead, it attracts a customs duty on importation, further adding to its cost, for the duty is imposed on the importer's cost. So when you see a pure maple syrup in your health food store, you know that you are looking at a very special sweetener, the only one which is also a food; and for that, there is no price comparison.

Margarine Numerous health problems associated with too many saturated fats in the diet have brought greater awareness in the choice of unsaturated fats, an awareness which is growing with increasing numbers of people suffering from heart attacks and hypertension. Butter is one of the foods to suffer, but its loss has been margarine's gain. Although margarine has been known for over a century, being originally made in 1870 in France from beef fat, it was only in this century that vegetable oils were used in its manufacture, to provide an alternative to butter. But even then, the process by which these oils were rendered solid for table use (hydrogenation) effectively saturated them, thereby negating their primary advantage. In the 1970s, scientists evolved a method (inter-esterification) by which margarine could be made solid without saturating its oils. This method is now in common use, resulting in margarine becoming the health-food counterpart of butter, as recommended by most health practitioners. But this practitioner is an exception. My preference is to avoid those foods with added vitamins, preservatives, antioxidants and chemically extracted oils — in general, to avoid manufactured foods. In the optimum health diet, bread is only occasionally eaten, being a portion of only one or two meals a week, so the preference should be to have the most nourishing spread on the bread — this is unequivocally avocado, nature's fruit source of natural fats. Alternatively, raw nut butters can be used, almond and cashew butters being far superior to peanut butter. In cooking, cold-pressed oils can be substituted whenever margarine or butter are recommended in the recipe. So, only for those whose habits addict them to a yellowish thick spread over their bread, should margarine be the alternative to butter for the sake of their health.

Milk Powders These cannot be regarded as health foods, but are included to shed light on oft-expressed misunderstandings. When asked if they drink milk, many of my patients have replied, "no, never". In subsequent dietary discussion, it is revealed that they use skim milk powder in their drinks or full cream milk powder in their cooking. While not intending to deceive, they actually fall victim to industry's deception in making believe that some magical health properties attend milk in its liquid or powdered form; and that skim milk is even more so. Please refer to Stage 6 for more about the "menace of milk", for its contributions to child and adult colonic, bronchial and respiratory problems are legion. Milk powders are potentially more dangerous because they hoodwink the consumer into a false sense of safety, yet they often result in greater concentrations of milk entering the body than if liquid milk were used. Do not believe that because fat is removed all problems associated with milk in the diet are corrected, for the casein (milk protein) is no less of a problem for the rennin-devoid human stomach to catabolise. Soya powder as soya milk is a far better product to use; even goat's milk or goat's milk powder presents somewhat of an improvement on cow's milk in any form.

Nuts The "eminent" nutritional scientist from Harvard University who is quoted throughout America as saying: "If you eat nuts, you are nuts" is rather quiet these days. Not that he has undertaken further research into foods to discover that nuts are, indeed, one of the richest and most nutritious natural foods available to man (he could have read that in Genesis 1:29), but recently he lost a very expensive court action for slandering the health-food industry. In so doing, he gained his most valuable nutritional education and, maybe, will now eat nuts more often than at Christmas. That people should limit their intake of nuts to the Christmas period or when they drink hard liquor is indicative of the general level of ignorance of this important nutrient source.

Nuts are seeds of large trees, packed with all the nutrients needed to produce another tree of the species. As food for man, nuts are highly concentrated sources of most valuable nutrients. Possessing minimal water (around 5 per cent only), they contain high concentrations of major nutrients, making nuts one of the most economical food sources per nutrient content. When compared with meat on a cost and nutrient basis, nuts win convincingly. The protein quantities are similar to meat, but nut proteins are easier to digest, being present in simpler peptide chains, therefore easier for the gastric juice to catabolise. The fat content of nuts averages 1½-times to twice that of average meat (yet equal to that of bacon), but nuts possess far greater quantities of unsaturated fatty acids than meat. Whereas meat contributes to man's cholesterol problems, nuts are totally free of cholesterol. Most meats are completely devoid of carbohydrate and dietary fibre (among the many causes of constipation and hypoglycaemia), whereas nuts are rich in complex carbohydrates, especially fibre. Nuts are richer than meats in calcium, phosphorus and magnesium (the vital bone-building minerals); they are also richer in potassium and iron. As with meat, nuts contain no vitamin C, so must be eaten with foods rich in this digestion-assisting vitamin. Nuts are also excellent sources of B-complex vitamins.

Being so low in moisture content, nuts have excellent storage qualities. So long as they are held in a cool, dry spot, they can keep fresh in sealed containers for many years. The problems which beset nuts when exposed to high temperatures are rancidity and weevil infestation. Rancidity occurs when fatty acids are exposed to atmospheric oxygen, a slow process of combining which is rapidly accelerated by heat. This danger is created when nuts are roasted or baked, especially when they are fried with other fats (which have often been reheated, and are therefore potentially carcinogenic); simultaneously, vitamin destruction occurs and some of the amino acids are coagulated. In commercial processing, chemical deodorisers, preservatives, dyes and bleaches are employed, significantly altering the organic nature of nuts — not a pretty chemical picture! Common salt is then sometimes added to compound a dietary felony, but salt induces thirst and the more people drink, the more profit is made by the beverage industries (which display a frightening disregard for human health).

Most popular of all nuts are almonds, and rightly so, for they are among the most nutritious and certainly are the most alkalising. Then come cashews, Brazils, pinenuts, pistachios, hazelnuts and walnuts. Peanuts are legumes, not nuts, but are not as easily digested as nuts; however, many people buy them because they cost less (you get what you pay for!) Macadamia and pecan nuts are classified as concentrated fats, rather than proteins, due to their exceptionally high fat contents and comparatively low protein values — 71 per cent and 7½ per cent respectively.

If nuts are too hard for some people to chew, the use of a grinder or blender offers an excellent solution. Buying nuts in the shell can ensure a fresher kernel, but it is uncertain how old the stock might be or what quality it is. Most people prefer to buy kernels from health food stores with a large turnover, thereby ensuring the freshest stock — although nuts crop only once a year, the method of their storage is a major determinant in their freshness, refrigeration being the best method. Almonds are offered as "naturals", with skins retained, or blanched, slivered or sliced, with the skins chemically removed. It is therefore best to buy naturals and to skin them just before eating — many people eat them with skins intact, but a better flavour is obtained when skinned, due to the tannic acid present in the covering. To remove almond skins, steep them in boiling water for two minutes, rinse under cold water, then the skins will pop off (the boiling water will not affect their nutrients in that short time). Cashews always come clear of their skins, for these are removed at the same time as shelling. There are two methods of shelling — the African and the Indian. The African method is by far the better, for it is largely hand-laboured, retaining most of the nuts' freshness, nutrients and flavour. The Indian method is by roasting the nuts, causing the shell to split, and then extracting the kernel, leaving the nut nutritionally poorer for the prolonged heating (it is also softer and less flavoursome). African cashews are always the best to ask for, although they are often a little more expensive.

Nut butters make nutritious spreads for breads, crackers, etc. They are not intended as replacements for nuts in the diet, for they do not have the full protein values of the whole nuts. To be ground into a butter, nuts must be mixed with a moderate quantity of oil, otherwise they would become far too hot in the grinding process and would not be ground into the smooth paste for which people ask. Usually peanut oil is used and, if the processor is highly reputable, it will be cold-pressed oil. Large processors, not concerned with health foods, will possibly use cheaper oils, which will most certainly be chemically extracted. This is the main reason that health food stores sell nut butters at higher prices than supermarkets, for the supermarket brand rarely matches the quality.

Phenylalanine This is one of the essential amino acids, required by the body for its manufacturing of the hormones adrenalin and thyroxine, as well as the colouring (melanin) in hair and skin. Amazingly, it is one of the two essential amino acids (tryptophan being the other) to have recently surfaced in researches for natural nutrients with therapeutic properties. Phenylalanine has been discovered to provide the body with natural stimulation, overcoming lethargy and depression, and to induce a balanced feeling of natural well being, when taken in therapeutic dosages of up to 2000 mg in special cases. A usual dose of 1000 mg will assist most people through emotional troughs, all the while providing only vital nutrition for the body with absolutely no side effects. This style of research presages a great change of direction in therapeutic treatment and a timely departure from drug dependency. However, care has to be taken that, when this nutrient becomes readily available on the local market, the health-conscious consumer chooses the natural, rather than the synthetic phenylalanine. The natural product is extracted from fibrin and albumin protein sources and is denominated "L-Phenylalanine". Its synthetic counterpart is chemically similar, but organically inferior, being synthesised from alpha-acetaminocinnamic acid and denominated "DL-Phenylalanine". The synthetic product will, of course, be cheaper.

Pollen Bee pollen has been known to possess remarkable nutritional, healing and therapeutic properties since before recorded history, yet medical science remains largely unaware of it. Drawn from the flowers of many plants, pollen comprises the male sperm cells which are deposited in the hive as food by bees. After being robbed from beehives, pollen is gathered by the apiarist and sent for dehydration into a fine powder (for use in making pollen tablets); some being granulated for therapeutic use as is. Bee pollen is possibly one of the richest foods ever known and is closely guarded in the hive by the worker bees, so its extraction can be far from easy, giving some reason for the very high cost and low quantity of this item.

A chiropractor and friend of mine had suffered for years from hay fever. Each springtime was misery for him. Although a leader in his profession, he could not overcome his constant sneezing, nose-drip and irritating sinusitis. Early one spring, I asked him to do me a favour and take two tablets thrice daily of pollen. He did, and within ten days his hay fever had virtually disappeared. He was astounded and proceeded to recommend this "miraculous" treatment to all his chiropractic patients with hay fever. All had partial or total improvement. Pollen is indeed most effective in building up the body's resistance to hay fever by antibody growth — an important tip for medical doctors who will no longer need to resort to drugs for relief. Other benefits ascribed to bee pollen, although not as yet proved, include the arresting and elimination of breast cancer, correction of prostate disorders, improvement of digestion and nutrient assimilation by the soothing of any inflammation in the gastrointestinal tract. The invert sugar contained in pollen is rapidly assimilated from the human gastrointestinal tract, thereby giving prompt nourishment to stimulate muscular action. This can be most beneficial to athletes and is also utilised by the bowel and rectum to improve peristalsis and minimise constipation. Bee pollen is known to stimulate reproductive glands of the body, by which life expectancy is increased, as is attested in the Soviet Republics of Central Asia; it also feeds the skin's glands to improve skin tone and appearance.

Very little further reading on pollen is available; few health or medical books even make reference to it. However, in 1978, Keats Publishing of Connecticut released an excellent little book entitled, *Bee Pollen and Your Health*, by Carlson Wade, the famous American health researcher. Most of the current research into bee pollen and its therapeutic properties are presented therein.

Protein Supplements The health food market offers many varieties of protein supplements. These are usually in powder form, although wafer and tablet varieties are also available. Some offer 70 per cent protein, others go higher — some as high as 95 per cent. Great care should be exercised in selecting a protein supplement to ensure that its ingredients are totally digestible; otherwise, the purchase price can be wasted. A supplement of such a high protein concentration will be quite expensive and must be suitable to the body for value to be obtained from the financial outlay. Unfortunately, most protein supplements are based on milk powder and, while milk is a complete protein, the human stomach has difficulty in catabolising it without prior coagulation. There is a strong tendency for this high concentration of milk protein to stimulate the stomach into manufacturing huge quantities of mucus, some of which will find its way into the respiratory system to create discomfort, maybe havoc. Concerned and knowledgeable health food manufacturers are recognising these problems and developing non-milk high protein supplements, usually based on soya protein, with added lecithin and methionine to provide a suitable balance of essential amino acids. A protein food must contain all essential amino acids to be its most effective — a shortage of one or more will render the body unable to assimilate the others by the proportionate degree.

Protein supplementation implies additional protein concentration, intended for people who are performing above-average muscular work (such as in sports, body-building or manual labour), thereby requiring a protein intake beyond the normal capacity of their stomach to handle in general food form. Supplementation is not intended to replace normal protein food intakes — only to "add to". These supplements can be made more effective by adding to them a dessertspoonful each of brewer's or torula yeast and powdered lecithin; some people go further and add a raw egg yolk or two (do not use the white, for it is indigestible when raw). Care should be exercised in taking only as much supplementation as the body requires, for protein cannot be stored; too much, therefore, will only overtax the liver in breaking it down into fat and carbohydrate for storage and future use.

Rice Bran Syrup When whole grain rice is trapped in a refining mill, it is stripped of its outer garments to be paraded before the world in its nude, white body. Thus it is offered as white, refined rice and sold to people around the world who mistakenly believe they are getting a nourishing food. But there is more nourishment in the "clothes" (bran) they left behind. Rice bran is so rich in alkalising minerals that it is actually better to eat the bran than the white rice. When we compare the nutritional properties of whole grain rice with polished (refined) rice, we find that far more than half the nutrients are contained in the bran. The only major nutrient to escape this separation is protein, for only 6 per cent of original protein is in the bran — but the protein in the white rice cannot be properly metabolised with such a deprivation of other essential nutrients. Of total nutrients in whole rice, the bran contains 70 per cent of the fat, 67 per cent of fibre, 40 per cent of calcium, 60 per cent phosphorus and iron,

49 per cent potassium, 68 per cent magnesium, 75 per cent vitamin B_1, 40 per cent vitamin B_2 and 65 per cent vitamin B_3, plus almost 100 per cent silicon. It is this silicon, plus the vitamin B_3, which gives rice bran such a potent therapeutic role. By a low-heat process, rice bran is converted into a syrup which is used to great advantage for people suffering skin complaints (psoriasis, acne, etc.). It is also valuable for mental and emotional patients, or as a good general uplifting tonic.

Salad Dressings Special inclusion of this category in Health Foods has been necessitated because so many people ask about various salad dressings and mayonnaise — whether they are nutritious, fattening, contain cholesterol, and what they can safely add to their salad to give it extra flavour. True, many of today's fresh foods seem to have less natural flavour than we remember from the pre-war days — this should convince us to return to organic agriculture! The added flavour for a salad can come from a little lemon juice and/or apple cider vinegar, or a light sprinkling of cold-pressed oil; some prefer a dusting of vegetable salt on their salad. All these are suitable in small quantities, but some people like to go further and add a virtual combination of all these — and this is what forms the bases for good salad dressings, the types sold in health food stores. Their common ingredients are cold-pressed soya oil, distilled water, sea salt, honey, lemon, apple cider vinegar and selected spices. To this base, the addition of puréed tomatoes, a little dried garlic and vegetable gum makes a healthy French dressing. Alternatively, garlic and other spices can be added to the base ingredients to make Italian dressing. Another variety is obtained from adding only selected dried herbs to the base, resulting in herb dressing. And by adding egg yolks to the base, mixing thoroughly and allowing to set, we have a delicious and nourishing soya mayonnaise.

Certainly, people dedicated to eating only natural foods will not agree that these salad dressings are needed — and if they enjoy their salad without them, so much to their credit. But many people prefer the extra flavour, especially those recently weaned from the modern diet of processed and highly flavoured (artificially) foods. They, at least, have a range of healthy dressings from which to choose, and to make in their kitchens if they prefer. People who regard their health as being at least as important as their car (who would never consider putting anything but the ideal grade of petrol into the car's fuel tank), should avoid buying the commercial salad dressings beckoning from supermarket shelves. To make a check of the labels will not reveal the total picture: that solvent-extracted oils have been used, as has malt vinegar, common salt, town water (with its full load of chemicals), plus chemicals of colour, preservation and flavour (including monosodium glutamate). This hotch-potch of unnatural ingredients can be conveniently disguised when the strong flavour of malt vinegar is present, permitting cheap and often unstable ingredients to be included. With these must be added a chemical stabiliser "to protect flavour", the label will sometimes admit. And the chemical used is often the same as that used in most frozen foods, a potentially dangerous compound called EDTA (ethylene-diamine-tetra-acetic acid), which has the effect of destroying many of the mineral nutrients (such as calcium, manganese and zinc). Although EDTA is officially described as having a *"low toxicity"* (why have any toxicity?), it is also used as a scouring agent and metal cleanser, among other things, in industry. Perhaps this will make us realise that these manufactured, preserved and frozen "foods" are best avoided, especially these days with so much fresh, nourishing food available.

Salt On numerous occasions throughout this book, salt has been revealed as a dangerous ingredient in the human diet. The body will extract all the sodium chloride

(NaCl) it needs from fresh vegetables, especially celery, beetroot, carrots and tomatoes, together with dried fruits, egg yolk and brewer's yeast. Adding common salt or sea salt in cooking or to table food is inviting health problems and inducing an unnatural thirst which interferes with protein catabolism. But the reason for its inclusion here is to debunk the theory, again, that salt in certain forms can be a health food. It is only healthy to the bank accounts of the salt processors. Whether it is in one of its many macrobiotic forms, or as simple sea salt, it should be excluded from human intake in this crude form. Sea salt does have some external therapeutic benefits, such as bathing sore eyes, and in this practice it is far better than common table salt. By its very nature, NaCl is hygroscopic — it attracts and absorbs moisture. If not treated, it will clog and fail to pour. So a chemical must be added to permit free-flowing. Common salt is usually mined from ground deposits and has mixed with it the chemical sodium silica aluminate, a by-product of refining bauxite into aluminium — hardly a suitable substance for human ingestion! By contrast, sea salt is dehydrated from the ocean and to this is added merely 0.5 per cent magnesium carbonate, a part of dolomite and a highly suitable compound for human digestion (in fact, it is the only component of domestic NaCl with nutritional properties).

Many forms of commercial "vegetable salt" offered on the health food market possess varying amounts of sea salt, averaging 50 per cent. This, of course, helps maintain a low cost price, but the compromise is not commendable. Vegetable salt should only comprise the concentrated and powdered extracts of vegetables and other suitable plant substances, such as herbs, grains, yeast and dried fruits. Together, these provide a powdered seasoning which can also be used as a winter broth base, free of added NaCl. Dr Bernard Jensen of California developed this combination and discusses its merits on many of his world-wide lecture tours. He is one of the many nutritionists now advising strongly against the use of common salt in the diet, recognising this habit as fundamental to the increase in hardened arteries, gout and arthritis, to name but a few health problems on the increase today.

Seeds Whereas nuts are the large fruit-seeds of trees, by which the tree will provide for the propagation of its species, seeds are classified as the propagation fruit of smaller plants. They are therefore endowed with significant nutritional properties which have been recently "rediscovered". Yet there are many modern esteemed nutrition and health text books among whose pages not a word of mention is given to the nutritional properties of seeds — implying that a far wider appreciation of these latent forces has yet to be recognised by the medical establishment. Of particular interest to us now are those seeds with proven dietary benefits — pepitas, safflower, sesame, sunflower and linseed. Most notable nutritional aspects of these seeds are their high protein values, together with generous amounts of most other major nutrients to guarantee their wider future recognition as vital concentrated foods for every race of people, particularly those currently suffering from malnutrition, whether it be the underfed people in Zaire and Bangladesh or the overfed people of America and Australia.

Pepitas are Mexican pumpkin seed kernels, grown today just as they were over a thousand years ago by the ancient Mayans, who first recognised their nutritional benefits. Pepitas are the propagating seeds of giant gourd-type pumpkins which grow prolifically throughout the Yucatan, the peninsular state of Mexico which juts out to separate the Caribbean Sea from the Gulf of Mexico. Today, native Mexicans gather the huge vegetables and manually extract their seeds, just as was done by the Mayans. The kernels (pepitas) are then extracted by mechanical hulling (a faster process than the Mayans employed!), they are washed in chlorinated water to remove any bacterial attachments, dried and ready to eat. Pepitas provide one of the richest sources of natural protein available in any whole food (29 per cent); they are also the richest source of phosphorus and of iron in any whole food (1144 mg and 11.2 mg respectively per 100 g pepitas). With a nice balance of B-complex vitamins and of minerals, pepitas are a veritable gold-mine of nutritional wealth just awaiting "discovery" by conventional dietitians and medicos.

Sunflower seeds are probably the most familiar of all edible seeds, being the tightly packed core of those glorious sunflowers growing prolifically throughout temperate climates around the world. No parrot ever read a book on nutrition, yet its instinct directs its flight to sunflower heads to voraciously feed upon the seeds. (In fact, sunflowers grown around an orchard or grain paddock will keep parrots away from maturing fruit or grain, for they far prefer sunflower seeds.) Many varieties of sunflower seeds have been propagated, the larger kernels being used for edible purposes, the smaller for crushing into edible oil. No other treatment than decorticating (hulling) is necessary for the kernels to be ready for human consumption. While not quite as high in protein, phosphorus and iron concentrations as are pepitas, sunflower kernels are well above average in these three nutrients (24-26 per cent, depending on variety, 837 mg and 7.1 mg per 100 g respectively). Sunflower kernels are very rich sources of B-complex vitamins, especially B_1 at 1.96 mg and B_3 at 5.4 mg. Their potassium is also high at 920 mg per 100 g.

Sesame seeds are probably the oldest of all cultivated seed crops, having been recorded growing wild in biblical lands. They have featured in Arab writings and have been highly regarded as a food throughout Asia since ancient Hindu days — and possibly earlier. Their hard husk must be removed prior to consumption, for it is abrasive on the intestines and rather bitter, due to its high concentration of oxalic acid. The husk is also very rich in calcium, iron and vitamin B_1, but these are unfortunately non-extractable by human digestive means. The calcium is used to combine with the oxalic acid, when sesame seeds are eaten whole, to protect the kidneys from the strong acid; but this causes the formation of sharp crystals of calcium oxalate which develop into urinary "gravel" and stones. Sesame seeds are reputed to be one of the richest sources of calcium, but this error must be corrected, for the kernel (the only edible part) offers only 110 mg — a reasonable amount, but insufficient to be regarded as "rich". Although sesame seed kernels are a reasonably nourishing food, they do not rate as highly as the other seeds, except in vitamin B_3, in which they are as rich as sunflower seeds.

However, sesame seeds provide the most highly prized of cooking oils, for it has the finest flavour and the highest boiling point. From the health viewpoint, this latter quality is important, for it indicates that less molecular restructuring takes place in sesame oil than any other. Another important and highly regarded use of sesame seeds is in the production of tahini. This Mid-Eastern "butter" is merely sesame seeds ground to form a thick paste for use on breads, as a salad dressing or as a base for a savoury dip. It is quite nutritious, when only pure raw sesame seeds are used, but loses some of its potential nourishment when the seeds are roasted prior to grinding. If this has been done, it will be noticeable by a darker variety of tahini; it will also be a little cheaper, being easier to grind when roasted. Tahini is usually imported from Israel or Lebanon.

Safflower seeds have similar nutritional properties to sesame, rather than to sunflower. The plant has a smaller and more orange-coloured flower than sunflower and is grown almost entirely for its lipid properties. Safflower oil possesses the highest linoleic acid content of any edible oil, being one of the most polyunsaturated. The nutritional value of linoleic acid rocketed to prominence in the late 1960s when a series of medical and scientific journals grasped the findings of researchers who proved how this fatty acid was of benefit by lowering serum cholesterol levels in laboratory animals and humans. From virtual obscurity (except in Egypt and surrounding countries where safflower has been known for centuries), safflower oil became a best-seller within a few years. This is no wonder, with its linoleic acid content averaging 72 per cent. Nearest to it is sunflower oil with 63 per cent, corn oil 53 per cent, soya oil 52 per cent, wheat germ oil 50 per cent, sesame oil 42 per cent. (Peanut and olive oils have higher levels of oleic acid, a mono-unsaturated fatty acid; not as useful to the body as linoleic.) Linoleic acid was also discovered to promote an improved availability of calcium to the body's cells, thereby virtually acting as a vitamin — some scientists refer to it as "vitamin F". Another valuable source of linoleic acid is linseed oil. Linseed is the seed of the flax plant and has a valuable therapeutic role for people suffering from colonic problems, but is otherwise rarely used for edible purposes.

Slippery Elm Powder   This is one health food which is not needed today, in fact, we are better off without it, ecologically speaking. The powder is ground from the white inner bark of a variety of beautiful American elm tree (*Ulmus fulva*). Obviously, the removal of this inner bark will kill the tree, a 15 metre beauty which is already being decimated by Dutch elm disease throughout North America. Many extravagant and unsupported claims have been made for the properties of slippery elm powder, from creating a spontaneous abortion to renewing the lining of the gastrointestinal tract. The active property of the bark is a mucilaginous matter which, when mixed with water, can provide a delightfully soothing coating for the entire alimentary canal — from the throat to the anus. Any ulcerated, irritated or inflamed component can be benefited from slippery elm powder, for it has the same effect as linseed. So why not take linseed? Virtually whatever slippery elm can do, linseed can do for the relief of gastrointestinal problems. Let the elm trees live — and let us live without slippery elm powder. Even better: eat only nutritious foods, properly combined and sensibly prepared, thereby avoiding gastrointestinal problems totally.

Soap   While certainly not a health food, in the strict sense, soap is a much misunderstood commodity that can exert a definite influence on the health of the skin. Avoiding the chemical aspects of soap and its functioning, we shall consider the two styles and why one is to be greatly preferred over the other. The original styles of soap were made from vegetable oils, usually coconut. Then competition, chemicals and commerce entered the scene and varieties were introduced with differing perfumes, consistencies, colourings and physical characteristics. As chemicals became more abundant and easily synthesised, they became cheaper; so the more chemicals could be used, the lower the cost of the end product. Now we find that most soaps available through general outlets contain a relatively high percentage of chemical ingredients. Some are even devoid of vegetable oils, using instead animal oils or fats (stearic, palmitic and/or oleic acids). So soap in which chemicals or animal products are used is incompatible with healthy living techniques.

Soap made from pure coconut oil, or a mixture of coconut and olive oils, without any form of chemical addition, is by far the best for human skin. Some varieties have the addition of wheat germ oil or peppermint oil — these are quite acceptable and, in fact, improve the lathering and fragrance of the soap. Olive oil is used when liquid soap (such as Castile) is required. This is an excellent shampoo — far superior to any chemical-based shampoo. In 1972 when in Acapulco, I "discovered" a pure coconut soap in the market, selling very cheaply, for it was locally made and unpackaged. This soap was found to be ideal for washing the body, washing clothes, shampooing; and it lasted for longer than the commercial soaps supplied on board ship. This same soap is now being packaged in Texas and is available in many countries, thanks to American initiative. The sole purpose of body soap is cleansing; it should not injure the skin in any way. Those suffering from any skin ailment can often discover how easily chemical-based soaps are guilty of this; they should be especially careful in their choice.

Spirulina One of the oldest and, botanically, simplest of all foods has recently been rediscovered. Spirulina is a tiny marine lifeform, visible as green-blue algae, and yet is a whole food. It is a sea vegetable, known by the general name of plankton, found throughout the world's oceans where it provides the primary natural diet for most of the higher forms of marine life. With its highly efficient photosensitivity, spirulina cells reproduce rapidly to provide a veritable never-ending source of nourishment, so long as its basic nutrient needs are met, foremost of which is carbon dioxide (returning oxygen to the atmosphere, as do all plants). Since its recent discovery (in 1964) by Western scientists, spirulina has undergone more research than almost any other food in the history of nutrition. It was rapidly recognised as the potential answer to an ever-increasing shortage of world food supplies. Spirulina has been found in inland lakes, growing there as readily as in the ocean, and is now being extensively cultivated in the Mexican highlands, Japan, Israel and Thailand, with farms now being established in the USA. It is the most easily grown, harvested and produced "whole" food currently available. As its production increases, so will its cost diminish, until eventually it will also be the least expensive form of food available.

Spirulina can be constantly harvested — one of its wonders. Next, it is pasteurised at 70°C for up to twenty minutes. It is then spray-dried so that it can be offered as a fine powder or compressed into tablet form. Its nutritional properties are eye-opening! Protein content varies from 50 per cent to 70 per cent of the dried powder, including all essential amino acids and most of those classified as "non-essential"; twenty-one in all are contained in spirulina. Its relatively high concentration of methionine and moderate offering of lysine suggest that spirulina is an ideal protein supplement for those who erroneously depend on beans and other legumes, or on grains, for their primary protein supply. Spirulina offers an almost immediate energy source to the body, for its carbohydrates are primarily in the form of glycogen, saving the body the time and energy of converting from starches and complex sugars (polysaccharides), as would be required from land plants. Spirulina is also credited with containing the entire B-complex vitamin group, in high concentration, especially vitamin B_{12}. This much sought-after nutrient has twice the concentration in spirulina (150 μg per 100 g) as in liver. It is also rich in vitamins A and C, as well as all known minerals, especially calcium, iron, phosphorus, potassium, magnesium and zinc.

Current total production of spirulina is estimated at just under 1000 tonnes annually, but demand is certain to accelerate this. Spirulina is the most space- and time-conserving crop ever known. It requires no soil, only open sea or enclosed pond systems to double its weight every few days. It can produce the same amount of protein as soya beans in one-twentieth (5 per cent) of the surface area, needs virtually no processing and has an unlimited shelf life, on present indications. Meanwhile, for people who seek protein supplementation with minimum processing, free from animal or legume sources, spirulina is ideal.

TVP: Textured Vegetable Protein In the 1960s when meat became expensive and soya beans were cheap, a resourceful food processing organisation in Illinois, USA, completed its extensive research and developed a non-meat protein food to look and taste just like meat. They called it "Textured Vegetable Protein", registering the name, which today still belongs to A.D.M. — Archer Daniels Midland Co. Being addicted to meat as their only reliable source of protein, many people sought to have their "meat" but be free from the health problems then associated with meat — for we were then in the midst of the fashion of blaming animal foods solely for the heart problems raging throughout the Western world. And cholesterol was the guilty party. Many people endeavoured to develop a new diet, without meat. For them, TVP became the vital transition which led many to a natural foods diet. For others, TVP was a tasty, occasional alternative to meat; for some, it was a fun food by which to fool their guests who thought they were eating meat. Processed meat manufacturers and hamburger makers had a field day — TVP was so much cheaper than meat and they could use it as an "extender" without diminishing the protein value of their meal (that was only to comply with government regulations — the processors really did not care so much about nutrition, nor did most of the consumers). So TVP became established; and it still sells, stimulated by increasing prices of meat with no increase in the price of TVP.

The nutritional properties of TVP derive from soya beans. The soya flour undergoes cooking, mixing and extruding to provide the various shapes and sizes in which TVP can be purchased. In the mixing process, flavourings, seasonings and colourings are added to compose the desired finished product. The processing methods are kept highly secret, but it would appear that the primary flavouring used is glutamic acid, by which the "beef" flavour is obtained. To what extent chemicals are used is unknown, but we do know that the final product is highly acceptable as a meat alternative to most people. It is devoid of cholesterol and almost fat-free. When cooked, its average protein concentration is 16 per cent and this includes the added methionine, necessitated by soya beans' natural deficiency in this essential amino acid. Thus, TVP contains a reasonable balance of all essential amino acids, making it a complete protein food, although not to be preferred over nuts or seeds.

Tryptophan One of the eight essential amino acids, tryptophan has recently been discovered to have another important property. When taken in megadoses, it will relax the brain, calm the muscles and induce restful sleep. In the course of normal utilisation within the body, tryptophan is converted into vitamin B_3 by the liver if sufficient other B-vitamins are present, but only after the body's primary needs (blood clotting, nourishment of digestive and optic systems, and the brain's action of using it to synthesise serotonin) have been satisfied. Vitamin B_3 nourishes both brain and nerves, while serotonin works between the two as the neuro-transmitter, the natural chemical which relays messages between nerve cells and the brain. The nerve system in most people is being constantly overworked, thereby creating one of the major causes of insomnia. Tryptophan ensures that the brain sends messages to the nerves to calm down, and it appears that the more serotonin, the more the nerves are sedated and the sooner sleep is induced. Not enough research has yet been undertaken to define categorical guidelines as to how much tryptophan is required, for this aspect of its use is relatively new. However, being a vital nutrient and with the liver ready and capable to convert excesses to B_3, tryptophan has never been found to create a problem with excess intake. For this reason, tryptophan tablets usually come in 500 mg size, allowing 2–4 to be taken before bed (at least half an hour before) without any adverse side-effects — only benefits. Contrary to drug-type tranquillisers, tryptophan is a food component and certainly non habit-forming. Yet, it should only be required occasionally — if insomnia persists, recognise that some nervous or emotional problem has yet to be confronted.

Wheat Germ   To obtain white flour from wheat, the mill first removes the germ of the grain, then the husk. Both of these are sold separately to health food stores, as there is an avid market for them among the aware minority of the population. The unthinking majority persists in buying the deprived white flour and its products, hoodwinked by the manufacturers into believing they are being adequately fed on this high-starch, low-nutrient partial food. And what is not used locally is exported to "under-developed" countries in a vain endeavour to overcome their malnutrition problems, when in reality, white flour only contributes to their malnutrition and under-development.

The embryo of wheat grain is the germ — that flaky, light brown product sold as wheat germ. It is somewhat similar to wheat bran in shape and colour, just a little larger and certainly tastier. Wheat germ contains twice as much protein as bran, 50 per cent more oil and 350 per cent more vitamins B_1 and B_2. Wheat germ is lower than bran in iron and fibre, as well as in B_3, yet is higher in these than are most other foods. But the problem with these nutrients in bran is their difficulty of access, due to the cellulose toughness of bran, which is why most people eat it. The purpose of this comparison is to emphasise that it is generally better to eat wheat germ than bran (the lower fibre content of 3 per cent in wheat germ is adequate for the diet in which reasonable quantities of fresh fruit and vegetables are included). A very special advantage of wheat germ is its vitamin E content; it comprises as much as 3 per cent of the oil content, or about 260 mL per 100 g wheat germ. Wheat germ is so easily eaten and digested that most of the nutrients become readily available — 26 per cent protein, 50 per cent complex carbohydrates, 990 mg phosphorus, 10 per cent iron, 1000 mg potassium, 336 mg magnesium, 2.2 mg B_1, 1.3 mg B_2 and 9.5 mg B_3. These are the major sources of nutritional richness; a very impressive list. Weight for weight, wheat germ has only a few more kilojoules than medium-cooked beef steak; but due to its greater density, more kilojoules will be obtained from meat than wheat germ of similar volume.

Wheat germ should not be cooked if its optimum nourishment is to be gained. Certainly its use in baked goods will improve their nutritive value more than the use of any other ingredient, but wheat germ's two most unstable vitamins, B_1 and E, lose much of their value through cooking and oxidising. Wheat germ is best eaten as part of the breakfast cereal, so long as it is not cooked, but only soaked by whatever liquid one chooses to use (apple juice or soya milk are best). Heat does more than destroy part of the wheat germ oil — it induces rancidity which can totally destroy the germ itself, rendering it unfit for human consumption. Rancidity occurs when oils become oxidised and is particularly prevalent among polyunsaturated oils (wheat germ oil contains 50 per cent linoleic acid, the major polyunsaturate). For this reason, wheat germ should only be bought fresh and always stored in the refrigerator in sealed jars, thereby excluding heat and free oxygen.

Whey Powder   Whey is the serum of milk, the liquid residue after the making of cheese or butter, after the coagulation of protein and settling of fat. Thus, whey is very short on both protein and fat — in fact, its primary nutritional attribute is its high level of sodium, much of which is combined with chloride to provide a natural source of salt for those who might be low in both these minerals, generally the older people whose bodies are becoming stiffer, blood thicker and digestion difficult. Whey powder will benefit people with bowel problems, for it contains bacteria which are in harmony with the colon's acidophilous baccilli. Many health writers ascribe to whey all sorts of miraculous properties, some of which might be correct, but none of which appear to be substantiated. It is not an item that I have found of special benefit in my practice, other than for the aforementioned few.

White Willow Bark Since before Christ, the dried and powdered bark of the white willow tree was used by the dwellers of northern Africa, central Asia and Europe as a means of relieving pain and reducing fever. The active ingredient has been analysed to be salicin, a glucoside, soluble in water and converted into salicylic acid in the stomach. Cost-oriented manufacturers have realised that a less expensive way of obtaining this pain-reliever could be developed without gathering and processing willow bark, so they synthesised salicylic acid in the laboratory. Soon a faster pain reliever was developed from acetylsalicylic acid, now known as aspirin, but this has subsequently proved to be responsible for stomach irritations and some forms of kidney disease, with other probable iatrogenic problems now being investigated — it is also potentially addictive. Health-conscious people have recently tended to veer away from aspirin, with a consequent return to white willow bark powder. In recent years, white willow bark has been used in America with beneficial results in the relieving of pain, reduction of fever and inflammation, as an astringent for the control of internal bleeding, as a diuretic for rheumatic and gout sufferers and, in some instances, for the relief of stomach problems, many of which are manifested as "heartburn". The tablets are usually prepared in 300 mg or 500 mg potencies of the compressed powder, but for most instances where pain relief is needed, this will not be found sufficient since salicin is a milder form of analgesic than aspirin. For temporary pain relief, at least 1000 mg, maybe to 1500 mg white willow bark would be required initially — since it is neither a drug, nor habit-forming, such a quantity is generally regarded as safe. It is important to remind pain sufferers that the cause must be discovered and corrected to obtain permanent relief and avoid future occurrences.

Yeast, Dietary Forms We draw the distinction between dietary yeasts and baker's yeast. The former have been pasteurised to stop growth and inhibit any bacterial action within the yeast; baker's yeast is still alive and growing (held in check only by refrigeration), feeding avariciously upon B-vitamins to increase its growth (instead of supplying B-vitamins, as do dietary yeasts). Once baker's yeast is used in manufacturing and heated to bake the product, its action has been killed. Dietary yeasts include the well-known brewer's and torula varieties in powder form, plus flaked yeast, usually marketed as "Savoury Flaky Yeast". Brewer's yeast is either grown especially for dietary use in large vats or, more economically and frequently, gathered as the residue of beer brewing. This explains its variations in colour and flavour, resulting from whatever variety of beer the yeast is gathered from. Torula yeast is usually cultured on cellulose, with a similar nutritional pattern and growth rate. Yeast is one of the oldest forms of plant life on earth and is the most rapid in reproduction, increasing at the rate of doubling every half hour (hence its need for closely controlled supervision). Yeast is one of the richest foods known to man, being so concentrated that it can only be digested in small quantities. Its general concentration of protein, B-vitamins and minerals establishes it as a valuable therapeutic food for a host of diet-oriented problems, from diabetes and hypoglycaemia to pellagra and stress.

Torula and brewer's yeasts vary a little in their nutrient properties and should be therefore recommended in accordance with the patient's need. Torula is low in sodium (15 mg per 100 g, whereas brewer's yeast has 121 mg), and is best suited for people with hypertension or any other problem related to a high sodium intake. Torula also has approximately double the fibre and calcium contents (3.3 g and 424 mg per 100 g) found in brewer's yeast, which could be an important consideration for those who seek increases of both items in their diet. The only important nutrient registering a higher concentration in brewer's yeast is magnesium — 231 mg, compared to 165 mg in torula yeast. Other nutrients are somewhat similar for both, averaging as follows: protein 39 per cent, fat 1 per cent, 1170 kilojoules, 38 per cent carbohydrate, 1733 mg phosphorus, 18.3 mg iron, 2000 mg potassium, 15 mg vitamin B_1, 4.6 mg B_2 and 40 mg B_3. Neither yeast contains anything but a trace of vitamins A or C.

Other than the nutritional aspects of the two yeasts, the choice would lie with their flavours. Some people prefer the stronger taste of torula, others the slightly sweeter and saltier taste of brewer's yeast. Either yeast can be added to cooking, as many health and recipe books recommend, but this will cause the reduction of some vitamin content. The best way to take dietary yeast is in a cool drink with fruit juice, vegetable juice or soya milk. The savoury flavour of yeast flakes is created by the addition of common salt during the process in which the flakes are formed under heat. This creates a tasty form of yeast, but its nutritional properties are lowered in the process. For those who prefer to avoid the flavour of yeast, yet do not want to be deprived of its nutritional values, brewer's yeast tablets are available, offering a convenient and compact way to take this supplement when travelling or at work. A few people manifest physical allergies to fungal foods, so for them, any form of nutritional yeast is taboo; they should be looking to other supplements or concentrated foods with somewhat similar nutritional properties.

Yogurt Continuing the previous advice to those people who are allergic to fungal foods, it is suggested that they also avoid yogurt, kefir or any cultured dairy product. Yogurt (sometimes spelt "yoghurt", "yoghourt") has been in use in the human diet since before man's recorded history, as have many of the previously mentioned health foods. But it is only in the decade immediately preceding World War II that the medical establishment began to recognise yogurt as offering certain valuable therapeutic properties, especially for colonic problems. Yogurt has since been gradually elevated beyond the limitations of general interest, into the realms of a therapeutic food. Many people still buy it for its smoothness, its pleasant and refreshing taste, while others now buy yogurt for the health benefits they derive (or feel they derive) from it. Yogurt will suit most people and is one of the best ways to take milk, for those who seek to rely on milk nutrients in their diet. But yogurt offers more than milk, for it has effectively coagulated the milk protein, by-passing the limitations of the human stomach (past infancy) which has become devoid of rennin. In yogurt are also found helpful bacteria (*Lactobacillus bulgaricus*) which, in moderate quantities, are beneficial in supporting the work of human colonic bacteria and in counteracting the presence of foreign, disease-spreading bacteria which may be induced into the colon by unsuitable foods and/or drugs. But when eating yogurt, do not fall for the misconception that if a moderate amount of something is good for you, a lot of it is better. This excuse for gluttony never works, emphatically not with yogurt, where too much *Lactobacillus bulgaricus* will inevitably give rise to an internal "star wars", with the stronger invader overcoming the normally placid host. Such a diminution of the colon's normal bacteria can result in temporary bowel dysfunction (which a moderate amount of yogurt would normally rectify) until native bacteria effectively repopulate. A suggested maximum daily ingestion of yogurt is 100 mL (a little less than 4 fl oz).

These days, when so many women go out to work, and find insufficient time to undertake normal domestic duties, sales of commerical yogurts have increased enormously. But these yogurts are rarely comparable in taste, texture or nutritional properties to home-made yogurt. Worse still, commercial yogurts are often injected with setting agents to hold them firm for transportation — gelatine, agar agar, or other setting agents have been found in many such yogurts. But these are not as bad as the sweetening and flavouring agents often used to cater for the growing modern addiction to sweetened foods. Many processors use cane sugar or fruits preserved and sweetened with sugar in their yogurts. Such yogurts compare poorly with the home-made style developed by experience, with patience, love and care. The method is simple — bring the milk just to the boil (prolonged boiling will spoil the delicate flavour), pour it into suitable containers and as the temperature reduces to around 45°C (so that you can place your finger in it without burning), add a little yogurt saved from a previous batch. Then maintain this constant temperature (it can drop to 40°C without any problem) for 4 to 8 hours, until it has set; then refrigerate to stop bacterial action. Practice will indicate the quantity of "starter" yogurt to use, for it will depend largely on the nature and age of the milk. If no starter yogurt is available, use a package yogurt culture as per instructions — then save a little of this batch for future yogurt making. The best way to keep new yogurt steadily warm is in an electric yogurt maker.

By far the best milk to use is whole, raw goat's milk. Nutritional properties of goat's milk are superior to cow's milk, as is commonly realised, and the raw milk is likewise more nutritious and easier to set than pasteurised milk. The fresher the yogurt, the better it is for you (another reason why home-made yogurt is superior to commercial varieties), for the value of the bacteria will diminish with age. Some people have used soya bean milk with success, although such a yogurt is more difficult to make and often quite bitter.

In terms of actual nutrients, yogurt has the effect of concentrating those in the milk by 10–35 per cent. This is especially evident in the protein measurement, offering the maximum increase of around 35 per cent over liquid milk, or around 5 per cent by weight of total product. In skim milk yogurt, the reduction of fat allows a further protein increase — up to 6 per cent of the total yogurt being protein. But, of course, the primary benefit of yogurt is the considerable increase in its ease of digestibility, when compared to liquid milk of any type.

Herb Teas

Mention a hot beverage and most people turn to tea (China tea) or coffee. Up to a few decades ago in America and in the British Commonwealth, hardly an alternative was available even if desired. But circumstances have changed and the change is growing, thankfully. Health consciousness, together with the infiltration of many European and Asian cultures into English-speaking society, has been accompanied by many varieties of new foods and drinks, among which is a vast range of herb teas.

For centuries, herbalists have been aware of and have dispensed a vast array of dried herbs for preparation as hot beverages — we call them "teas", although the word more accurately refers to the east-Asian shrub from which the leaves are plucked, fermented, dried and prepared into a hot beverage. So what we now call "herb teas" have been in use for ages, both for therapeutic purpose and to enjoy as a drink. With the modern emergence of the health-food concept, precipitated by so much "junk" and processed non-food now available, herb teas have attracted a rebirth of interest, both as "alternative" medicines and alternative taste sensations. They are eagerly sought by those who know of their many virtues, cautiously approached by those either addicted to convention or prepared to experience something different.

As earlier discussed in this book, addiction to tea and coffee drinking can lead to subsequent kidney disorders due to the presence of strong oxalic acid in the beverages. This is the major precursor to kidney stones and urinary gravel, as well as the more acute variety of irritations and inflammations of the eliminatory organs. But to find alternatives to tea and coffee has presented a horrifying experience for many people to contemplate. Decaffeinated coffee is not an answer, for this only removes that emotionally and mentally damaging drug (which is also in tea). It does nothing to deactivate oxalic acid; instead, the decaffeination process introduces new chemicals to the brew — a potential danger to the body. Cereal coffee substitutes are now readily available through health food stores, offering pleasant beverages without harmful side-effects (but neither do they offer any therapeutic properties).

So the answer lies in herb teas. With these, the dual purpose is achieved — with such a vast range of varieties and flavours, pleasant-tasting beverages with beneficial therapeutic properties can be chosen and prepared just as easily as conventional China tea. As a bonus to this, many herb teas offer valuable therapeutic properties by aiding the body's natural recuperative powers to overcome a wide range of discomforting symptoms. With such value to human well-being, herb teas should, of course, be encouraged by governments and health commissions everywhere — perhaps they are in many countries, but in Australia they are taxed as though they were luxury goods. Most varieties are subject to import duty and *all* varieties (whether local or imported) have a sales tax of 20 per cent imposed as though to give price advantages to coffee and China tea, both of which are favoured with sales tax exemption. (Concerted approaches to the Commonwealth Government by the health food industry proved costly and useless!) In spite of their comparatively high prices, herb teas are proving more popular, as is to be expected when people come to realise their many advantages.

The following general guide includes the most popular varieties of herb teas, together with some of the popular blends which are beneficial to health and enjoyable to drink.

Alfalfa Tea   One of the most popular herb teas, obtained from dried leaves of the deep-rooting alfalfa (lucerne) plant, with the occasional addition of stems and flowers, depending on the harvest time. Alfalfa tea provides vital alkalising benefits for hyperacid stomachs in two ways — it tends to control the flow of hydrochloric acid and to aid the action of gastric enzyme, pepsin. This is of considerable assistance to people converting from meat-eating to vegetarianism, for they would otherwise experience an excess of hydrochloric acid until the stomach readjusts to the reduced needs of plant proteins. Arthritics also benefit by the alkalising of food residues aided by alfalfa tea, as do food allergy sufferers, but such relief will not be permanent unless appropriate dietary changes are forthcoming. For maximum benefits, alfalfa tea should be drunk hot and between meals.

Alfalfa-Mint Tea   The addition of peppermint to alfalfa is a favourite blend for helping to settle disturbed stomachs after an over-rich meal. It also refreshes the palate and, for this reason, is an excellent hot drink first thing in the morning. As a cool drink, alfalfa-mint is found to be most refreshing on a hot, steamy day, either by itself or as a basis for a fruit punch.

Aniseed Tea   A small annual, the anise plant is found both wild and cultivated in most parts of the world. Its seeds give a characteristically sweet taste when chewed, a habit which has been adopted by most races since pre-biblical times when dwellers of eastern Mediterranean lands (of which the tree is native) found digestive relief from anise. They probably did not realise that anethol, the oil contained in and released by crushing the seed, aids pancreatic enzymes. Aniseed tea is brewed from the crushed seeds with boiling water, and must be served hot for the oil to be of maximum benefit. The palate will also be refreshed from this beverage, as will the respiratory tract, especially if the hot cup is held near one's nostrils to inhale the refreshing (and blockage-clearing) aroma. The refreshing and digestive qualities of aniseed are also highly beneficial in herb tea blends, especially for a nightcap.

Chamomile Tea The German, rather than the English chamomile, is the more popular variety of flower used in America and Australia. Hot water applied to the dried flowers provides a mildly sweet, very pleasant and popular beverage, found to be both relaxing and alkalising. As a natural relaxant, chamomile tea induces a calming effect upon the central nervous system, helping to relieve tension, confusion and cramping. It is not a sedative, nor is it habit-forming, making it highly beneficial for business people and for women during their menstrual cycles. Children are found to greatly benefit from this tea (especially those who are hyperactive), both before school and before bed. As chamomile flowers contain phosphates of the alkalising minerals calcium, potassium and magnesium, this tea offers a digestive aid when too much rich food or poorly combined food are ingested — it should always be served both before and after a large party! For the relief of painful sunburn, a cool bath can be most beneficial when chamomile tea (complete with the soggy residue) is added. Chamomile tea also makes an excellent hair rinse, bringing a special lustre and nourishment to the scalp; the oil extracted from chamomile flowers is even richer and an excellent scalp tonic, especially after washing the hair.

Chicory Rarely used by itself, chicory is highly regarded as a suitable coffee substitute when mixed with roasted cereal grains such as barley and rye, and/or with beans such as carob and soya. Some brands of cheap coffee also use chicory as an "extender" — this is one of those rare occasions when cheapness is best! The yellowish rootstock is the part of this plant used, for it has the therapeutic benefits of providing vitamin A (from its carotene) and choline, thereby greatly aiding liver functioning and cholesterol breakdown in the arteries.

Cinnamon Tea The sweet, spicy flavour of cinnamon rates it as one of the most popular of the aromatic spices. It is the dried inner bark of a huge tree, native to India, but now found in most tropical countries. Cinnamon is a favourite food flavouring and, although not strictly a herb, its use in herb teas always adds flavour. It offers little in the way of therapeutic properties, although many people attest to its ability to clear the head and improve the level of thinking — some using it as a beverage, others in their bath water. A most delightful herb tea blend of cinnamon with dried hibiscus flowers (a ratio of two whole cinnamon sticks with eight dried hibiscus flowers, brought to the boil in a litre of water and simmered for ten minutes) produces a most refreshing beverage, either hot or cold.

Cloves Rarely used on their own, cloves offer a valuable component for herb tea blends. A spice, rather than a herb, the clove is a dried flower bud of a tall, evergreen tropical tree. It is a favourite kitchen flavourer with a characteristic sweet spiciness, especially familiar to anyone who has suffered from toothache. As an age-old nerve soother, the influence of cloves can be of benefit throughout the gastrointestinal tract, from the mouth to the anus, but especially in the vicinity of mouth and throat. Cloves are traditionally soothing after a highly spiced meal, especially when curry powder is used. For countless years, cloves have been used as a preservative, even for embalming. When blended in a herb tea with orange peel and rosehips, it gives a delicious fruit-and-spice effect. Alfalfa can also be added for improved digestive benefits and energy.

Comfrey Tea Dried leaves of the comfrey plant rate among the most highly recommended healing herbs ever known. Its dried root is also used for healing properties, but this, of course, kills the plant, whereas leaves can be picked progressively as the plant grows. Comfrey is a perennial plant which likes plenty of moisture, reflected in its deep green leaves. It is in these young leaves that the nitrogenous compound allantoin is found; but when the leaves are old and oxidised, allantoin diminishes (so be careful when buying comfrey tea to ensure leaves are green). Allantoin is amazingly beneficial in reducing scar tissue and minimising adhesion formation within the body, as well as aiding in the oxidation of uric acid (the arthritis-forming residue of meat metabolism). Comfrey tea can aid in the stimulation of the appetite for those suffering from anorexia nervosa; being rich in iron, it offers nourishment for anaemics and is an excellent beverage for coeliac sufferers. Once the tea has been brewed, the soggy residue should be saved for soaking in your next bath, for this will help to improve skin-tone, especially if any blemishes or sores are present, so long as they are already closed (any open sores must be first disinfected before closing as comfrey heals skin quite rapidly — calendula is the ideal herbal antiseptic).

Comfrey-Alfalfa Tea The blending of alfalfa with comfrey will aid the nutritional properties of both by supporting the body's ability to absorb iron, stimulated by the iron that is in this blend. Alfalfa also enhances comfrey's alkalising properties, making this a valuable blend to drink between meals.

Comfrey-Mint Tea Another alkalising blend, this combination is particularly beneficial for arthritics. Both teas work towards neutralising uric acid residues, but of course their benefit is maximised when combined with an alkalising diet, free from common salt. Comfrey-mint tea also provides that bonus which is characteristic of both peppermint and spearmint — it refreshes the palate, making it an ideal early-morning beverage, especially for people past the age of forty.

Dandelion Tea To so many people, this plant is a weed; but they should be mindful of Emerson's advice that "a weed is a plant whose virtues have not yet been discovered". Thanks to herbalists, dandelion's virtues are now well known and respected, both for its therapeutic properties and as an alternative to tea and coffee. The entire plant is used by many herbalists, although the tea is usually brewed from the root. As with chicory, it is a valuable source of carotene (for vitamin A) and of choline (for improved cholesterol distribution). The choline, plus many alkalising salts (calcium, potassium, iron, etc.), benefits both liver and gall bladder in their vital role of handling fats within the body and aiding the detoxifying role of the liver. Sufferers from hepatitis can greatly benefit from dandelion tea. But it is not a tea with limitations — dandelion can be used as a general body tonic, for its influence also extends to supporting kidney function, bowels, bladder and skin, these being the hard-working eliminating organs. Acne and allergy problems often respond to dandelion taken regularly between meals.

Dill Seed This is another spice with important therapeutic properties when used wisely. The seeds develop when the yellow flowers of this common annual plant fall in early autumn. They are rarely used on their own in a herb tea; the seeds are usually crushed and added to other herbs or spices to provide a blend which is highly beneficial to the digestive tract. They combine well with aniseed, both containing anethol oil to aid pancreatic digestion. When blended with chamomile and hops, these two spices produce a herb tea which aids the digestion and soothes the nerves of the gastrointestinal tract. Such a blend will be highly beneficial for those who have had a large meal too soon before retiring — a warm cup of this combination will help induce relaxation and pave the way for a restful sleep.

Equisetum Tea To some, it is known as "shave grass", to others, "horsetail grass", but this perennial plant is common throughout the northern hemisphere. The entire plant is used for important herbal benefits, for it is nature's richest source of silicon oxide, a vital cell salt. Its silica is combined with calcium and magnesium to give compounds of great therapeutic benefits to the skin, hair, tooth enamel, toe nails and finger nails. Internal cell tissue is also benefited, for silica provides special support for the eliminating organs. Equisetum is a strong tea with marked astringent action, so care must be taken in its use. So strong is it that it has been known to dissolve urinary gravel and kidney stones, or at least soften them for ease of passing. It can also soften and dissolve thickened tissue within the body, such as fibroids and adhesions. It is one of the most potent herb teas in general use and one should, therefore, be careful not to overstimulate the body with its punch.

Eucalyptus Tea Although native to Australia, this tree is now found on every continent. Its leaves, although not strictly a herb, are used by many herbalists with success in preparing concoctions for clearing blocked respiratory passages. The tea also aids bronchial sufferers, relieves the throat after coughing and helps to normalise the temperature of anyone suffering from fever.

Flax Tea Known also as "linseed tea", this beverage has a unique and special virtue — its mucilage. The ripe, brownish seeds are crushed and pressed to extract their oil for making linseed oil, a rich source of linoleic acid (the most valuable polyunsaturated fat). The seeds are boiled to obtain the mucilage which is so prized for soothing inflamed and irritated intestines, especially the bowels. It also soothes the bladder, kidneys and urinary tract, conferring significant relief from irritations created by oxalate crystals as gravel or stones. When dry or sluggish bowels induce constipation, or when bowel or intestinal surgery induces sluggishness, flax tea offers relief by lubricating the colon and supporting the recovery of its normal action.

Fenugreek Tea Native to the Mediterranean region, fenugreek was one of the herbs used by the first master herbalist of our times, Hippocrates (in no way did he practise allopathy, as it is regarded in later medical practice). The ancient Egyptian priests and healers also used fenugreek — for its many therapeutic virtues as well as its culinary properties. Indians soon discovered the sharp taste of fenugreek and began using it in their curry mixes. It is this same pungency which deters many people from using fenugreek as a tea, but they should persevere if the therapeutic benefits of these leguminous seeds are to be felt, rather than take harsh antibiotics or other drugs. During the early acute stages of any of the respiratory tract infections (bronchitis, influenza, sinusitis, catarrh, suspected pneumonia, etc.), fenugreek tea will help the body to produce perspiration, dispel toxicity and shorten the period of fever — take up to four cups daily and reduce as condition improves. To improve flavour, a few drops of lemon can be used, but no other addition, for during such treatment, no form of food or nourishment should be taken (fasting and fenugreek will allow the body to correct these respiratory problems in a few days, but if your illness persists, consult your health practitioner). Fenugreek offers the cell salt, iron phosphate, which aids in overcoming hypertension and recurring inflammations. It also contains lecithin, thereby aiding the body's fat absorption ability. In this context, fenugreek is a valuable beverage for teenagers suffering from acne; aided by its vitamins A and D, this tea works to stabilise skin and hormone functioning. This in turn will help to overcome teenage lethargy. Fenugreek also helps overcome headaches and is thus a valuable herb tea and should always be a part of the larder.

Ginseng Tea Much has already been said about ginseng in our discussion on health foods and their properties. As a tea, ginseng has a milder effect than when taken in tablet or powder form. It is, therefore, suitable as a general tonic to overcome lethargy. Women often find it highly beneficial in normalising menstruation and for easing childbirth. It is also highly regarded as a good, general blood tonic. As it has the property of stimulating the pituitary gland, it is not recommended for people who are already highly active. It should certainly never be given to children, unless under professional guidance.

Hawthorn Tea A popular hedge-plant native to England, the hawthorn was imported to America soon after colonisation. Later its therapeutic properties were given great impetus by a booklet (now out of print) written by that pioneer of healthy living and organic agriculture, J. I. Rodale. He recognised and made extensive use of the therapeutic properties of the hawthorn berry in his early years when he learned of his weak heart and the probability of a short life expectancy (he died in 1971 at the age of 72 after a very active and rewarding life). By its influence in helping to regulate the action of the heart muscles, hawthorn berries are beneficial in normalising blood pressure, soothing the nerves in the heart region, overcoming stress-induced nervousness and generally toning the major blood vessels. These are the therapeutic properties of the crushed berries, when infused as a tea and drunk regularly. In tablet form, hawthorn berry has even stronger properties, more suited to the extremely hypertensive businessman, especially when insomnia is an accompanying problem.

Hibiscus Tea One of the most beautiful of tropical flowers, the hibiscus is not just a pretty face! When the flower dies, it may be picked and dried, for it offers both a delicious flavour and important therapeutic properties when it is infused in a tea. With about 200 species of hibiscus, it is impossible to list all the therapeutic aspects, so we shall consider only that variety used in American and Australian herb teas, *Hibiscus sabdariffa*, from the West Indies. All varieties of hibiscus offer the characteristic deep red hue when made into a herb tea, but this one is also a mild diuretic and nerve nourisher. It is not usually used alone but is blended with rosehips and peppermint. Both hibiscus and rosehips are excellent sources of vitamin C, with hibiscus also abundant in minerals iron and copper, both of which are more readily absorbed in the body with the aid of vitamin C. Therefore, this tea blend is a vital blood nourisher as well; in turn acting to dispel lethargy. It is an excellent blend for creating the start to a happy, bright day.

Hops Tea Rarely taken on its own, hops are found in some of the most effective herb tea blends, where their phosphate salts act in concert with a suitably selected herb. Cultivated extensively throughout much of the world (Tasmania is famous for its vineyards), hop vines are prolific growers, producing a cone-like fruit, harvested for beverage-making. The major therapeutic property of hops is its calming effect on the nerves which, of course, is why most people drink beer; but as a herb tea, the same nerve toning is possible, without the detrimental effect of alcohol reducing one's level of consciousness. There is a tendency for people to become addicted to drinking hops (even without the alcohol), so be careful not to make it too strong or drink it too frequently. (Perhaps it is this addiction to the hops in beer which contributes to a country's endemic lethargy!) This is why we find hops as part of a blended herb tea. An ideal blend with hops is chamomile, aniseed and dill seed — one of the herb tea blends devised by this author and marketed under the name of "Dreamtime". It is a most effective blend for relaxing the nerves (particularly of the stomach before a meal), and improving the functioning of the respiratory tract. This beverage can be taken about half an hour before a meal (drunk either warm or cooled) to improve the appetite and aid digestion; or it can be drunk before going to bed, to relax the digestive tract and help overcome insomnia. It also assists in overcoming flatulence and abdominal cramps.

Horehound Tea   This herb needs no cultivation, for it is generally found growing as a weed in most temperate countries. Because of its natural bitterness, it is not a popular herb tea, although as a fermented beverage, with added sweetening, it still attracts a substantial following. Being such a powerful beverage, horehound tea has been effectively used for many centuries to counteract colds and coughs so it tends to be regarded by many as a folk remedy. Leading herbalist Dorothy Hall, in her recently published *Herb Tea Book*, says of horehound: "[it] is often blended with foenugreek, licorice and thyme as a bronchial tea to help loosen heavy mucus. Horehound tea does not cure a cold, but it does speed up the eliminatory process and powerfully tones the mucus linings of the respiratory system".

Jasmine Tea   A traditional mark of Chinese hospitality, jasmine tea is one of the most pleasant-tasting of all herb teas. Jasmine is a small vine which favours warm climates; it is indigenous to China, but is now cultivated in most warm climates. Its deep green leaves and highly fragrant white flowers are both used for tea-making when dried, producing a tea with an interesting colour and a delightful taste. Tradition has it that dried jasmine flowers, when decocted, calm the nerves, whereas their fragrance has the reputation for sexual stimulation, a rather curious paradox. The truth probably lies between the two, for jasmine appears to have no special therapeutic properties, nor stimulatory benefits, beyond those responsive to the imagination; however, it does offer a very pleasant and satisfying herbal beverage.

Juniper Tea   Juniper is an evergreen shrub with the capacity to adapt to most climatic conditions by altering its growth height from as low as a metre to over seven metres. It produces a cone fruit, rather like a berry, which is dried and crushed for making into herb tea. It has the ability to stimulate the secretion of hydrochloric acid if the stomach is not producing sufficient, thereby acting counter to alfalfa tea. Juniper tea is an effective diuretic, being highly beneficial to sufferers of gout, water retention and for those with sluggish kidneys. However, care must be exercised in choosing strength and quantity of juniper tea, for it can become an irritant to the kidneys and urinary tract — it is not recommended for those suffering from kidney problems, nor for pregnant women. It is certainly an excellent herbal corrective for the easing of cystitis attacks, where the aggressiveness of juniper tea will attack and remove the irritants and assist in counteracting the infection, but it should only be taken during the day of a severe attack and no longer.

Lemon Balm Tea   Native to the Arab part of the world, this perennial is now more widely cultivated as a culinary herb. It is often known merely as "balm", although the prefix is becoming more popular since the lemon fragrance (deriving from any part of the plant being crushed) is its predominant attraction. By inducing the body to perspire profusely, lemon balm tea aids with temperature regulation in hot climates. Hence its high esteem with Arabs. It is also a beneficial digestive aid and mineral balancer, thanks to its own balance of sodium and chlorine. This implies a special advantage for people tending to suffer cramps after excessive perspiration. Many people attribute to lemon balm the property of improving the memory and level of comprehension by clearing the brain. This is probably achieved by a calming of the nerves which would follow its diaphoretic action of inducing perspiration. In this domain, it can also counteract hysteria, depression, headaches and dizziness arising from mental confusion and uncertainty (in a word: worry).

Lemon Grass Tea   One of the most popular of all herb teas, due to its highly refreshing flavour, lemon grass has very little to commend it therapeutically, beyond its ability to refresh the palate, sparkle the eyes and act as a mild pick-me-up. For many people, this is quite enough to justify their drinking this tea, a further justification being that it is so easily grown, cut, dried and stored, enabling one to become quite self-sufficient with just a small garden and lawn. Lemon grass can be effectively used as part of a blend of herb teas, especially with horehound or one of the other less pleasant teas which are taken primarily for their therapeutic properties.

Licorice Tea   Originally found growing wild in southern Europe and central Asia, the licorice plant is now cultivated in many more countries, especially in North America. A hardy perennial, licorice (sometimes spelt in its original form of liquorice) has become famous for its sweet taste and black colour. Its most common use in confectionery is covered earlier in this Stage, so we shall now only consider its qualities as a herb tea. In this realm, licorice is growing in popularity each year, for people are finding its gentle laxative action to be far preferable to harsher herbs or drugs. With it, they get the bonus of a delicious-tasting beverage which is also very pleasant on the throat. Its pleasant after-taste always leaves the throat feeling clear and the voice smooth and resonant, making it ideal for singers and orators. Licorice tea is also regarded as being a source of iron salts, which can be important for those suffering a form of anaemia or lethargy.

Linden Tea   Both varieties of this tall tree, the European and the American, are alternatively known as lime trees. Their flowers, leaves and bark all have therapeutic properties which have been recognised for centuries. In the main, linden tea offers benefits similar to chamomile, but with more strength, especially the American variety. For general consumption, the European variety is recommended for its calming, anti-depressant effect; the American variety should only be taken under professional direction. However, even the European variety should not be taken over long periods, for it could tend to slow the heart beat too much. Chamomile is the safer tea to drink.

Maté Tea   This is a herb tea we can do without. A native of South America, maté leaves provide a popular indigenous beverage, a long-established habit of the natives in the central regions of the continent. It is a very strong, bitter beverage, not unlike coffee or cola in many respects — it stimulates the heart and muscle action by the effect of its caffeine. It should also be avoided because of its oxalic acid content, for the burden this places on the kidneys and urinary tract is painfully known to every sufferer of gravel and kidney stones.

Nettle Tea   No one with childhood memories of severe nettle stings would believe that, in later life, they would be writing about the health-giving virtues of such an "obnoxious" plant. But that only goes to prove how much we change as we mature. For indeed, nettle leaves that sting can also provide some valuable therapeutic properties, once they have been cut, dried and desiccated. Iron and phosphorus contained in nettle tea will stimulate the blood circulation, providing vital aid for those suffering from low blood pressure. These minerals also enrich the blood to overcome anaemia. However, care must be taken to regulate the quantity of nettle tea consumed, avoiding the overenthusiasm which can result as a consequence of improved energy and blood tone. This tea must be avoided by those hyperactive and tense people who are probably suffering from temporary or permanent hypertension. Many people have found that drinking nettle helps to overcome diarrhoea.

Papaya Tea As the name implies, this is a herb tea made from the dried and desiccated leaves of the tropical plant called "papaya" in North America and "paw paw" in the South Pacific. This tea has the reputation of aiding digestion, but is most beneficial in its ability to kill most types of intestinal worms. A poultice made from the soggy residues of papaya tea can also be used effectively to dress festering wounds or tropical ulcers. The tea has a rather bland flavour, but is not intended to be consumed for its flavour — it is primarily a therapeutic beverage.

Parsley Tea There is probably no more nutritious plant than parsley. It is one of the richest natural sources of calcium, iron, potassium and of vitamins A and C. And even when it goes to seed, valuable use can be made of it by drying the plant and the seeds for later use as a herb tea. Parsley tea is an excellent source of nourishment for the heart, liver, kidneys, blood and nerves — it is more a tonic than a tea in its vast range of therapeutic and nourishing benefits. It is a powerful diuretic, being highly beneficial to arthritics in the excreting of uric acid — of course, its benefits will be largely negated if a dietary change to avoid further production of uric acid from meat intake is not simultaneously undertaken. Parsley tea has also been effectively used to overcome dropsy, asthma (in conjunction with halting the drinking of milk) and coughs induced by mucus accumulation. A shampoo of this tea is also an effective scalp cleanser, especially for removing lice and similar infestations.

Peppermint Tea The common, wild mint usually found in moist, wooded regions of the world is the peppermint. It possesses the strongest menthol flavour and aroma of all the mint family, characterised by their dark-green, pointed leaves. Even when dried, these leaves possess the menthol stength, and a very refreshing herb tea can be brewed from them. The menthol oil is retained in the dried leaves and released by boiling water into the herb tea brew; but when the dried leaves are "instantised" (to comply with the modern syndrome of fast foods and drinks) the menthol oil is destroyed, leaving behind only the flavour (which often has to be artificially stimulated to be strong enough). So do not buy instant peppermint tea if you seek more than mere flavour.

Peppermint tea offers some valuable therapeutic benefits from its natural menthol oil — settling the stomach when rich or over-abundant food has been consumed; counteracting heartburn (which occurs from the same cause); settling headaches and nausea if the tea is consumed as soon as these commence. Menthol also refreshes the palate, and if taken as soon as a cold starts, it can materially aid in its clearing, accompanied by adequate vitamin C. Thus, peppermint tea works well with rosehips and hibiscus to offer an excellent "anti-cold" blend, which simultaneously works to calm the nerves of the solar plexus and clear the head, nose and throat. In fact, peppermint blends well with most herb teas, alfalfa being another favourite and valuable combination (see Alfalfa-Mint Tea).

Raspberry Tea The wild raspberry vine is a common nuisance for most landholders around the world, but for herbalists, it is a valuable plant. Its leaves possess important therapeutic properties which can be pleasantly and readily obtained when brewed into a tea. For men, this is a mild blood tonic and a pleasant beverage; but for women, particularly during and after pregnancy, raspberry leaf tea is most beneficial. With its balanced offering of iron and copper salts, with vitamins A and C and folic acid, this tea strengthens the pelvic muscles when they are under added stress from an enlarged uterus. A cup of very warm raspberry tea is also highly beneficial each morning during early pregnancy to lessen morning sickness and help avert a miscarriage; during the final stages of pregnancy, it will help to reduce labour pains (when frequent cups can be consumed). Following childbirth, a continuation of the morning cup of raspberry tea will help tone the abdominal muscles and ligaments to aid in their recovery. Such care will significantly contribute towards the maintaining of a trim abdomen when combined with sensible abdominal exercises, and will avert the later discomfort of a uterus prolapse.

Rosehips Tea Few people realise that the rose bush has a fruit. It is the deep red bulb which forms beneath the flower, ripening in autumn when the flowers die. All rose bushes produce this fruit, but the most therapeutically useful are found on the wild briar rose bush, far more common to North America and Europe than to Australia. Seeds of the rosehip are extracted, dried and crushed to make the beverage many people have come to recognise as a rich source of vitamin C. However, this nutrient is bound in a resin-clad coating which needs boiling water to dissolve — in so doing, a little of the vitamin C is lost, but ample remains for it to be of important therapeutic value. As the vitamin C is in the presence of iron and vitamin P, its value (and that of the other two nutrients) is enhanced, combining to make this tea of benefit during a cold and a valuable circulatory tonic for the bloodstream. It is, therefore, an excellent beverage for a daily stimulation of energy, supported by a similar benefit to the nervous system by the stimulation of adrenalin within the body. For this reason, it should never be taken within a few hours of bedtime. These properties are enhanced when rosehips are combined with peppermint and alfalfa teas in a blend — an excellent trio by which to overcome the afternoon slump or a general lethargy induced by low blood pressure or poor circulation. Leading herbalist Dorothy Hall often recommends rosehips for people seeking to break the coffee addiction.

Rosemary Tea Probably no herb is more widely known, or has such a variety of uses, than rosemary. "Rosemary for remembrance", "rosemary for the hair", for seasoning and flavouring, for the garden — all these have been attributed to this evergreen shrub which has been a "must" in the garden since early Roman and Greek days. It is a favourite culinary herb, being highly esteemed for use in pâtés. As a garden plant, rosemary is both attractive and aromatic. For herb tea use, one is tempted to pick its leaves fresh, but this will not provide as valuable a herb tea as when well-dried leaves are used from wild rosemary. Therapeutic uses for rosemary tea are threefold: for the digestion, circulation and hair. Experience shows that rosemary helps improve liver function, in turn improving the production of bile in the gall bladder, thereby improving general digestion. Improved circulation is achieved because rosemary tea slightly raises the blood pressure. The combination of these two benefits will improve brain functioning, especially memory cells; it will also minimise halitosis (bad breath). Rosemary oil is renowned for nourishing the scalp and offsetting baldness — rosemary tea, in aiding blood circulation, also helps from within. A strong decoction of the tea can be used as a shampoo and hair rinse. Some herbalists credit rosemary tea with the ability to relax the muscles, others with the ability to relieve headaches — both are sometimes effective, but this appears to be an occasional, rather than a general property.

John Lust, in his brilliantly researched *The Herb Book*, warns against too much rosemary tea "because of the genuine danger of poisoning". He does not state a reason, so one should perhaps be a little more than casually aware of any adverse reactions from drinking large and frequent quantities. The occasional or daily cup or two is unlikely to create a problem, but can be of benefit in the three categories listed above.

Sage Tea It is more than coincidence that sage follows rosemary in alphabetical order, for they are very closely related in therapeutic properties. Sage is best known as a culinary herb, highly favoured as a poultry stuffing. But as a tea, it has even more important properties, particularly in its ability to settle the nerves (especially in older people) and to reduce fever or excessive perspiration. It aids the memory by inducing a calmness through which memory cells find the best medium of expression. Again, this works well for older people. For sore throats, sage tea proves to be an effective gargle. For mothers of recently weaned infants, sage tea (especially when cold) will help stop the flow of breast milk. It is also a proven hair tonic and found in many home hair care kits. Sage and rosemary are often used in blends, both as oils and teas. Together, in a herb tea, aided by peppermint, they offer a tasty and beneficial blend, especially for aiding the digestion of pie-eating ockers!

Sarsaparilla Tea This favourite drink of Hopalong Cassidy was once considered an acceptable non-alcoholic beverage to order at the bar of a hotel. Little did those who resisted alcohol realise that what they were doing was improving their virility and cleansing their blood. As a herb tea, sarsaparilla root has these properties, being highly suitable for both sexes. It is a proven hormone stimulant and balancer, having been most useful (together with a highly alkaline diet and relaxed nerves) for women seeking to become pregnant and for both men and women with lowered sexual virility. Male prostate problems and female menopausal depression also usually respond to two cups of this tea daily. It also has a reputation as an effective blood purifier and a diuretic, working on eliminating uric acid, thereby minimising gout and arthritic conditions.

Spearmint Tea Similar in most general aspects to peppermint, spearmint belongs to the same family of menthol herbs. Its leaves are rounder in shape are not quite so dark a green as those of peppermint — spearmint has, in fact, a slightly sweeter taste than peppermint. Being the less powerful of the two mints, spearmint is more favoured as the domestic garden variety, found growing prolifically in most backyards. Children far prefer the spearmint freshness to the stronger flavour of peppermint, a preference probably stimulated by the advertisers of chewing gum. This makes spearmint tea an easy means of introducing children to herb teas and a way of improving their appetite if they become finicky about good food. The refreshing aftertaste of spearmint tea can be beneficial in overcoming indifference to food. Therapeutically, spearmint acts as a diuretic and also has the ability to relieve flatulence induced by overeating or unsuitable food combinations. Spearmint tea can be served cold in warm weather as a delightful refreshing beverage, either on its own or with other herb teas or fruit juices. It makes an excellent base for a delicious fruit punch.

Thyme Tea Although one of the commonest garden and culinary herbs, thyme is not so extensively used as a herb tea. However it should be more highly regarded in this role. Its most volatile property is its powerful antiseptic oil, called thymol, a major component of the high oil content of this herb. Thymol and menthol (a minor oil component) are released by boiling water, exuding a strong aroma which will deeply penetrate the respiratory tract to bring relief to congestive and bronchial conditions, as well as to sore throats and laryngitis. These oils also relax throat muscles and vocal chords, indicating their benefit to singers and public speakers. These relief measures also aid in overcoming headaches, but do not make a habit of drinking thyme tea — it is too strong for that and should be consumed only occasionally.

Valerian Tea This fragrant herb grows to around a metre in height and is so common throughout north-eastern United States and Europe that it is sometimes regarded as a weed, but only by those evidencing ignorance of its powerful therapeutic properties. Valerian tea is universally regarded as the most valuable natural sedative and mild tranquilliser of all herb teas. Being stronger than chamomile, it should not be given to children, unless they are exceedingly hyperactive. Whereas chamomile flowers are used, it is the rootstock of the valerian plant which provides the means for relaxing overtired and overused muscles, organs and nerves, this ability deriving from its phosphate salts of calcium, magnesium and potassium. Muscular spasms and cramps also respond well to valerian tea, as does bile stimulation in the gall bladder — care should be exercised in the amounts taken, in case too much bile is produced, in which case nausea will develop. In general, valerian tea is not addictive, in fact its smell turns more people off than on. But it is most effective in inducing relaxation in overworked and overstressed bodies. Valerian has no relationship with "Valium", the trade name of the tranquillising drug diazepam.

The foregoing list of common herb teas, outlining their characteristics and therapeutic virtues, is intended as a guide only. It should not be used as a replacement for professional advice when recurring or acute pathological problems prevail. A persisting problem of discomfort reveals the need to correct the cause. Herb teas are not intended for this role, but a considerable amount of other guidance is offered in this book; all health problems being related to dietary, emotional or structural disharmonies.

Most people enjoy drinking herb teas as they are brewed. Others prefer the addition of a sweetening substance or lemon to the brew. If a sweetener is chosen, be sure to avoid refined sugar — raw or coloured sugar is little better. Honey is a slight improvement on all of these, but the best sweetener to use is pure maple syrup (refer earlier this Stage for supporting reasons). It is wise to keep a range of suitable herb teas in your cupboard, both for personal use and for your guests. The foregoing list will provide a basis for enlightened choice. Most people include in their choice alfalfa, mint, chamomile, comfrey, dandelion, fenugreek, licorice, spearmint, together with blends including hibiscus, aniseed and dill seed, and sage. Happy, healthy drinking.

STAGE TWELVE

Fasting:
Abstinence Makes the Heart Grow Stronger

I have four good reasons for being an abstainer — my head is clearer, my health is better, my heart is lighter and my purse is heavier.

Thomas Guthrie (1803-1873),
Scottish clergyman

Perhaps the Reverend Mr Guthrie was more concerned with abstaining from one particular vice than with the discipline of total abstention. Nonetheless, his reasons are no less applicable, no less timely in support of what is about to be unfolded.

This is the astounding story of how the human body can live without food for a certain period of time. It is the revelation of a secret withheld from man because all animals which employ it with continual success cannot convince man of life's simplicities, so predisposed is he toward the seeking of complexities. This is the story of the *fast* way to health. If you want to speed up, slow down. If you want to eat more, eat less. If you seek better mental command, stop thinking. If you seek greater virility, abstain from sex.

The secrets of these apparent paradoxes lie in the body's vast latent powers of recuperation, if only they would be utilised. To abstain from sex, for a time, is to allow the body's virility to recover; when coupled with a programme of improved nutrition following a fast, astounding results will take place. Likewise in achieving mental control, work potential and food enjoyment.

To stop thinking for a few days, or weeks, is the most difficult thing imaginable — even thinking about it proves how difficult it is for man not to think about it! Yet, when the brain is allowed to rest for longer than a mere few consecutive hours of sleep, the recovery of total consciousness gives rise to mental and psychic abilities previously unexperienced.

We all enjoy our food. If you do not, then you are a foremost candidate for a fast. But we can enjoy our food even more when our taste buds are cleansed, our bloodstream detoxified and our appetite restored to optimum sensitivity. Only fasting can achieve this efficiently and effectively. Then we shall live longer and in this way eventually be able to eat more than those who immoderately overeat at every opportunity.

Man cannot possibly continue to live at a demanding pace without availing his body and mind of the opportunity for total rest. And sleep cannot always provide that rest. The multiplicity of dreams which entertain one during the night are testimony to this. The body must be taught to unwind, allowing the mind to become detached for sufficient time to facilitate the recovery of its better command of individual life and expression.

The thorough "house-cleaning" which is automatically undertaken during a fast is the best investment in time humanly possible. The word, "fast", seems quite paradoxical in relation to our modern rate of living. It implies a total antithesis to our general living pace, requiring that one submit to a gradual slowing down of the body through complete abstention from food, maximum rest and no thinking.

"Fast" derives from the old Teutonic *faestan*, meaning to make fast, observe, be strict. And this is exactly what it implies. But what rewards await the discoverer!

The Physiology of Fasting

However great the variance between different schools of healing may be, all agree that the body needs rest at regular and adequate intervals. Overactivity implies inadequate rest, preconditioning illness. But rest must be more than the mere prostration of the body — it must be thorough physical and mental inactivity.

An ideal night's rest will be achieved if the stomach is empty and the brain clear of thoughts. With both body and brain relaxed, with no tension in muscle groups, discomfort in the gastrointestinal tract or disharmony in the mind, a restful eight hours sleep will see a remarkable change develop. Renewed vigour, enthusiasm and growth have taken place; even minor detoxification has occurred so that valuable cleansing has also improved the health by a small degree. It is this latter undertaking which is developed further when fasting.

Whereas medicine generally induces a swift reaction from the body, fasting allows a slow, natural cleansing to develop. Fasting for health requires a total submission to rest. This enables most of the body's energy forces to be directed towards the vital job of detoxification and cleansing. Such process, which commences each night in sleep, is greatly reduced during daily activity when energy is directed into channels of muscular expansion and contraction, together with the removal of by-products of muscular activity such as lactic acid and pyruvic acid. Energy directed into these avenues cannot be used for the cleansing of accumulated toxic build-ups. This suggests that an important reason for total rest is cellular detoxification.

When we eat or engage in activity, food must be broken down into component nutrients, then built up into cellular tissue or energy supply. The residue must be gathered and thrown out. The body recognises these priorities and thus acts to direct all energy into the nourishing and muscular activity fields as the most vital avenues of need. Therefore, if too much food, or food containing disproportionate amounts of unusable matter, is constantly ingested, or if too much activity, with inadequate periods of relaxation to cleanse the action areas is undertaken, toxicity will accumulate within the body until it results in discomfort and illness.

These illnesses initially manifest as acute symptoms of toxaemia (e.g., a cold). If ignored or suppressed, they usually intensify in time, developing into more chronic pathologies (e.g., pneumonia). Under the guidance of a health practitioner experienced in the science of fasting, great benefit will derive from a short fast in the acute stage. In the chronic stage, longer fasting will be needed. Even so, varying degrees of irreversibility may reduce fasting's detoxifying effect, but it will still provide a far greater pathological benefit than can ever be achieved from the administering of drugs.

Fasting permits the continuation of the brief cleansing period that takes place during sleep. It allows the body to enact its cleansing priorities in a far more successful manner than we could consciously direct them. For this reason, fasting demands total submission and an absolute minimum of energy usage, enabling every kilojoule of available bodily energy to be directed into the area or areas requiring greatest attention. With no food in the gastrointestinal tract and with no tension in the muscular or nervous systems, all available energy is directed into cleansing action.

No food is consumed during fasting. The body lives on its stored reserves, for it is by the gradual breakdown of these that most detoxification occurs. Fresh air and pure water are the only substances to enter the body; even then, only sufficient water to allay the thirst is required. This might vary from a large glass a day to a litre or more, depending on the condition of health, previous dietary and drinking habits and prevailing temperature and humidity.

The body will adequately live on its energy reserves for much longer than most people believe. Until such time as these are consumed, fasting can continue, although the need to continue should be determined by a practitioner experienced in the supervision of fasting. Once the reserves have been consumed, starvation sets in and the body commences to consume its structure, breaking down muscle tissue and organs. (This ultimately leads to death.) Yet fasting — of itself — causes not death but a new awakening (more about that to follow).

Most people can fast for many days without risk, but this should not be undertaken without the supervision of a practitioner. Such supervision generally requires no more than two or three visits per day as the fast develops, but this guidance will allay any fears which might otherwise develop as this new situation involves the body. It is thus best to fast at a health institute, away from the home environment and influences, where constant care and guidance can assist nature's work.

The duration of the fast should be spent in bed, rising only to make an occasional short walk and use of the toilet and bath. As the fast develops, the body becomes weaker — a combined result of diminishing energy and muscular inactivity. This weakness is desirable to facilitate the best results in the most efficient manner.

People fast for many different reasons and their purpose is often a guide to the most suitable duration of the fast. If fasting for rejuvenation reasons, shorter fasts of one or two weeks are the usual. For health reasons, especially if chronic pathologies are present, much longer fasts can be undertaken. The longest known to this writer is 105 days, conducted in Mexico some years ago. Yes, that is 105 days without any food, but it should be pointed out that this was a very heavy woman with a huge cancerous growth on her chest, who just wanted to die.

She was Spanish, a sufferer who could find no relief in her country from the pain of a rapidly spreading cancer. Told of a doctor then in practice in Mexico City, she determined to visit him and fast so that she could die without pain. For she was told that death would be her only release: "medical science had no hope for her". Well, nature did. On the 98th day of her fast, a very thin and weak lady saw something she would never have believed possible — the huge, cauliflower-like growth just imploded, it caved in and fell apart, for its entire substance had been remitted from the body during those long weeks of fasting.

After such a long fast, the recovery period was most tedious and very slow. But she lived. Another "miracle" of nature: no miracle when nature is allowed to do its thing! This lady was still alive when the writer visited the doctor a few years ago — he had recently been in contact with her. She was back in Spain, happy, fit and well and totally committed to following a healthful diet after such a traumatic experience — almost literally "born again".

As the cleansing action takes place during fasting, toxic residues are eliminated in many different ways. The body uses the most expedient means as its disposal. The bowels and bladder are employed very sparingly during fasting; in fact a urination once each day or each second day, depending on the amount of water consumed, is quite usual. A bowel movement as rarely as once a week is not uncommon when fasting, some people not having a bowel motion at all after the second week of the fast.

Elimination through the ears, nose, mouth and pores will continue constantly during fasting. The toxicity on the tongue is especially noticeable, taking the form of a concentrated "furriness" such as often develops at night and greets one's look into the mirror in the morning. When fasting, this coating on the tongue is a good indicator of the progress being made by the body's detoxification efforts. If it becomes too unpleasant, the tongue can be lightly scraped with an inverted spoon, but the coating will eventually pass of its own accord if left alone. However, comfort is a vital consideration during fasting; hence the recommendation of scraping with a spoon if any distaste exists.

It is interesting to note that soon after any food is taken, the tongue's coating greatly diminishes or disappears altogether. For this reason, it becomes apparent that no food should be taken during the fast, for it would reverse the body's eliminating programme. Fasting is a controlled extreme in metabolism, which is the reason for it to be undertaken and terminated properly and with great care. The reintroduction of food can be the most important aspect of the fast.

"Partial Fasts"

It is no more possible to have a partial fast than it is to dig a partial hole. Man is either fasting or feeding. To undertake a partial *diet* is what people imply when they talk of a partial fast. The famous "grape diet" is properly termed, for it implies a monotrophic diet of nothing but grapes. But it is a food intake and definitely not a fast. So "grape fast" is just as inaccurate as using similar terminology when on grapefruit or oranges or any other single food for a specific period. The body must be either metabolising nutritional intakes or breaking down inner reserves. It cannot do both simultaneously, for the one is the reverse of the other.

The idea of eating one food for a predetermined period has certain advantages. It can facilitate some valuable cleansing of the gastrointestinal tract because it is being used less. Of course, this would not apply if the "single food" were hamburgers or frankfurters! One simple fruit at a time, such as watermelon or grapes, facilitates the most efficient digestion, but it does not always provide an adequate balance of nutrients. However, this latter point is not so important if the programme is intended for a short period, for it often follows a long habit of overindulgence when far more nutrients (and toxins) were ingested than could be appropriated or expelled.

Fresh fruit or vegetable juices for one or more days provide a satisfactory alternative to fasting if the time is not convenient to allow for total rest. Even so, it is wise to reduce one's activities as much as possible during the period of juice-taking. This will allow more effective inner cleansing to be undertaken between intakes. Such periods of cleansing are possible because the time required in the gastrointestinal tract for a single type of juice is far less than would be demanded by a more complex meal. This regimen is, therefore, an excellent one for busy people, especially those whose work involves them in business entertaining at mealtimes and/or stressful conditions.

The best time to undertake a juice diet is over a weekend, if one works hard during the week. For some people, the weekend sees them expending more energy than during their working week, so it is better for them to have their juice days during the week. For people who are overweight, a day or two on juices each week provides an excellent weight-reduction period which can materially assist in normalising their body weight.

Preparing for the Fast

The reduced diet and juice diet are both of considerable benefit in preparing the body for a fast. They will assist the stomach to prepare for lower intakes of food and will marginally condition the fatty tissues to prepare to give up some of their bulk and stored toxicity. In this manner, the actual fast will become far more beneficial and is often for a shorter duration than might otherwise be required. The general guide is for the person to refrain from all concentrate foods the week before a fast is planned, eating only fruit or vegetable salads, reducing to juices only during the final three days before fasting.

It is not uncommon for a person to have a deep-rooted fear of fasting. Invariably they have been conditioned by friends and relatives to believe that unless food is eaten every day and often, starvation will overtake them. Most people equate an empty stomach with starvation and, although quite well-meaning, often upset a faster, even though they have never undertaken a fast themselves.

The initial experience with fasting will allay these fears. The "virgin" faster will soon discover that it is only a matter of relaxing and enjoying, for the body soon adjusts to the fast and the mind certainly revels in the temporary disassociation from material concerns. After two or three days, the body loses it appetite for food and the feeling of emptiness disappears, enabling one to detach the mind from a preoccupation with food.

This is not possible to the same extent on a partial diet. As soon as the food has left the stomach, that familiar feeling of emptiness returns. This signals the commencement of the final catabolism of the food and then the cleansing action slowly begins. But this will be thwarted with the intake of the next small meal, so we have a stop-and-go system of feeding and cleansing, neither of which is very thorough. For this reason, the partial diet is best undertaken for limited periods of days, rather than weeks. It is certainly a good training in fortitude, provided it does not give rise to frustration and tension.

Often, a more suitable form of partial diet is to totally miss one or two meals. This is especially desirable after a day of excessive or rich food. To miss the next breakfast and, desirably, lunch, will allow a clearing of the gastrointestinal tract and elimination of toxic matter, rather than its storage, as would occur if more food were to be ingested. It will also encourage the return of the appetite which is always rewarded by the real enjoyment of eating.

Fasting Facilitates Fertility

A curious aspect of our Western society is the number of marriages in which infertility prevails. This problem has many aspects, varying from simple impotence to all the complications associated with fear and anxiety. It can generally be related to four basic factors — tension, malnutrition, physical deformity or obstruction.

Tension is all too characteristic of Western civilisation. (Its relative absence in the "underdeveloped" countries must be some sort of clue to their overpopulation!) Everyone is aware of the need to learn how to relax, but few practise it. The mere suggestion to relax is usually futile. It would be far more beneficial to show them how to relax and have them feel the resulting benefits. In this regard, no better method exists than fasting.

A second factor affecting fertility is malnutrition. But how does malnutrition relate to couples in affluent countries? In spite of the abundance of modern foods offered to man, many are quite low in nutritive value. This may lead to a condition of malnutrition, which is often not discovered until the adoption of a natural foods diet following a fast. The contrasts in vitality and virility following full recovery from the fast, compared to the conditions which prevailed before it, prove the point. In cases of infertility, the agreement of both husband and wife to undertake a fast has frequently resulted in the reward of their own child being born within the following year or so.

Quite obviously, many of the beneficial effects of fasting would be dissipated if one were to return to a conventional diet following its completion. It is important that the fast be employed as a break in old habits and a preparation for the new, the embracing of the natural foods diet which is so ideal for man's needs.

Not only must the dietary habits change, but other habits also must be corrected. Smoking and alcohol are known nutritional inhibitors. While their effects may not be so readily apparent normally, when it comes to the special demands on the body required for conception, there may be just not enough nutritional reserves to facilitate the action. The period of total abstinence during fasting is the ideal opportunity for refusing to return to those pernicious habits. And, of course, it should be realised that when on the natural foods diet, free of stimulating and thirst-producing components, there is no longer the urge to smoke for relaxation and to drink alcohol for either relaxation or thirst quenching.

A special word of advice concerning sexual intercourse and fasting. This act should be assiduously avoided during the period of the fast and until the body has recovered its full strength thereafter. Otherwise, it reduces the amount of energy available for detoxification, directing it to the revitalisation of the sexual organs at a time when such stimulation would be a definite setback to the fasting process.

How to Fast

No one would consider undertaking a journey to a new land without some care in its planning. Fasting implies such a journey so it, too, should be carefully planned to remove much of the fear of the unknown, felt by so many people.

Although many excellent books are available to give the proposed faster some guidance, it should be realised that the full experience of fasting can only be acquired by actual involvement. When one reads of the experiences of other "travellers", a form of general guidance is the best one can expect to acquire. This will be greatly improved if, when undertaking the same journey, we are accompanied by one who has great personal experience to guide us. And so it is with fasting, especially for the first time. Thereafter, we are more familiar with the journey and can relate our experiences to those of experts, whose written works will be understood more clearly.

Probably the most experienced practitioner in fasting anywhere in the world is Dr Herbert M. Shelton of San Antonio, Texas. His supervising of more than 40,000 fasts over half a century must constitute a record. Unfortunately, his age (he was born in 1895) has caused him to discontinue practice in recent years.

Second only to Dr Shelton, in terms of the number of fasts supervised, is Dr Carlos Arguello, a Nicaraguan who has practised extensively throughout North and Central America after receiving his training in the United States and interning with Dr Shelton. (I have, in fact, studied with both practitioners — Shelton in San Antonio and Arguello in Florida and Nicaragua.)

Australia's leading authority on fasting is Dr Alec Burton of Sydney, with whom I have both studied and fasted. However, the centre with the reputation for supervising the greatest number of fasts is the Hopewood Health Centre, just west of Sydney at Wallacia. They have three highly qualified practitioners who have achieved considerable success in aiding nature to restore people's health when their bodies are allowed to totally rest.

As a convenience for those who recognise the need to fast and are seeking a suitable location at which to undertake it, the following is a list of those practitioners whose work this writer has had an opportunity to observe. At the time of writing, addresses were correct; however, prospective patients should check before making the journey.

Hopewood Health Centre, Greendale Road, Wallacia, NSW; phone 047.738401.
Natural Health Society, 131 York Street, Sydney, NSW; phone 298656.
Dr Alec Burton, "Hygea", Cobah Road, Arcadia, NSW; phone 6531115.
Dr Carlos Arguello, Apartado 814, Managua, Nicaragua, Central America.
Dr Stanley Bass, 3119 Coney Is. Avenue, Brooklyn, NY, 11235, USA.
Dr John Brosious, 18207 Gulf Blvd., St Petersburg, Florida, 33708, USA.
Frances Cheatham, The Shangri-La Natural Hygiene Institute, Bonita Springs, Florida, 33923, USA.
H. Jay Dinshah, "Suncrest", Box H, Malaga, New Jersey, 08328, USA.
Dr William Esser, Esser's Hygienic Rest Ranch, P.O. Box 161, Lake Worth, Florida, USA.
Dr Robert Gross, Pawling Manor, Hyde Park, NY, USA.
Dr David Scott, P.O. Box 8919, Cleveland, Ohio, 44136, USA.
Dr Keki Sidwa, "Shalimar", First Avenue, Frinton-On-Sea, Essex, England.
David Stry, Villa Vegetariana Spa, Box 1228, Cuernavaca, Mo., Mexico.

It must be emphasised that this is not intended as a comprehensive list of fasting institutions and practitioners, merely a list based on the writer's personal travels. Elsewhere throughout the world, such centres and practitioners are functioning, but specific names and addresses are best obtained through telephone directories by calling local health organisations, vegetarian societies, vegan societies, natural hygiene societies, etc. In England, on mainland Europe, in India and South Africa, qualified practitioners should be found available to supervise fasting, all of whom would be known to such organisations.

I strongly urge anyone contemplating a future fast to make preliminary contact with a qualified practitioner, thereby giving him time to thoroughly understand the case history. In many ways this will be mutually beneficial. Fasting practitioners are more usually found among chiropractors, osteopaths, naturopaths and homoeopaths, than among surgeons or physicians. Naturopaths are the most likely practitioners, for in many such courses of study the subject of fasting is taught. Otherwise, it is left to the qualified practitioner to gain a knowledge of the subject when in practice and not all are prepared or disposed towards this end. Those who are, certainly make the best consultants.

When to Fast

The ideal time for the commencement of a supervised fast is when the body's temperature rises a few degrees. Then a state of crisis prevails. This is indicated by feverishness, headache, muscular pains or general debility accompanying the rise in temperature. It is then that the body is working hard to throw off an accumulation of toxic matter from within. Elimination will come very easily from such natural preparation. Should that occasion prove inconvenient in terms of pressing social or vocational involvements, one should then just take two or three days off to undergo a short fast until the crisis has subsided with the elimination of excess toxicity. If a supervised fast of longer duration can be undertaken, vital benefits will be achieved by a remarkable cleansing of the entire body and a reharmonising of body and mind.

To suppress such acute elimination crises as just described is to compound them into some future chronic illness which becomes more deeply rooted within the body by interfering with its natural functioning. Many is the case in which a person has taken antibiotics to suppress a cold or influenza (both of which are classic cases of acute toxic elimination) only to find that a few months later they are suffering from bronchitis or pneumonia.

At a time of acute enervation drugs severely complicate the condition by their interference with natural body chemistry, giving rise to iatrogenic effects (drug-induced diseases). Gout, arthritis, arteriosclerosis and cancer are just some of the more chronic conditions which would not develop if earlier toxic crises were allowed to run their courses and were subsequently avoided by reverting to a natural foods diet.

It is rare for a person to develop a cold when living on the ideal diet, but it can occur. If all other factors influencing health were likewise ideal, it would be impossible for a toxic accumulation to develop. But when living in smoggy cities, harsh climates or amid emotional tensions, the occasional toxic build-up is inevitable. An immediate fast of one or two days will soon correct this.

A wise person, even on an ideal diet, will plan to fast for one day a week, or each two weeks, or each month, as his lifestyle dictates. This is a sure guarantee that the highest level of health is maintained. Such a fast day is set aside to be a day of total rest and is the most valuable investment in health a person can make. Its cost is absolutely nothing, thus showing enormous profits for the investment.

At the very least there is no reason to avoid fasting one day a month. Everyone, no matter how busy, can find the time. It is far more convenient than to go visiting or travelling, for it involves doing exactly nothing. It is far cheaper than paying for health insurance or dining out on a multi-course meal. That monthly fast day should be set aside as, say, the first Saturday or Sunday in each month. No finer way could be found to spend a "sabbath"; no closer could you get to your Maker than by such practical respect for "His image". How much better it is to *be* a sermon, than to preach one!

Fasting and Obesity

Although all people possess the same type of gastrointestinal tract, considerable variation exists in the concentration and proportion of components of their digestive juices. Likewise, metabolic rates vary from person to person and variations exist in the individual utilisation of energy kilojoules. Thus a meal which could be fully utilised within the body of one person might induce the accumulation of some body fat in another.

Relating these differences to the enormous variety of meals people eat, it is easy to see why such a wide range of body weights can be found within one race of people living in the same environment.

For some, the accumulation of excess body weight is a severe problem. Many chemical and processed-food manufacturers have made fortunes from the exploitation of these fatty abundances. Yet all such attempts at control fail when the individual refuses to recognise the need to exercise moderation in quantity and discrimination in the quality of the food upon which he feeds. Fundamentally, obesity reveals a failure to learn how to live in accordance with one's body type and one's purpose. Yet this omission is very easily corrected.

A vital part of the re-education programme for overweight people is the expedient of well-planned fasting. No other method of weight normalisation is as speedy or as health-inducing as such fasting. Obese patients have been known to lose as much as ten kilograms in the first week of their fast, although the average loss is generally in the range of three to six kilograms. The loss in the second week will be some 25 per cent less as the body approaches normality. Weight loss for a slimmer person during fasting is, of course, considerably less.

The special bonuses which usually accrue from fasting to reduce body weight make it the most exciting slimming programme ever conceived. Detoxifying will relieve pressure on the organs, especially the heart, which can take a veritable new lease on life from the experience. Digestion of foods will later show marked improvement, together with the alleviation of such diseases of affluence as diabetes, hypertension, ulcers, anaemia, asthma, etc. No, these are not merely random diseases chosen to enforce the point; they are all proved symptoms of immoderate living which respond to the process of fasting. All the aforenamed practitioners testify to repeated successful case histories.

Breaking the Fast

Every practitioner agrees that a most important aspect of the fast is the manner by which it is broken. The reintroduction of food to the body becomes more critical the longer the person has fasted. Imagine how much intensive care was demanded of the practitioner whose patient stopped the 105-day fast and began the long process of rebuilding on food.

In general terms, the duration of the fast is equalled by the period required for rebuilding on a gradually developing food programme. If one fasts for a week, then another week must be allowed for the gastrointestinal tract to return to normal acceptance of a full meal; if the fast is for a month, then another month should be allowed for full restoration to a balanced diet. Remember, fasting is a reversing of metabolism.

The reintroduction of food when the fast is to be terminated should commence with a fruit juice. Of course, it should be freshly squeezed and, preferably, from organically grown fruit. Oranges, watermelon, grapes, apples or pears are the most suitable fruits to juice, the selection depending on seasonal availabilities and the patient's wishes.

Quantity and manner of consumption of this first meal are vitally important. If the fast is comparatively short, say up to two weeks, up to 200 mL of juice can be taken; if a longer fast, the quantity should be reduced to 125 mL. If the fast has been undertaken to correct digestive problems, the initial juice should be diluted with a smaller quantity of pure water. Whichever case, the juice should not be drunk from a glass. It should be sipped from a spoon and "chewed" before swallowing. This ensures proper ensalivation for best digestion.

Following the initial juice, the patient should rest in a reclining position with the head and shoulders higher than the stomach. This first food intake will be like nectar of the gods and he will remember it for a long time as the best meal of his life. The rest will help him enjoy it and facilitate its easier digestion as the metabolic processes revert to normal.

It is generally best to break the fast in the morning. The first juice can be followed by another, in two to three hours, a little larger in quantity. Whether or not it should be again diluted for the long faster will be determined by the practitioner, based on the response to the initial juice by the patient's body. Likewise, the number and frequency of juices that first day will also be decided by the experienced practitioner.

The first solid meal should be of fresh fruit without any concentrates. Two apples or pears, 250 g of grapes or a slice of watermelon or wedge of paw paw — any would provide a suitable choice. Following at least one and a half days on fruit, vegetables can be introduced in the form of a whole salad or a blended salad, depending on the patient's chewing ability. All such decisions are best left to the practitioner, guided by the patient's wishes and his responses to the previous meal.

When the patient can easily handle fresh fruits and vegetables, concentrated protein foods can be introduced. The first should be up to 30 g of nuts or seeds, again depending on the patient's chewing ability as to whether these are blended or given whole. They should be given with either oranges or a raw vegetable salad. In fact, for the entire period of recovery from the fast, no cooked food should be given — it has diminished nourishment potential and induces overeating, as experience always proves.

Following the one-day fast, no special feeding care has to be taken. The breakfast would normally constitute fresh fruit, ideal especially on this occasion. Likewise after a two-day or three-day fast, a fresh fruit breakfast is ideal, but care as to quantity is very important. Only two pieces of fruit, or no more than 250 g, should be consumed. A period of short rest thereafter should be mandatory.

Reinvolvement in physical activity after a fast should also be undertaken with discretion. Muscular energy has to be redirected from its fasting involvement and this is not done immediately. After the body has been reconditioned to the acceptance of food, it is wise to engage in a certain amount of activity, but only while sufficient energy prevails. Once the slightest feeling of tiredness intrudes, the body must be allowed to relax. It will require many days for the body to be able to engage in fluent activity after a fast of two or three weeks; a week or more if the fast extended over a month.

Never rush the recovery processes. Some people are inclined to become anxious and impatient for a rapid restoration to full energy after their fast. They must realise that their body is virtually being born again and the speed with which it develops full facility should be allowed to proceed naturally. Not only can the body fully recover its energy, it can develop greater potential for work and expression after the fast than was previously the case.

The Spiritual Fast

The two most ancient religious groups, the Hindus and the Jews, uphold the importance of fast days in their religious observances. Such occasions are intended to benefit both body and psyche, to bring them into better harmony and thereby nearer their Krishna or God.

Pious members of these religious groups ensure that on their fast day they not only abstain from food, but also from work. By resting, they observe proper fast days. This is in marked contrast to some other religious groups which observe "Lenten fasts" and put on weight. All they do is to abstain from one type of food, but substitute another, the different flavours of which generally inspire overindulgence. Obviously, their use of the term "fast" is a misnomer.

Muslims also have different ideas about fasting. During their month of Ramadan, orthodox Muslims consume neither food nor drink between the hours of sunrise and sunset. However, their intake during the hours of darkness often more than compensates.

The true spiritual fast is the one which is accompanied by meditation. It is not easily achieved if the body has any critical pathological problems, for the crises and/or withdrawal symptoms from food would detract from the desired physical and psychological state.

Meditation is used in effect to dissociate consciousness from the body, to elevate it into super-consciousness, the "overself"; thereby associating it with psychic awareness. This achieves the restoration of perfect harmony between psyche and body, permits the development of conscious psychic awareness and attunes the individual to his purpose and his environment in a natural, reliable manner.

Before any significant progress can be achieved in elevating the consciousness from the physical level, the gastrointestinal tract will need to be emptied of all but the final traces of refuse. This generally requires two or three days, during which one can engage in short meditations to quell the emotions and dispel any fears.

With more and more time spent in meditation during each day of the spiritual fast, by the end of the first week the candidate is ready for further development. At least for the first of these fasts, it is important to be under the care of the practitioner, but he should be acquainted with your intentions and thus will not disturb you unless it be for a regular morning check-up. Throughout the second week of the fast, that morning contact will probably be your only touch with physical consciouness.

The experiences sought by many young people with the use of addictive drugs are as nothing compared with those obtainable by means of the spiritual fast. The extra time is more than amply repaid by the experiences awaiting those who would know the secrets of life. Furthermore, the fast offers the added benefit of cleansing the body and creating no negative after-effects. No other method of investigating the psyche can be as rewarding.

It must be emphasised that only if it is the intention of the faster to undertake esoteric spiritual experiences will such be accorded him. Very few people are aware of this faculty, so to most who fast, no such intensity of beauty awaits them. Yet everyone will find that a new lightness, an inexplicable tranquillity, will enrobe them during a fast of reasonable duration. As Doctor Shelton puts it:

"The freedom and ease that one experiences during a period of abstinence from food often enables one to discover new and previously undreamed-of depths to the meaning of life."

But that is as far as most people go. Even so, it will reveal how much more they can enjoy life when this new-found harmony embraces their total being. Under such circumstances, it is so much easier to adapt to the world, to life and to its other members, to love life and every part of it.

Indeed, as one comes to learn the true meaning of life, both in general terms and in relation to individual purpose, every thought, every action is recognised for the full responsibility it implies as a representative of its author. The realisation, not only that everything has its purpose, but more significantly, that that purpose is the acceptance of a very special responsibility, is a measure of true initiation into the secrets of the inner self.

STAGE THIRTEEN

Therapeutic Diets for Common Illnesses

Throughout the history of this planet, man has been smitten by many forms of disease. Up to a century or so ago, most of these were related to either malnutrition or lack of hygiene. In the twentieth century, world sanitation has improved considerably, consistent with improvements in habits of human hygiene — externally. But internally, the position is different.

Many governments, groups and individuals will be offended, possibly, when told that the present state of human health evidences greater internal deterioration in hygiene than ever before. Although nowadays people wash more often, they also use more breath sweeteners, body deodorants and chemical purifiers than ever before. Just what is going on inside? Something must be rotting!

The Body's Disharmony

It is that the modern diet has become so far removed from man's pristine requirements that his bodily systems are just not coping. Digestion, absorption, assimilation, utilisation and elimination are all taking place, but with lowered efficiency and under stressed conditions. The fault is no longer lack of food, but inadequate nutrition, a breakdown in natural hygiene, a failure to live in accordance with nature's laws. And so at variance are modern man's living habits that to isolate and endeavour to correct them is to imply to the individual that a grave personality fault exists.

This fault is related to the persistent belief that processing is necessary for modern dietary needs. But this same processing diminishes the potential nutritional value of the foods it is supposed to be "improving". Hence we find many and varied cases of human illness caused not by insufficient food, but by overeating. Such illness still gives rise to malnutrition, although it is now manifested in widely varying forms. We have a far greater range of illnesses afflicting man today than ever in his history so we can no longer close our eyes to the causes by pretending they will evaporate and not upset the establishment created by government and commerce.

As has been explained in detail earlier in this book, every form of illness is traceable to one cause — disharmony. This might have its foundation in dietary problems, in emotional conflict, in skeletal areas or in the mind. All of these aspects of human construction and expression exert an influence on the total being we know as man, but generally one aspect will predominate. If the area of weakness is structural, a chiropractor or osteopath is usually the practitioner with the special skills for diagnosing and correcting the problem. If emotional, a competent counsellor should be sought. If the disharmony lies in the regions of the mind, a wide range of specialists is available, including neurologists, psychiatrists, sociologist counsellors, not to forget metaphysicians who can be of special help if the problem is a spiritual one.

Finally, if the problem has its roots in the dietary domain, the specialist has to be a nutritionist. But there are many areas of diet where the person can effectively become his own nutritional consultant. For this reason, the following dietary guidance is offered to those sufferering from specific symptoms (often, erroneously, called "diseases"). Not every known problem condition will be listed, but rather those which specifically and readily respond to dietary correction. Many conditions also respond to other forms of relief treatment, such as herbs, Bach remedies, homoeopathy, and so on, but they are not within the scope of this book.

In listing the following symptoms, no attempt will be made to describe or to diagnose. It will be assumed that sufferers will be aware of their condition and seek only the dietary guidance to overcome it. Such guidance, it must be stressed, is not intended to be either exhaustive or categorical. It is general guidance, found to be beneficial to most people suffering those symptoms. If the recommendations do not work, other factors must prevail and these should be investigated by a competent practitioner. One advantage of dietary correction is that, if perchance it does not work, it certainly does no harm. Sad that this cannot be said of all therapeutic suggestions.

Some Common Symptoms

Acne 1) Common minor skin eruptions (including eczema) indicate a dietary imbalance and/or an excess of protein which the body is not assimilating. This will usually imply the consuming of protein foods from unsuitable sources, generally too much animal protein. Gradual improvement will be obtained by reducing the amount of animal protein and increasing the amount of vegetarian protein (see Stage 6). Faster improvement will occur when food combining rules are adhered to (see Stage 9), even better when all animal foods, acid-forming starches (particularly flour) and sugars (particularly refined and raw) are eliminated from the diet. But the speediest results will be seen when a short fast is undertaken (see Stage 12).

2) Teenage acne is a particular problem when the body's hormones need freedom from interference by poorly combined foods, sometimes occurring when the youth "discovers" the new taste addictions of "fast foods". Correct food combining is very important here, as well as minimising animal foods, especially fatty foods. Speediest results will be obtained from a raw foods diet along vegetarian lines.

Certain herb teas and food supplements will be beneficial to those suffering from any form of acne. Dandelion, alternating with equisetum tea, is best for adults; fenugreek tea, alternating with equisetum tea, is best for teenage acne. One cup of each type of tea each day should suffice. The addition of lecithin (powdered or granulated or in tablet form) will prove highly beneficial. The most valuable of all sources of silica (the most beneficial mineral for the skin) is in rice bran syrup, but this is not always readily available. Alternatively, brown rice will help. Valuable supplements are dolomite, plus vitamins A and E.

Alcoholism The causes of alcoholism are manifold, but they can be put into two categories — nutritional and emotional. For many people with emotional problems, alcohol is a way of hiding from their realities and the necessity of facing them, of easing the pain, of not facing and overcoming their "insecurity", or of succumbing to the need for sensations. But alcoholism is also a symptom of dietary deficiency — no doubt one will exist once alcoholism prevails, but it often exists as a precursor to alcoholism. The usual deficiency area is in the B-vitamins. This is often caused by too many refined foods in the diet, too much sugar and salt. To rectify, replace the white bread with whole grain cereals (best to avoid bread and eat muesli, brown rice, buckwheat and the like), replace white sugar with dried fruits. Avoid tea and coffee; have fruit juices. Avoid salt, thereby reducing the craving to drink. Take megadoses of B-complex vitamins in the most potent anti-stress formulation available, so as to obtain at least 1000 mg of B_3 (with as high a proportion of niacin as can be handled without facial flushes creating anxiety). With this should be taken up to 5000 mg vitamin C and 1000 mg vitamin E (so long as no history of hypertension prevails). The amino acid, tryptophan, should also be taken (up to 2000 mg one hour before bed) to improve sleep and restore normal slumber patterns and revitalisation.

Allergies Entire books have been written on this subject — here goes for a paragraph! Most allergies are related to protein or to a poison. Drugs are some of the frequent causes; and foods which induce allergies are often treated as drugs by the body. Allergies are generally the body's heroic effort to eliminate, discard something it considers unsuitable, probably poisonous. Seek the cause and eliminate that item from the diet or from whatever treatment is being undertaken. Milk often causes allergies; little wonder, for few can handle it satisfactorily (see Stage 6). Replace it with fruit or vegetable juices, soya milk, nut milk or water. Wheat is a common allergen — this will be covered under "Coeliac". Obviously, when such foods or groups are recognised, their avoidance is wise, for many other foods are possible. Allergies can be easily masked, appearing to be one type of food, when they are actually something else — for instance, hay fever can be caused, not by pollen in the air, but by milk in the stomach. Allergies can manifest as respiratory problems, bowel problems, skin eruptions, intestinal swelling, and so on. Prompt relief will usually be afforded by taking alfalfa and pollen tablets and drinking alfalfa tea, then by not eating for 24–48 hours, drinking only alfalfa tea. Should the condition persist, a longer fast might be needed, in which case, supervision from a competent practitioner should be sought. Such a fast would be followed by a natural foods diet, accepting animal foods (if one cannot live without them) only when all symptoms have disappeared. If fasting is difficult, undertake an elimination diet of raw fruits and vegetables for at least three days, or if possible two days on fresh juices only. Most cases of allergy indicate hyperacidity, hence the highly alkaline fruits and vegetables to neutralise. Highly recommended vitamin supplements are B_5, A and C, supported by a well-balanced B-complex.

Anaemia 1) Common anaemia describes the condition of the blood where its red cells are insufficient and too small, being short of haemoglobin. This is usually indicative of inadequate iron intake — either from the food or inadequately absorbed although available. Iron and its role in health are discussed in Stage 8. It is a trace mineral and vital for energy supply to the muscles, so anaemic people are usually listless and low in vitality. They often experience severe emotional problems, among which depression usually prevails. Emotional disharmony (anger, stress, depression, and so on) significantly interfere with the body's ability to absorb many nutrients, especially the more difficult ones, such as iron. Not only are the nerves of the stomach and intestines then in disarray, but an emotional person usually does not chew food adequately, further inhibiting the absorption of whatever iron content it might possess. For these people, the intake of supplemental iron will do nothing, except perhaps induce toxicity. Their need is to handle the emotional aspect of their life first — anti-stress B-complex vitamins and/or valerian tea can help, but must be accompanied with improved self-command. The person suffering from inadequate dietary sources of iron is the easiest to assist. They need to include such foods as pepitas, parsley, nuts, other seeds, egg yolk, alfalfa sprouts and abundant other greens. Dietary yeasts, liquid chlorophyll, alfalfa tablets and iron tablets combined with vitamin C all offer vital supplementation. Adequate exposure to the sun's rays is also important. If constipation accompanies their anaemia, licorice tea is a valuable beverage for its gentle laxative properties and abundance of iron salts.

2) Pernicious anaemia differs from common forms of anaemia in that the bed blood cells are larger and contain more haemoglobin, but of an immature form. This also indicates lack of adequate iron but, more particularly, lack of the vitamin which provides another vital trace mineral — B_{12} — of which cobalt is a chemical component. The most suitable food sources of B_{12} are whole grains, alfalfa sprouts, green vegetables, egg yolks, cheeses and whey powder. Dietary yeasts are also worthwhile sources of B_{12}, being the basis of B_{12} supplements in tablet form. Liquid chlorophyll is a further valuable food supplement.

A fairly wide range of herb teas contain small quantities of available iron and copper salts of worthwhile assistance in building haemoglobin in the blood, copper providing assistance in the assimilation of iron. These teas include comfrey, dandelion, hibiscus, parsley, raspberry and rosehips. Kelp is an additional food supplement which will also provide nutritional benefit when anaemia prevails.

Anorexia Nervosa   Loss of appetite is a more common problem than often conceived. A temporary loss can be caused by any one of a host of circumstances, generally emotional and related to anxiety, sorrow, disappointment, fear, horror and the like. Genuine anorexia is a prevailing syndrome where psychosis, accompanied by hysteria, results in gradual loss of weight which, if not arrested, must result in death. It generally occurs in young women with a fanatical desire for slimness, but they are also emotionally immature and unstable. Care must be twofold — psychological and nutritional. Herb teas can be most effective in stimulating a dormant appetite — comfrey, fennel and ginger teas particularly. In chelated form for easy assimilation, the mineral, zinc, will also usually help to improve the acuteness of taste detection, the appetite being closely related to the sensation of taste. Smoking will numb taste buds, as will common salt, so these must be avoided. Fatty foods should also be avoided, for these can induce nausea. Fresh fruit and vegetable juices are often successful in reintroducing food. When solid foods are offered, keep them simple, attractive and natural. This system of reintroducing food is not unlike the process of breaking a fast, but a person who has fasted has a great desire to eat again — after anorexia, it returns gradually.

Arterial Problems   Both common forms, arteriosclerosis (hardening of the arteries in which the arteries become thickened and lose elasticity) and atherosclerosis (hardening of the arteries due to thick deposits of fat and cholesterol), are related to diet, activity and attitude. Both conditions will be exacerbated by hypertension (see p. 246), itself arising from similar causes. Inadequate exercise and emotional balance are characteristic of most modern people as they settle into their mature years (thirties and forties), when the effects of an unsuitable diet start to become evident. Most detrimental to arterial health are meat, poultry, sea food, eggs and dairy products, together with salt and processed and refined foods. Small quantities of these foods will generally not create problems, for the arteries can handle them, unless the intake becomes a flood. And this occurs in most diets, because up to 75 per cent of the average diet comprises the foregoing ingredients. Other factors known to contribute to these problems are smoking, alcohol and the use of aluminium, enamel or copper cookware (stainless steel is the only suitable metal). The ideal diet, as outlined in Stage 10, will maintain healthy arteries and prolonged good health. If the arterial problems are at their life-threatening stage (and many people refuse to do anything until this condition is reached), a series of short to medium fasts (see Stage 12) must be undertaken. The excuse of not having time for fasting and planning the dietary changes will not be accepted by St Peter! Early in the dietary change, it is most helpful to include at least a tablespoon of lecithin (either in a fruit drink or over a fruit salad) and to add liquid chlorophyll to fruit juice or water. Vitamins A, D and E are also most helpful supplements.

Arthritis One of the most common maladies of modern living, arthritis has become more prevalent during the past century in somewhat direct proportion to the increasing acidity of modern diets. The condition is characterised by inflammation of the joints, with which is related often rheumatism and gout. It now afflicts, in varying degrees of intensity, three out of every four Western people over sixty years of age and more than half those over forty-five. Once considered an old person's disease, it is now found in children and, occasionally, in infants. It is rarely inherited, but the dietary habits certainly are. Arthritis can become one of the most painful of diseases, but will not be fatal, although the accumulation of drugs taken for it can ultimately prove fatal. Drugs, at best, will only temporarily relieve arthritic pain; only dietary correction will relieve the condition to the extent that reversibility is possible. Some remedial action is possible when dietary changes are made and the earlier the condition is detected, the more complete the correction will be.

Arthritis is largely caused by the same highly acid diet that is responsible for arterial (see p. 228) problems (often the two sets of symptoms appear conjointly). The same general dietary correction applies — highly alkalising, with special emphasis on vegetable salads, alfalfa sprouts and parsley. Greatest improvement will be achieved by adhering to strict vegetarian principles, avoiding flour and sugar products. Beneficial supplements are alfalfa, dolomite and kelp tablets. Beneficial herb teas are alfalfa, comfrey, equisetum and parsley. In popular demand now is the tableted extract of the New Zealand green-lipped mussel, which has been proved to be anti-inflammatory, relieving painful symptoms until dietary changes are registered within the body. Without the dietary changes, however, the condition remains uncorrected and eventually the temporary relief will dissipate as the arthritis worsens.

Asthma Severe attacks of breathlessness, with difficulty inhaling and, particularly, exhaling, characterise asthma. Spasm in the muscles of the bronchial tree and swelling of its mucus lining trigger an asthma attack, but the causes are not so easily defined. Basically they are twofold — physical and emotional. Sometimes both causes are contributory, especially in children, for their body reacts more acutely to unsuitable intakes than does the adult body, and their emotional reactions are likewise more acute and spontaneous. Emotional problems revolve around feelings of insecurity, nervousness and hypersensitivity. These can be overcome by wise counselling for the patient and those closely related. Physical causes of asthma are often due to the body's rejection of cow's milk (sometimes goat's milk, as well). If this is not recognised and corrected, later rejection of all dairy products can develop. Cow's milk is the least suitable food for human babies and the older the child grows, the more dangerous this substance can become (see Stage 6). Hay fever and sinusitis, with intolerances to pollen and dust, together with other allergies, can develop if early asthma is not corrected. Medical palliatives do nothing to find the cause — at best they bring temporary relief to the symptoms. But the cause has to be negated and this can only be achieved through dietary correction and emotional balancing. A non-dairy diet is vital, absence from all forms of animal foods is desirable. Bread and flour products should be avoided. Diet must be based on abundant fresh fruits and vegetables, with nuts and seeds as primary protein foods, for these are the "mucus-free" foods. Excellent food supplements are dolomite tablets combined with vitamins A and D, plus liquid chlorophyll — both these are rich in magnesium. Alfalfa tablets and pollen granules or tablets are also highly beneficial during the transition-diet period. If an attack occurs, asthma will be rapidly diminished by a short fast, taking only a small amount of water as a thirst-quencher.

Backache Chiropractic is the primary professional care for backache, but if it continues to recur, we must look to more than a casual cause. Probably the posture is in need of correction; unsuitable or infrequent exercise could be the cause, so that stiffness occurs; obesity is often a cause (see p. 253); diet can also be unsuitable. The dietary problem will be related to insufficient minerals present in the food, or insufficient absorption of available minerals. Calcium, magnesium and phosphorus are the primary minerals related to bone structure and integrity, vitamin D the primary vitamin working with these minerals. Nuts, seeds, cheese (Swiss and cheddar), soya beans, parsley and other green vegetables should feature in the diet. Food supplements, such as dolomite, liquid chlorophyll, comfrey tablets and dietary yeasts, will be of vital benefit, as will multi-vitamin-mineral tablets. Herb teas with appropriate mineral content are also beneficial — these include alfalfa, chamomile, comfrey, dandelion and hops. Bad dietary habits, responsible for interfering with the body's absorption of these minerals are tea, coffee and cocoa drinking, meat, chocolate, rhubarb, common spinach — all of which are rich in oxalic acid, thereby binding calcium and magnesium. Sugar also leaches the alkalising minerals and must be avoided.

Baldness Far more prevalent in men than in women, progressive baldness can be overcome in most cases, so long as it has not caused complete top hair loss. It requires some determined care and attention, but men are rarely prepared to undertake this until it is almost too late. By contrast, women give their hair considerable care and this helps to explain why baldness rarely afflicts them. When the hair becomes light or thin, this care will improve its density, for both men and women, irrespective of age. The care must be given from both inside and outside. By undertaking scalp massage, with improved diet, plus emotional balance, balding can be averted. An inexpensive, round plastic scalp and body massager will suit perfectly. Stand beside the bathtub each morning before breakfast, bend the head lower than the heart (to facilitate a good blood flow to the scalp) and massage the scalp as vigorously as comfortable, first with the plastic brush, then with the fingertips. Be sure to also press the fingertips onto the scalp and move the scalp in all directions. All this works to loosen the scalp, keeping the skin supple and the follicles (through which the hair grows) open and useful. Plenty of exercise will also help stimulate blood flow to the scalp, especially if you rest between exercises by lying, head downwards, on a slant board. The hair should be shampooed no more than twice weekly and use only a pure soap or shampoo, as described in Stage 11. Do not use chemical hair dressings and keep the hair covered when exposed to dirty and dusty situations. Be sure the diet contains adequate polyunsaturated oils, avocado, wheat germ and green vegetables. A good multi-vitamin-mineral supplement, plus a B-complex vitamin will also assist. Silica is the important trace mineral for the skin and scalp and this is best obtained from the foregoing foods, plus rice bran (and brown rice) and equisetum tea.

Body Odours Not in itself an illness, body odours generally bring to a person's awareness the fact that something is wrong inside. Contrary to most people's beliefs, it is *not* natural to exude unpleasant body odours and to have to regularly apply perfumes and anti-perspirants to delude people into believing that you smell like a flower. Food residues and toxic eliminations do not all pass into the toilet. Many are exuded through the pores, the tongue and the eyes. Unclear eyes, bad breath (halitosis), stale underarms and crutch, malodorous feet are all symptoms that the diet is unbalanced and contains too many toxic residues. Most likely, too many acid-forming foodstuffs are consumed, including "fast foods", fried foods and others which are inadequately digested. In particular, the diet will be found deficient in B-vitamins, especially B_3, in calcium and magnesium. Prompt correction is possible by taking supplementary vitamin B_3, dolomite tablets and liquid chlorophyll (commencing with a dessertspoonful in a glass of cool water on rising each morning). Breakfast should be a fresh fruit meal, lunch a salad and dinner another salad and/or steamed vegetables with your protein concentrated food (as outlined in Stage 10).

Bronchitis Inflammation and congestion in the bronchial tubes is not a disease in itself, nor a separate symptom. It is an acute form of respiratory discomfort, similar to asthma and, for long-term eradication and total correction, is treated as for asthma. Fortunately, bronchitis is not as chronic as asthma when treated promptly. It induces malaise, anorexia, muscle pains, sore throat and fever. The fever should not be suppressed — those who take drugs to achieve this, effectively trap the mucus and toxicity instead of allowing it to be expelled by the fervent activity of the fever (see p. 240). Permanent relief will follow a short fast. Temporary relief is often obtained by drinking a herb tea blend of aniseed, dill seed, chamomile and hops. This will settle the respiratory tract, calm the nerves and induce a restful sleep. Eucalyptus and licorice teas are also beneficial, best taken in the morning.

Cancer There are many forms of cancer — now regarded as a disease of modern civilisation. In general, it is a malignant tumour, cultured by primitive, or wild, cells produced within the body as a consequence of severe interferences to the body's natural cell reproduction system. Causes of interference can be categorised into three groups: physical, chemical and emotional. Anger, hatred, frustration, insecurity and similar unbalancing emotions will disturb the body's biochemical balance. This imbalance transmits right down to cellular level, where it is further deranged by interactions between some of the 3000 and more chemicals in current use by food manufacturers and processors. Benign tumours can be deregulated and released into malignancies by severe or repeated physical abrasion. These are the general causes of cancer, simplified for general comprehension, but not inaccurate. They enforce the long-held knowledge of most naturopathic practitioners that cancer does not arise from bacteria, germ or virus — it is a man-made consequence of careless living. And it can be treated, usually with considerable success, by natural means. But in some parts of the world, Australia for one, no one, other than a registered medical practitioner, can treat a patient for cancer. Yet, with all its research and resources, medical science has not been successful in counteracting or eradicating cancer. Fortunately, advice can be given through a book, but not by personal consultation with a nutritionist and naturopath, in whose domain a form of correction may lie.

Some of the significant causes of cancer will first need to be removed from the diet of the sufferer (and of everyone, for cancer is now a major killer). These include excessive meat-eating (especially any preserved meats such as ham, bacon, sausage), any preserved foodstuff, caffeine (tea, coffee, cola), tobacco and fried foods. Anti-cancer foods, those which should be emphasised in the diet, include all raw fruits and vegetables (organically grown), raw egg yolks (free-range), natural yogurt, raw nuts (especially almonds), plenty of fresh sprouts, some whole grains (buckwheat and millet are best), small amounts of raw seeds. Green vegetable juices are highly beneficial, especially wheat grass (see Dr Ann Wigmore's book, *Why Suffer*, Hippocrates Health Institute, Boston, USA, 1964), liquid chlorophyll, celery and beetroot tops, comfrey and parsley. Other vegetable juices are also beneficial, including carrot, beetroot and potato. Of the fruit juices, grape is the most beneficial (see *The Grape Cure* by Johanna Brandt — numerous publishers). Fasting can be highly valuable in many types of cancer, but only under professional guidance; especially when laetrile (vitamin B_{17}) is included. General vitamin therapy includes megadoses of C and E — vitamins A and B-complex can also be vitally beneficial, again depending on the nature of the cancer and its location. A multi-enzyme digestive formula can also help. Brewer's yeast and wheat germ are the most beneficial food supplements, due to their high concentration of selenium. In conclusion, remember, this is a complex condition, best prevented by avoiding cancer-inducing habits and foods, as do sincere Seventh Day Adventists and Mormons, who are among the most cancer-free people in the world.

Canker Sores Most people at some time have suffered from the discomfort of a canker sore in the mouth. It is a spreading ulcerous sore inside the cheek, lips or on the gum, being usually initiated by the inside of the lip or cheek being inadvertently bitten or by irritation from a denture. From a slight swelling and inflammation, a sore develops, generally fed by stomach acidity. A persistent sore will indicate a hyperacid stomach, which can be rectified by a reduction in foods of animal origin, better food combining (see Stage 9) and relaxing after the meal. Drinking alfalfa tea between meals and before bed will also help, as will the taking of a good B-complex vitamin supplement — a daily intake of up to 1000 mg of B_3 and 1 mg of folic acid are most important, as are foods rich in these two vitamins (see Stage 11). Dolomite and liquid chlorophyll are valuable sources of the mineral magnesium, which is also highly beneficial for hyperacidity-aggravated canker sores. Calcium lactate tablets will rapidly help the area around the sore to heal, thereby speeding recovery.

C(o)eliac Disease This is becoming a very common symptom of malabsorption, yet until this century, was virtually unknown. The name implies a stomach disease, but the problem does not occur in the stomach; it is of the small intestine. Symptoms are abdominal distension, poor muscle tone with eventual wastage, diarrhoea, anorexia, weight loss, vomiting, leg weakness and anaemia. Not all of these symptoms necessarily occur at one time, for it is a progressively debilitating syndrome, often occurring in infants from six months upwards. The symptoms might disappear around age two, but unless care is taken, will generally reappear during late teen years. Societies of and for people suffering from this syndrome now appear in many countries, indicating the extent to which the problem has grown. An important function of these coeliac societies is in guiding sufferers to suitable foods and encouraging merchants and manufacturers towards providing an adequate range of foods free from gluten. Research has proved that the major protein in wheat and rye (gluten) is the offending nutrient in this allergy syndrome. Gluten is composed of eighteen amino acids, of which the most abundant is glutamic acid, a non-essential part of protein. So the sufferers of coeliac problems can adequately (indeed, must) live without gluten. But for them it is somewhat difficult to obtain replacement foods, unless they develop an understanding of the natural foods diet, from which bread, pasta, cookies, cakes and other processed products of wheat and rye gluten are absent.

For coeliacs, one of the worst offenders is the breakfast cereal, yet this is generally where the syndrome commenced. So addicted are people to the concept of stomach-filling breakfast cereals that they unthinkingly inflict this on their infants as early as they can, often as young as a few months. Highly processed wheat, rye and corn products cannot be enzymically handled at that age, even though the baby might have no difficulty in letting them slide down its tiny oesophagus. Starchy foods need the activity of the enzyme ptyalin, present in the saliva of children and adults, to commence starch conversion to sugar for starch's ultimate digestion. Ptyalin does not develop until the teeth have formed sufficiently — nature's way of guiding. (At this same time, rennin, the milk-settling enzyme in the stomach, commences to dry up.) Without ptyalin, starchy foods will not be properly catabolised, and the intolerance to those foods (wheat and rye) develops as an allergy reaction. By avoiding bread and cookies, cakes and breakfast cereals, these people are most fortunate — they have been forced to look for whole foods, primary quality and unprocessed. To seek rice cookies, millet cereals and the like is to pass up their opportunity for total dietary improvement. These processed grain products are a disgrace to the ingenuity of man.

Childhood Illnesses Although there are variations in symptoms, duration, susceptible ages and complications, the communicable illnesses most common among children can be grouped together for general consideration from the most practical viewpoint — the dietary influences on their development and correction. To a far lesser extent, adults are afflicted with some of these illnesses, and when this occurs, it can induce more serious complications. The more common of these illnesses are chickenpox, mumps, rubella (German measles) and tonsillitis. Less common today are whooping cough, scarlet fever, diphtheria, rheumatic fever, and the like. Each of these is regarded as an acute illness with a rather short incubation period during which their level of contagion can be quite high. General symptoms include debility, anorexia, fever, rash, persistent headache, malaise, cough, localised oedema, etc. Not all of these symptoms necessarily occur with each illness, but a majority will do so. The most common aspects of this grouping are their prevention and treatment. Personal and community hygiene are primary influencing factors in preventing the occurrence and spread of communicable illnesses, for the common medium they need is toxicity. Whether it be exposed sewers or unhealthy intestines, bacteria need rubbish in which to breed. Guaranteed avoidance of serious communicable diseases comes with adherence to the practice of eating only those foods natural to man, properly combined and consumed in accordance with guidelines set forth in this book. Too often, indulgent parents submit to pressure from their offspring to buy them sweets, biscuits, white bread, hamburgers and such junk items in place of natural foods. Next time your child asks for sweets, give an apple. Meat, poultry, seafood, cow's milk, salt, sugar, preservatives and the like are certain to create inner toxicity, which is conducive to the breeding of dangerous bacteria — whatever strain is breeding best at the time. So prevention comes with total dietary care.

Treatment is also largely dietary. When any of these illnesses strike, at the first symptom (even before spending time seeking to have it diagnosed), remove all food from the child and place him or her in bed on a short fast. The room should be cool and shady, with a good circulation of fresh air; plenty of pure, fresh water should be available for drinking as required — but no food, no stress, just a total fast (see Stage 12). Symptoms can thus abate within 48–72 hours. Nature facilitates this by diminishing the sufferer's appetite, making fasting easy. After the fast introduce fresh fruit juices and if desired vitamins C, A, E and P — potencies depend on illness and age, so be guided by your local naturopath (alternatively, contact the vitamin manufacturer who will have an adviser on hand). One to two odourless garlic capsules daily are also highly suitable. After two days on juices (vegetable juices being introduced on the second day), whole foods can be commenced, so long as symptoms have been totally eradicated (otherwise, remain on juices until this has been done). Fresh fruits and vegetable salads should be given without concentrated protein, carbohydrate or fat foods, until the patient has totally regained vitality.

These are general guidelines for the most effective, natural and rapid manner for overcoming childhood illnesses. They apply as effectively to adults, whose periods of fasting, juices and non-concentrate meals would often be slightly longer. Where possible, consult your health professional for specific guidance.

Circulatory Disorders Under this general heading come many syndromes related to the blood and heart. In general, the advice is to change to a natural foods diet, thereby discontinuing saturated fats and cholesterol-bearing animal foods. Eliminate salt and sugar from the diet and especially eliminate the excuse for not finding enough time to exercise. Casual activity is no substitute for a balanced exercise programme, vital to maintain muscle and blood tone; lung and heart muscles being of foremost concern (see Stages 3 and 5 for exercise guidance). Do not wear tight-fitting clothes, in fact, the lighter the better, allowing for the weather. Ensure the diet contains adequate nutrients (see Stage 10) and eat only at mealtimes, which are when you feel ready to eat, and relax afterwards. Many people with circulatory problems find these are merely the forerunners of more complex illnesses. Not all of these are physical — some are connected with emotional imbalance, boredom being a notable example. Rarely do people with active, interesting lives suffer from circulatory disorders.

Colds When the nose becomes very dry and the back of the throat is tender, it is reasonable to assume the onset of a cold. Left untreated, these symptoms will change to runny nose and eyes, slight increase in body temperature and a general feeling of lassitude. The cold might last for a few days or a few weeks (or months), depending upon what you do. The world "cold" is a misnomer. It is not something you catch, it is something you do — you have developed a crisis in your body toxicity level and it wants to overflow. Often stimulated by sudden temperature, diet or emotional change, a cold only needs these external influences to bring it on when your body needs to detoxify. A cold, then, is merely an overflow of toxicity because your normal organs of elimination cannot cope with the load. No virus or germ causes toxicity so much as unnatural living (especially eating) habits. And toxicity provides the medium in which bacteria love to breed — they are the secondary factor, not the cause. Reduce the toxicity level by abstaining from food and resting for a period — that is the only certain way to recover health. A short fast as soon as the initial symptoms appear (24–48 hours), will do the job; otherwise a longer period of abstinence and rest will be needed. If a total fast is impossible due to commitments, abstain from solid foods, drink fresh fruit juices and herb teas (aniseed, chamomile, eucalyptus and peppermint), minimise energy use to allow the body maximum energy for its inner cleansing work. Never resort to suppressant drugs, for they will only force the body to use more effort on a future occasion to detoxify — this is how influenza, tonsillitis, and sometimes bronchitis and pneumonia can develop and recur. Take only megadoses of vitamins C, P and A, plus a moderate amount of B-complex if you feel the need for supplements.

Colonic Problems If people ate properly, they would eliminate properly. But the colon is now the most abused organ of the body, indicating how unsuitable the modern diet has become. Problems with the colon range from constipation and diarrhoea to colitis, enteritis, spasticity, diverticulitis and the sometimes fatal, ulcerative colitis.

Many medical authors still write that causes of colonic problems "are unknown" and to them it reveals a need to search elsewhere than through a microscope. The answer gapes at them in the mirror — it is what goes in or what does not go into the mouth that affects the other end. Processed and refined modern (partial) foods, being devoid of so much roughage, create a great handicap for the bowel, designed as it was to operate on fibre-rich vegetables, fruits, nuts, seeds and whole grains. And what goes into the mouth in damaging quantities are the sugars, liquids and other manufactured "foods", including bread, snack crackers, jams, etc. They provide calories, some protein (incomplete) and starch, but little else. Meats and animal foods, dairy products and seafoods are consumed in far greater quantities than the bowel can handle, yet all these are totally devoid of fibre. Then chemicals are introduced to irritate the already inflamed colon, hastening its breakdown. To recover, the colon must be allowed to rest. Fasting is essential. Therapeutic help is gained from flax and licorice teas, if constipated; in general, natural yogurt, comfrey-pepsin tablets, whey powder and the like, but no treatment will bring about a quicker recovery than fasting. (Read the true story of near-death from ulcerative colitis by Dr Jack Goldstein in *Triumph Over Disease*, Arco Publishing, New York, 1977.) Recovery after fasting is as important as the fast itself (see Stage 12). Then, adherence to the natural foods diet will guarantee a healthy colon in a healthy body. Nothing is quite as comforting as the knowledge that we can go through life totally free of colonic problems.

Cot Death An excellent research programme was carried out by Dr Archie Kalokerinos into the mysterious sudden infant death syndrome (*Every Second Child*, published now in paperback by Keats Publishing, Connecticut, 1981). The results created a great deal of interest in the media around the world when it was shown that the death rate of Australian Aboriginal children had been startlingly reduced. Parents and infants in the programme took vitamin C and Dr Kalokerinos's theory was that a lack of vitamin C was a significant cause of cot death. This lack could have resulted from an inadequate nutritional level in infants or in one or both of their parents — smoking being a contributor to this. Noise is another damaging factor at birth, where peace, love and harmony are important to the newly born soul. More recently, Australian scientists have discovered large amounts of thiamine (a substance in vitamin B_1) in the bodies of children who have died in this way. But they have not yet discovered how thiamine is linked to cot death.

Cramps The old belief that cramps were caused by insufficient salt in the diet has no scientific substance; in fact, common salt can be a cause of cramps, for it is known to induce arteriosclerosis. Hardened arteries inhibit good blood circulation, inducing one of the major causes of cramps. Other causes include atmospheric cold, enervation and exhaustion, excessive activity too soon after eating, or going to bed too soon after eating. These are all factors contributing to poor circulation whereby the muscles do not have their waste products adequately removed, consequently going into spasm with sudden pain. Relaxation techniques can help, varying from meditation to drinking suitable herb teas (sage, rosemary, chamomile, valerian all help). A warm bath in which are soaked some rosemary and sage herbs, or epsom salts, will also help to relax tired muscles and permit better circulation through them. Moderate exercise is far better than inadequate or excessive, each of which can induce cramps. Whenever cramp occurs, apply a warm pack and gradually stretch the muscles in the opposite direction to their contraction.

Cystitis Inflammation of the urinary bladder is called cystitis, so named because the bladder is actually a cyst (a thin-walled hollow organ or cavity containing a liquid secretion). Cystitis occurs mostly in women, although men can develop it after an operation involving the urethra. Cystitis will only occur when toxicity is present in the urinary tract and associated organs, developing from an introduced infection or irritation. In women, it will often follow sexual intercourse and, if not treated promptly upon the initial feeling of discomfort, can work its way into the bladder, inducing an increasing level of discomfort. Nutritional therapy is easy and effective.

During the first few days of the discomfort, avoid solid food but drink plenty of liquid. Vegetable, watermelon and cranberry juices, plus specific herb teas are ideal. The most suitable herb tea is made from juniper berries and it should be drunk every 2–3 hours for the first day; followed by two cups only on the second day, replacing it with equisetum and parsley teas thereafter. As the irritation subsides, reintroduce solid foods, comprising fresh ricotta or cottage cheeses with parsley and alfalfa sprouts and a little other salad vegetables. Steamed buckwheat, rice and millet casseroles are suitable, for the body needs these whole grains to reduce the alkalinity of the bladder. So avoid fruit for these few days and until the body feels totally comfortable in that area. Then, it is important to embrace The Ideal Diet (Stage 10) to ensure that cystitis does not recur (as it has a tendency to do) and that the body's toxicity is minimised. Added relief during the cystitis attack will be obtained by supplemental vitamins C, A and E in megadoses.

Dental Caries Another major symptom of declining general health is the state of human teeth. No other animals need false teeth or expensive dental work because they instinctively eat food natural to their appetites, because the young are suckled through most of infancy and because they do not eat processed, mushy, sugary, denatured or chemically imitated foods. Dental caries afflicts everyone; and the incidence of dental arch deformity is rapidly increasing. If any convincing of human dental deterioration is needed, read Dr Weston Price's startling book, *Nutrition and Physical Degeneration* (The Price-Pottenger Nutrition Foundation, Santa Monica, California, 1977), which documents the photographic and comparative study he undertook in the 1930s before Western foods had totally destroyed good teeth around the world.

Dental caries, or tooth decay, is the gradual breakdown of tooth integrity from the many causes already mentioned, the most vicious being refined sugar. This poison adheres to tooth enamel and is so acidic as to actually eat into the enamel surface and create a cavity in the pulp of the tooth. Other factors contributing to decay are lack of supply or absorption of calcium, magnesium and phosphorus — the same minerals that are needed for good bone structure; but the teeth are affected first, so take care to arrest the deficiency before your skeletal structure commences to break and disintegrate. Decay often commences in infancy with cow's milk and its abundance of lactose which adheres to the new teeth. This implies another danger in drinking this unnatural fluid. Until weaning, infants should drink only mother's milk (if this runs short, alfalfa tablets will restore the supply). Goat's milk is an acceptable alternative, but only if necessary. Once weaning has commenced milk is unnecessary. Vital nutrients will then be derived from solid foods which exercise gums and teeth, so necessary for good formation. Foods rich in minerals essential for healthy teeth are nuts, seeds, soya beans, whole grains, natural cheeses, parsley, sprouts, aided by that versatile supplement, dietary yeast. Avoid the use of commercial toothpastes and powders (too abrasive); chew an apple at the end of your fruit meal, some cucumber at the end of other meals and massage gums regularly with fingers for the best and most natural tooth care, supported by a water brushing with a soft toothbrush. If you feel the need for toothpaste, use only herbal brands. Avoid fluoride in any form (see Stage 3 for its dangers). Cloves, their oil extract, and herb tea can provide prompt temporary relief for toothache, as can liquid chlorophyll.

Diabetes Mellitus Generally regarded as "a disease of abundance", diabetes is not an inherited syndrome, as is often supposed, but a consequence of severely overloading the body's digestive abilities. It is primarily a disorder of carbohydrate metabolism, induced by eating habits, themselves sometimes inculcated by over-indulgent parents. The syndrome enters the chronic stage before many sufferers realise, with progressive deterioration in the body's metabolism of other major nutrients. From an over-straining of its insulin resources, the body's digestive processes are impaired, often inducing further complications which can affect its every system. Conventional treatment offers, as one medical book puts it, "life-long control and care ... but no cure". And yet insulin was "discovered" some sixty years ago, its molecule synthesised twenty years ago! No more than an alcoholic can be cured of alcoholism while drinking, can a diabetic be cured (yes, it is possible in many cases) of diabetes while submitting to the addictions of modern eating habits. A hundred years ago, when refined sugar and cereals were expensive, diabetes was rare. The increase of the one parallels that of the other — and will continue until humans wake up to their gullibility and stop buying all those promoted, processed junk "foods". Many minor cases of diabetes have been unmasked by surgery, stress and infections, for all these syndromes are related. So we should look, not to the treating of an illness, but to the restoration of health to the body. No symptoms evidence this need more than diabetes.

In the treatment of diabetes, some specific needs must be met, but these extend to a total approach to general health upliftment as has been outlined throughout this book. Diabetics, unlike most sick people, should not be fasted, except under the closest of professional guidance and for short periods. They need to totally avoid refined foods, especially carbohydrates, to beware of the many hidden sources of sugar in canned, packaged, processed items, hitherto regarded as foods. They need to embrace a lacto-vegetarian diet (non-animal foods, except for some dairy products and eggs), eating frequent small meals, with particular emphasis on those foods rich in complex carbohydrates — whole grain cereals, fresh fruits and vegetables. Nutrients of special value are manganese (the most vital mineral in natural insulin production), zinc, B-complex vitamins and polyunsaturated fatty acids. The most important foods are alfalfa, brewer's yeast, parsley, buckwheat, wheat germ, nuts, seeds, cucumber (whole), celery and all green vegetables. Fruits are not a problem for diabetics, for their natural sugar, fructose, is easily catabolised without insulin, being a simpler sugar than sucrose. Diabetics must ensure they get plenty of vigorous exercise, avoid stress, maintain proper bowel activity and develop the habit of dry skin brushing morning and evening to maintain top peripheral circulation.

Diabetes can often be corrected. It requires time and diligence; but not as much time as it took to create. Even an apparently dormant pancreas can be induced to reactivate its insulin development. A patient of mine, one who had suffered from diabetes and all its complications for 35 years, after 18 months on the above diet found to his excited amazement that his pancreas responded so well that its latest test revealed it was now producing 50 per cent of his body's insulin needs. Continued dedication to his recovery can see him free of insulin injections in less than two more years.

Emotional Illnesses Under this general heading are included such common psychological disorders as depression, anxiety, nervousness, hyperactivity and all those disharmonious and unstabilising forms of illness which detract from human happiness and loving concern for self and others. Emotions are modes of expression by which we emphasise our feelings and register our relationship with our environment (human and material). They are largely reactions which can be either joyous or joyless. But they should be no more than temporary modes — many people cling to their emotions, become identified by them, use them for attaining influence over others, gaining sympathy, and so on. Emotions then become illnesses; they cause people to be less than joyous, to be other than their natural, healthy selves; they become ways of hiding, "cop-outs". Disharmonious emotions also indicate one is not living in the present, but is focusing the consciousness on the dead past or the imagined future, neither of which can be productive through an emotional attachment. Or maybe you are feeling lonely, insecure, afraid, grieved, ashamed, guilty, confused, embarrassed, jealous or apprehensive — these reveal the makings of disharmony, personal insecurity. Some people are on "power trips", seeking to exercise disharmonious control over others. Their emotional problems are generally expressed as anger, annoyance, frustration, hatred, impatience and/or hostility.

Occasional expression of any of the above emotions creates little problem. But the constant holding on to negative emotions will certainly induce a depth of personal disharmony that will give rise to any number of symptoms of illness. A vast majority of common illnesses, including allergies, arthritis, cancer, heart disease, hypertension, impotence and multiple sclerosis, have significant emotional bases to their development. But if these diseases do not manifest, acute emotional illnesses will invariably intensify into one of the other serious syndromes, grouped under the general heading of schizophrenia (see p. 256). Treatment to avert such chronic development of these entrenched emotions includes wise counselling and dietary changes to eliminate those items not coming within the scope of "Man's Ideal Diet", as outlined in Stage 10. Processed and refined foods are both nutritionally depleting and emotionally unsettling, as are animal foods — no better proof being needed than their incontestible influence in hyperactivity.

Foods for nourishment of the nervous system are those rich in the B-complex vitamins — nuts, seeds, soya beans, dietary yeasts, whole grain cereals, sprouts and green vegetables. Herb teas which best assist nerve balancing are chamomile and valerian. Thoughts which contribute best are those focusing on today as the most important day in your life, the only one in which you can achieve anything, especially "empire over the self", as Pythagoras would say.

Emphysema Similar to chronic (suppressed) bronchitis, with which it usually co-exists, emphysema is a response to persistent irritations, inflammation and mucus formation, inducing physiological changes in the respiratory tract and the lungs. Tobacco smoking is one of the major causes of such illness, hence its cessation is a major factor in recovery. The alternative is fatal. Failure to rectify the situation can result in pneumonia (see p. 255), probably the most severe warning the body will give. The condition is too entrenched for mild treatments, such as herb teas, to exert any significant influence during the early stage of treatment. There is only one permanent remedy — to let the body do its own correcting by undertaking a total fast for at least ten days (heavier people can easily extend this to some weeks). Such fasting must be done under professional care, resting in a relaxing environment where there is pollutant-free air. Simple breathing exercises should be undertaken each day, as indicated by one's vitality. Upon recovery from the fast, activities should be increased to include extended walking, ultimately leading to running and deep breathing, with light yoga a desirable addition to the programme. When recovering from the fast, vitamin supplementation can be beneficial — C, A and E being most needed. Herb teas, such as comfrey, fennel and rosehips, can then be effectively taken between meals. Two garlic capsules per day will also be of benefit.

Enervation The most common symptom of illness is never a subject for medical consideration; in fact, it is rarely listed in the index of even the most erudite medical text. The loss of vigour, depletion of nerve energy, is the condition known as enervation and the result of immoderate living habits. It implies inner toxicity and insufficient rest and relaxation which would otherwise allow the body to recuperate. So other means must be employed for internal house-cleaning. These include the elimination diet and fasting from time to time. Elimination diets allow you to attend to your regular daily functions while the body gradually restores its natural energy, so long as the level of daily activity is minimised. While on such a diet, no concentrated foods should be consumed — during the first stage, only raw fresh fruits and vegetables should be eaten; during the second stage only fresh fruit and vegetable juices. The duration of such a diet will depend on the intensity of the enervation and the amount of time one can allocate to a period of low activity, for the less energy used, the more benefit derived.

Epilepsy Epilepsy could have been included in our discussion on emotional illnesses, but it is something more than that, for it includes brain dysfunction and unconsciousness. The transitory nature of epilepsy has been a condition of human life since before recorded history and was once greatly feared as "demon possession". We know now that its origins are far simpler — either chemical or emotional. Metabolic problems can give rise to poisoning, hypoglycaemia, blood toxicity, all of which affect the nervous system and brain. They can induce tumours (see "Cancer"), especially when abundant foreign chemicals feature in the diet, thereby precipitating epileptic fits. Epileptics are among some of the most chronic sufferers of emotional illness.

Dietary treatment should recognise that epilepsy can be an allergy condition, triggered by foods, oral substances or inhaled allergens. Fasting, with the gradual reintroduction of foods, with careful observation of response, can soon reveal how to control this aspect of the problem. Malnutrition can be a cause. Magnesium is the nutrient most involved and hypoglycaemia (see p. 247) the syndrome most frequently associated with epilepsy. The natural foods diet will avoid these problems, being devoid of animal foods (which rob the body of magnesium and calcium), free from refined sugar and its products (which induce hypoglycaemia), and abundant in all desirable nutrients. Food should be especially sought from organically grown sources and the sufferer should be encouraged to produce his or her own food — farm life being so beneficial to epileptics. Extremes of emotional involvement and of temperature should be avoided; plenty of rest and relaxation should be ensured, for enervation occurs easily with epileptics.

Eye Problems From the early stages of eye malfunction to the ultimate stage (blindness), the eyes are seeking to give warning signs that something is unsuited to their proper functioning. This "something" will generally be found in the region of nutritional, environmental or emotional factors. Commencing with such symptoms as night blindness and conjunctivitis, the eye is telling its owner that avitaminosis A (lack of carotene in the diet) is becoming a problem. Lack of vitamin B_2 is partly responsible for the scaliness of conjunctivitis and the redness of the lids. The diet manifesting these deficiencies is doubtless lacking in most other vitamins and minerals and probably abundant in refined foodstuffs, especially sugar, flour, preserved meats — in fact, there will be too much animal food in the diet and probably too many drugs. If the tendency is there, the weakened eyes will probably develop cataracts or glaucoma, both conditions becoming increasingly prevalent, often resulting in blindness. A step towards this direction is the increasing need for contact lenses and corneal grafts in modern society. Glaucoma is a pressure build-up within the eye caused by thickening lubricating fluid or the overmanufacturing of intra-eye fluid because older fluid is not draining away properly. Cataract is the degenerative opacity of the lens — the area immediately behind the pupil thus becoming cloudier. Some of these advanced degenerative conditions are irreversible, although a corrective diet, with vital supplementation, may halt the deterioration. In milder cases the corrective diet, accompanied by exercises, will bring about definite improvement.

The corrective diet for better eye nourishment is no different from that for better total health. It is the Ideal Diet expounded in Stage 10. But for the eyes, special emphasis must be given to the inclusion of those foods richest in vitamin A — parsley, carrots, sweet potatoes, apricots and all yellow, green and red vegetables and fruits. Many of these foods are, fortunately, rich in vitamin C, which is also needed in large amounts. With these foods, such supplements as vitamins A and C are needed, in potencies up to 15,000 mg of C and 50,000 i.u. (15 mg) of A, daily. Poisons to especially avoid are tea, coffee, and nicotine, all of which reduce vitamin effectiveness and are particularly dangerous when eyes are frail. The drinking of carrot juice and rosehips herb tea will assist in supplying vitamins A and C respectively, and is better than taking vitamin supplements in such strengths. Eye exercises are also highly beneficial in the early stages of deterioration, but be careful not to strain the eyes. Reading small print, especially on a moving vehicle, can create undue eye strain, as can prolonged watching of television.

Fever   Rarely an isolated symptom, a fever will generally indicate an accumulation of toxicity, of which the body is unable to rid itself through its normal channels of elimination. It could also imply that one or more of those channels is blocked. So the body endeavours to throw out the accumulated toxicity through its pores and nose. The heat created within the body by increased pumping of the heart, raises body temperature a few degrees above normal. With the resultant depletion of energy, it is most unwise to further tax the body, so be prepared to rest in a cool room, with nothing to eat until the fever abates. If it does not begin to subside within 24 hours, call your health practitioner. Generally the fever will have run its course within that period, if fasting was begun as soon as the fever became apparent. Then, on the second day, drink fresh fruit or vegetable juices. Continue drinking only juices and water for another day or two, until the body temperature returns to normal and solid food is needed. But do remember to look for any other symptoms which might be associated with the fever, such as a sudden chill, the ingestion of poison, the onset of a contagious condition, or similar symptoms. If in doubt, be sure to seek professional advice, especially in implementing whatever change in living habits (usually diet) is needed to save the body from further efforts to normalise itself.

Frigidity and Impotence   The normal sexual appetite of the healthy person does not need a book to guide its best expression. That is one of the most natural actions of the living body. Yet in more and more people, sexual dysfunction is becoming a problem that detracts from their happiness. Frigidity in the woman rarely accompanies impotence in her male partner — if it did, they could call a truce! The rather common problems of frigidity and impotence can usually be traced to emotional or dietary sources. Emotional problems demand suitable counselling and today it is not difficult to find psychologists who specialise in this area, so widespread is the need. If the sufferers would undertake their own analysing, their gain in self-satisfaction would support their recovery, for so much in the emotional arena is related to assumed inadequacy and low self-esteem. Related to these are the problems of marital discord, anger, guilt, fear, expectation and, perhaps the basis for so many marital and partnership problems, communication breakdown. Many of these areas, together with a very common lack of sex education, can be remedied by wise counselling.

The dietary influence in sexual dysfunction extends beyond nutritional deficiencies into the regions of toxicity and related pathologies and to the inhibiting influence of destructive habits. The average diet of processed "foods" will induce vitamin and mineral deficiencies, detracting from one's vitality and virility. This is compounded by the increased level of toxicity and enervation from which many disease syndromes arise. Among these are herpes simplex (a painful problem when related to the sexual regions), diabetes, vaginitis, muscular disorders (dystrophy, M.S.) and cancer, especially if a mastectomy has been performed. Toxicity-inducing habits, such as drug-taking (smoking, alcohol, tranquillisers, some oral contraceptives) can similarly reduce vitality and virility. The Ideal Diet (Stage 10) will certainly rejuvenate one's energies, especially if supported by an appropriate fast. Initial dietary supplements can be most helpful, such as vitamins B_6 and E, chelated zinc, together with ginseng and sarsaparilla in tablet and herb tea form.

Gall Bladder Problems These are usually of one or both common occurrences — gallstones (cholelithiasis) and inflammation within the gall bladder (cholecystitis). The medical names indicate the presence of cholesterol, its role being the basis of the formation of bile acids in the liver; but often too much cholesterol is present in the body (only of meat-eaters) for the liver to utilise. Some of the excess finds its way into the formation of gallstones. Other factors attend gallstone development, these also being related to the presence of excessive steroid compounds and saturated fatty acids. But it is difficult to glean a full picture, since an amazingly small amount of research has been undertaken on gallstones, considering how common the problem has become. Gall bladder inflammation is believed to derive from similar causes, but with irritation occurring within some of the tiny folds in the gall bladder, with or without the presence of stones. Salmonella bacteria are usually associated with this irritation, implying that unsuitable foodstuffs have been consumed.

Relief treatment for gall bladder problems should be undertaken immediately they are suspected. It is difficult to isolate gall bladder-induced pain from other types of indigestion pains. General symptoms are abdominal distension, excessive belching, some feeling of nausea and possible biliousness. If these symptoms become worse a few hours after a fatty meal, indications are gall bladder problems. Natural remedies should be implemented for, even if the gall bladder is not at fault, they will convey general benefit to the body with no side-effects (the risk always attending drug therapy). Importantly, the diet should be primarily vegetarian, with the additions of yogurt, cottage and ricotta cheeses and an abundance of lecithin. Fresh pears and grapefruit (and their juices) are highly beneficial, as is the drinking of dandelion tea. If the sufferer can consume it, linseed oil (can be taken in capsule form) is an excellent supplement which can relieve pain from the gall bladder region and has even been known to dissolve gallstones or reduce them so they can pass into the intestines for elimination. Drink two tablespoonsful, preferably early morning, then lie on left side for an hour. If the stones are stubborn, you will need to double the amount of linseed oil and the time to two hours. Additional supplements of benefit are lecithin tablets, choline, inositol and biotin tablets, vitamin A+D+E tablets and the drinking of fennel tea. Under professional guidance, a fast can be most beneficial.

Goitre This common name refers to the nontoxic goitre, an enlargement of the thyroid gland due to a deficiency in the production of thyroid hormones, mainly thyroxine. Iodine sufficiency and utilisation determines adequacy of production of these hormones which, in turn, influence the body's metabolic rate and growth rate. Thus, an inadequate dietary supply of iodine will cause this type of goitre, regarded as "endemic", for it becomes relatively common in people from regions where iodine is deficient in soil and foods — generally inland areas, where fresh seafoods are not so readily available. Certain drugs are known to be responsible for blocking iodine utilisation in the thyroid, including some types of analgesics, lithium and even megadoses of iodine. These goitres usually occur at puberty or during pregnancy and should not be removed, for they respond well to an adequate increase of iodine (see Stage 11) from the diet. Also beneficial are ginseng tablets and tea. The swelling should then gradually disappear.

The more toxic counterpart, the goitre known as the condition hyperthyroidism, can occur either from an excess of iodine or from emotional disharmony or both. This results in an increase in thyroxine and an elevation of the metabolic rate. Symptoms are hyperactivity, muscular weakness, nervousness and weight loss, even though the appetite is high. Surgery should be avoided, for removal is not the answer. Dietary correction is achieved initially through supervised fasting, then a closely supervised pure vegetarian regimen. Avoidance of anxiety, stress and old frustrations which might inhibit recovery should be ensured. Dietary yeast is a valuable supplement, as are vitamins C and B-complex.

Headaches Included in this group are the common headaches of minor inconvenience and short duration stimulated by a vast range of causes, plus the intense and most painful of headaches, migraine. There are so many possible causes of headaches that space does not justify their enumeration. Should the cause be of a structural nature, the chiropractor is the practitioner with the correct techniques for its rectification. Stress and other emotional causes can also benefit from wise counselling. Dietary and chemical causes will rapidly respond to corrective measures because headaches are acute warning signs, generally indicating that the diet is too acidic. Foods to be eliminated are those of animal origin, plus all cereals and flour products, sugar, salt and alcohol. Meals should always be of moderate size, for large meals can create alcohol in the stomach from premature fermentation (sugar will do this rapidly — see Food Combining, Stage 9). The resultant headache can be identical to a "hangover", even though alcoholic beverages might not have been consumed. Some of the less obvious causes of headache can include an unsuitable pillow, overtiredness, boredom, loneliness, frustration, confusion, allergy to a particular food, constipating chemicals in foods or those used agriculturally or in storage techniques. Some of the natural techniques for relief are running, hot-and-cold showers, massage, music, a vacation, sexual intercourse and, most effective of all, abstinence from food — the short fast. An old therapeutic aid to recently appear in health food stores is white willow bark, a natural source of salicin (see Stage 11), used for centuries as a pain reliever and food supplement.

The foregoing considerations apply to migraine just as much as to general headaches. But special consideration has to be directed to migraine sufferers, for their prolonged and more intense pain, with its recurring nature, indicates a persisting disturbance to cranial circulation. Chiropractic treatment over a short period will usually be most successful in rectifying the disturbance. If the condition recurs, it is advisable to next look into the emotional and/or psychic domains. Some valuable guidance in these areas will be derived from a deeper investigation of Stages 4 and 5 of this book and from the studying of the best-selling book by Ken Keyes, Jr., *Handbook to Higher Consciousness* (Living Love Publications, St Mary, Kentucky, 1972). Ken has become a personal friend of mine and is a man who has elevated himself from the misery of being a polio cripple to a level of joyous living rarely seen on this planet. We have both shared the misery of migraine and the freedom of a total recovery by knowing how to elevate one's centre of consciousness. No truly happy and adjusted person ever became a victim of migraine! Dietary assistance for migraine is identical to that for common headache — emphasis on an alkaline diet, supplemented by alfalfa-mint, fenugreek, thyme and rosemary herb teas, dolomite and vitamin E tablets and liquid chlorophyll. No holes need be drilled in the head, as was done by the Chinese, as far back as 2000 B.C. to "allow the demons to escape", unless the head happens to be solid and too dense to comprehend that these conditions are self-inflicted!

Heart Disease One of the major killers of modern times, heart disease is actually the end-product of a long series of personal health abuses. By the time the symptoms become so deeply rooted as to inflict upon the heart conditions which are intolerable enough to stop its functioning, we may be certain that many of the body's systems have so deteriorated that they too could have stopped. Various experts attribute heart disease to all manner of causes — saturated fats, cholesterol, hypertension, refined sugar, emotions, tension, obesity, indolence, smoking, and so on. And they are correct; but it is not just one of these causes, it is many of them, for they all indicate an unstable, disharmonious lifestyle. The commonly accepted, long-established approach to heart disease is to pour vast resources into searching for cures within today's conventional lifestyle. With such injurious eating habits — in fact, so many of our habits are counterproductive to healthy living — it is impossible to protect people from their own undoing. A primary fault lies with those in established medicine who undertake to guide people to counteract heart disease, when they, themselves, are seemingly oblivious of some of its causes. This could not be more strikingly (nor sadly) exemplified than by the untimely passing of one of the founders of the National Heart Foundation of Australia in 1979 — from a heart attack, so the press stated. He, like most victims, had no warning. Yet, even those to whom the body gives warnings, such as recurrent hypertension and sudden chest pains, take little positive action to avert the ultimate calamity.

Positive action to avert heart attacks is no different from that required to attain an optimum level of general health. One must eliminate unnatural living habits and adopt instead those habits which will ensure good health — a natural vegetarian diet (as outlined in this book), correct food combinations, adequate exercise and so on (see Stage 3). There should be no excuse for following patterns adopted by others (even one's parents — for they need help now too), if they are detrimental to our health. If the heart has been weakened by poor living habits, special care should accompany the change in lifestyle. The most valuable is to undertake a supervised fast as the ideal means of breaking with the old, unsuitable traditions (see Stage 12). When back on healthy food, a juice day each week is an excellent habit, and fresh juices during other days provide ideal vitamin and mineral boosters — carrot, celery and beetroot juice being among the best. Herb teas with special properties for the heart are chamomile, hops, valerian, parsley and hawthorn. Vitamin supplements for daily support are C, to 3000 mg, and E, to 1500 mg (but must be reduced if a history of hypertension or heart damage exists); B-complex vitamins are also very beneficial for restoring nerve control. Food supplements of benefit include liquid chlorophyll, dolomite, hawthorn berry tablets, dietary yeasts (torula preferably, because it is lowest in sodium) and lecithin — in fact, all supplements and foods that are predominantly alkaline, except for sodium.

A major cell salt for heart disease sufferers is magnesium sulphate and foods most abundant in this are nuts, seeds, soya beans and their products, and greens. On this special diet, it is best to minimise or even avoid grains. Cold-pressed, polyunsaturated oils are beneficial if used in moderation — linseed, safflower, sunflower and wheat germ being best. Be sure to avoid common salt, alcohol, tobacco, tea, coffee, cocoa, chocolate and cola drinks. Caffeine, contained in the last five items, is extremely dangerous for the heart. If possible, avoid drinking water containing added fluoride, for it is a known heart weakener. Avoid animal foods, for their high levels of saturated fats and cholesterol are highly undesirable, as is the uric acid residue they induce within the human body.

This diet plan has some aspects in common with the Pritikin Diet, the latter having been more recently developed to assist those with insufficient strength of will to undertake the needed dietary and exercise reform on their own. But the Pritikin Diet is not recommended for anything but a transition period. It is only and essentially a therapeutic diet — one should not live on it for more than a few months, at the most. It is too deficient in polyunsaturated fats and essential protein foods (nuts and seeds), to name only the major inadequacies, insofar as its suitability as a maintenance diet is concerned. Yet, many people have followed that diet with benefit for a short time, with sought-after weight loss and improved blood circulation as important gains. However, these same people have found that their energy levels remain low, inhibiting their return to active life. A low kilojoule diet will help the heart to recover, but it cannot support an active life (which a happy one always is). The Ideal Diet, espoused in this book, is designed to provide adequate kilojoules for the body's use, but not an excess for unwanted storage.

H(a)emorrhoids Also known by the common name of "piles", haemorrhoids are actually varicosed swellings of the haemorrhoid veins, located near the anus. As they have no valves by which to transmit pressure further along the system, these veins react by swelling and becoming inflamed if the pressure is not eased. Exacerbation of the problem can result in bleeding and/or the formation of a thrombosis. These symptoms are warnings that the pressure build-up must be rectified. Since it is usually caused by constipation, or other colonic problems (see p. 234), correction of the latter will bring a two-fold benefit. Some of the other common causes of haemorrhoids are obesity, hypertension, emotional tension, anxiety, and the most common problem of all — a diet of unsuitable foodstuffs. Particularly offensive in the diet are refined, processed items, especially sugar and flour. Noticeably deficient in the diet are fresh, raw vegetables and fruits. Thus rectification is easy and enjoyable. Plenty of activity and exercise will be greatly beneficial (too much sitting is another minor fault); plenty of vegetable juices, pure water and suitable herb teas are also very important. Most suitable herb teas are chamomile, flax seed (linseed), nettle and valerian. Foods rich in magnesium (see p. 106) will help shrink haemorrhoids. Dr Airola also recommends vitamin B_6 (25 mg) after each meal. Pollen granules or tablets will greatly assist in the healing of this and most anal problems.

Hepatitis This general name applies to those inflammatory conditions of the liver manifesting as various forms of necroses (dead cells), thereby impeding normal function of this vital organ. A variety of acute and chronic forms of this syndrome can be found in various people with differing backgrounds. But in general, the condition is one of enervation (often stress induced), wherein the body becomes suddenly anorexic and feverish, with nausea, malaise and a yellowishness appearing in the eyes and through the skin. It can be a most debilitating illness with a protracted recuperation period. In elderly people, it can be fatal, but rarely so with younger sufferers. Total recovery can require up to six months, but if no drugs are used and total rest is undertaken, recovery can be completed within a month. The ideal treatment is a total fast for at least the first week, followed by fresh vegetable and fruit juices (avoiding those rich in vitamin A; preferring apple, orange, pineapple, watermelon, and all green vegetables). Thence to a raw fruit and vegetable diet for the next week, again without concentrated foods, with the exception of those low in fat, such as dried fruits, potatoes, skim milk yogurt, ricotta or cottage cheeses, whole grains and plenty of sprouts, any of which should be eaten in moderation. Suitable herb teas are dandelion and fennel, with valerian if anxiety develops. No amount of rest can be too much — forget about the worry of losing bodily strength, that will return when health has been recovered. Meanwhile, allow the body to devote all its energy to cleansing and recovering itself.

Herpes Generally listed among the viral diseases in medical books, the two most common forms of herpes are *herpes simplex* and *herpes zoster*. The former manifests as cold sores and fever blisters, filled with a clear fluid, and a little inflamed. The latter is a different form and more related to chickenpox, but commonly called "shingles", however its skin eruptions appear along sensory nerve pathways over the body, generally in the thoracic region. Both conditions can be most uncomfortable, especially *herpes simplex* when it develops around the genital regions. There are some common factors between these syndromes and other so-called viral, infectious or germ-induced "diseases": they all arise from internal toxicity and enervation. So herpes, as with the others, can be speedily rectified by appropriate detoxification, the most effective being fasting. Juice diets and "detoxification" diets of fresh fruits and vegetables only, will also do the job, but each at a slower rate. In cases of herpes, because the skin and nerves have been affected, supplementary vitamins A+D+E, supported by C and B-complex, should be taken when back on solid food.

For people who are very selective in their diet and who choose foods with special care, vitamin supplementation need not become a regular practice. But when a particular area of weakness occurs, the therapeutic support of prepared vitamins can be most beneficial. Vitamin-rich food supplements can also be of particular assistance; in this case, dietary yeasts, wheat germ, lecithin and rice bran syrup (which is not easy to obtain outside the USA) will be most rewarding, due to their important vitamin B content and the silicon value of rice bran (obtained to a much lower degree, but still very useful, in unpolished rice). The richest source of silicon in herb teas is found in equisetum — a worthwhile aid to herpes (and all skin problem) sufferers. Great care should be exercised in choosing soap — avoid commercial chemical-based brands, selecting only those made from pure coconut oil or with added wheat germ oil.

Hiatus Hernia Of the many openings in the diaphragm between the thorax and abdomen, the most important is that through which the oesophagus passes to join up with the stomach. There is a loose attachment between the oesophagus and the diaphragm, but in many older people, this tends to weaken, with a resultant tearing between the oesophagus and stomach. The opening (hiatus) at which this occurs, gives rise to the name of hiatus hernia, an uncomfortable, but by no means dangerous, problem, unless haemorrhaging occurs. The weakness inducing the formation of the hiatus hernia can be precipitated by a heavy, unnatural physical movement, occurring more frequently in women than in men, largely due to social habits — as they grow older, women are inclined to do more constant physical work (around the home) than do retired men. But the weakness must be attendant for the hernia to occur; and these weaknesses are the consequence of deficient dietary habits over long periods, together with lack of adequate muscle tone from effective exercising.

Natural methods of correcting the hiatus hernia and of minimising its discomfort are not to adopt the bland diet that is often suggested, for this is even more constipating and devitalising than the normal (poor) diet. To minimise gastric acid activity and the unpleasant burning of regurgitation, reduce foods which make heavy demands on production of hydrochloric acid in the stomach. Ideally, totally eliminate meat and animal foods from your diet, for they are the offenders. Pay special attention to food combinations, thereby allowing the hydrochloric acid to be its most catabolically effective. Avoid all refined flour and sugar and their products and do not drink either with meals or while food is in the stomach. Eat smaller meals, even if it is necessary to eat four or five meals in a day. All these factors are significant in contributing towards overcoming hyperacidity, thereby allowing most comfort when a hiatus hernia is present. Drinking alfalfa tea is beneficial to stabilising the gastric juices; mixing peppermint tea with it will also stimulate digestive effectiveness with its menthol oil, helping to settle any accidentally overloaded stomach. Should gastric reflux occur during sleep, prop up the bed head by 20 cm or so, for this condition is highly responsive to posture. It is not a condition to take lightly, but should be treated with care, as suggested here, to avoid secondary problems, such as anaemia, ulcers, or constipation-induced haemorrhoids.

Hypertension Increased blood pressure is one of the most common symptoms of modern living, affecting around half of Western populations, but it is not regarded as hypertensive until readings indicate appreciable increases above average. Usually, only Westerners can afford hypertension, for it is surely one of the many symptoms of affluence. It is also a foundation for many serious health problems, particularly heart disease. Most medical texts state that some 15 per cent of people are hypertensive, but they err in basing their comparisons on average blood pressure measurements for Westerners. In so doing, they confuse "average" with "normal", for normal has now been left far behind. The older the person tested, the greater the difference between average and normal, for it is not normal to record more than a minimal variation for age (it is just as "normal" to record a slight decrease for age). Modern Westerners will invariably show an increase in the readings as their bodies reflect the abuses of modern living, with hardening arteries, thickening blood, increasing toxaemia, impaired kidneys, defective metabolism, increasing body weight and emotional disturbances. Common early indications of hypertension include recurring headaches, agitation, flushed face, nose-bleeding (a common safety valve), dizziness and ringing in the ears. A normal range of blood pressure readings should be 100/70 to 115/80; slightly below the low end of the range is often found in healthy people, reflecting their inner calm. A reading set above the upper end should be regarded as hypertensive and a warning that corrective action is needed. To accept medication or any treatment specifically intended to reduce blood pressure is to be oblivious of nature's intention. What is needed is a rectification in lifestyle, a return to more natural living habits, following which, the blood pressure will automatically adjust downwards. You could not have a better indicator; medication only falsifies the readings. Major factors contributing to hypertension are non-vegetarian foods (animal and sea foods are high in saturated fats), salt, spices, coffee, tea, chocolate, alcohol, cola, stress (both expressed and suppressed). Dietary factors most beneficial to overcoming hypertension are lecithin, buckwheat and wheat germ, together with the Ideal Diet, as outlined in Stage 10. As soon as the sufferer can devote the time away from work to undertake a fast, this will be found most beneficial; meanwhile, juice dieting will be a valuable therapy, for up to a week at a time, using greens, carrots, grape and watermelon juices. Beneficial herb teas are hawthorn berry and fenugreek. Hawthorn berry tablets are also very helpful as a dietary supplement. If supplementary vitamins B_3 and C are also taken, this can hasten the recovery process. Remember to eat smaller meals, lose weight and relax more (yoga could be a very valuable discipline). Skin brushing and regular exercise also help.

Hypoglycaemia The pandemic of low blood sugar has swept the Western world this past decade to become the most fashionable syndrome ever in medical history. Its virtue, for so many people, is that it is an excuse for tiredness — a real cop-out, without being fatal. Dr Abram Hoffer of Victoria, Canada, estimates that 50 per cent of Westerners are victims of this problem, the root cause of which is not dietary inadequacy (that is a considerable factor in its development), but boredom. Disinterest, indolence, laziness, lethargy are all symptoms of the problem. For so many of these people, life has lost its excitement and purpose. They need help, first with their diet, then with their mental and spiritual approach to life. Their diet has been centred around animal proteins and refined carbohydrates, plus the drinking of stimulating beverages, all of which contribute towards energy levels which fluctuate between very high and very low. This also induces emotional instability, leading to fears, uncertainty and lack of personal confidence. Dietary changes must include the basic Ideal Diet, but with emphasis on whole grains and a little less fruit. Meals should be a little smaller than usual, with a mid-morning and mid-afternoon snack of either a herb tea (rosehips, ginseng, nettle being best) or a piece of fresh fruit and a few dates or figs. Nothing should be eaten after dinner, to avoid gastric action disturbing the sleep. Vitamin supplements are similar to those suited to sufferers of heart problems (see p. 243), plus megadoses of B_{12} (at least 100 μg daily). To attend to the emotional bases of hypoglycaemia, we must turn to wise counselling to guide the person onto the most suitable life path, where life's fullest meaning can be expressed, by which means the satisfaction from successful and purposeful living will be harmoniously derived. (Refer to my book *Secrets of the Inner Self*, Angus & Robertson Publishers, Sydney, 1980.)

Indigestion The most common of all symptoms in the daily habits of man and in the study of nutrition, indigestion is the overt message from the gastrointestinal tract that something fed into it is unsuitable. Many people seek to silence this valuable warning device by antacids or other remedies, without recognising the call to seek the cause. This habit is as dangerous as hearing a noise in the engine of your car and blocking your ears — it will be quite costly! Likewise with health, for so many health problems arise from ignoring the intestines' call for help. Attention to natural dietary guidance includes selecting suitable natural foods, combining them in the best way for easiest digestion and living harmoniously so that digestion is not impaired by disruptive emotions. Guidelines are provided throughout this book.

Infertility Frigidity and impotence are two frequent causes of infertility and these have already been considered (see p. 240); but for many couples, infertility remains a problem even with the absence of the others. Assuming there is no anatomical reason, fertility can be caused by the enervation/toxicity syndrome resulting from unhealthy living habits. Many couples have found that a fast of moderate duration, taken during their vacation and under professional supervision, has produced remarkable results for their reproductive systems (see Stage 12). For men, two of the important minerals to aid virility are zinc and manganese, supported by vitamins A and B_6 — foods rich in these nutrients are listed in Stage 11. Herb teas which help both males and females are red clover and ginseng, plus the extract of the Chinese herb dong quai.

Insomnia Disturbed sleep or difficulty in going to sleep are rather common problems among people today. Where previously people worked harder physically, today they work harder mentally and emotionally, but with seemingly far less sense of achievement or purpose. To aggravate this syndrome, most people are fairly inactive and are not getting sufficient exercise. Although they go to bed exhausted mentally and emotionally, they are physically under-utilised, thereby in conflict with a primary requirement for balanced, innervating sleep. This is achieved best when all systems of the body have been used and are ready for rejuvenation. Sleep is the need of all beings whose bodies run out of energy — it is the process of recharging, of innervation. A night's sleep can be handicapped by a stomach full of food, for although a heavy meal is known to make one sleepy (due to blood being withdrawn from the brain to aid digestion), this is only a temporary feeling, for once the food passes out of the stomach, the body becomes energetic again. Many people are not relaxed sufficiently before bed — they assume that sleep is a direct alternative to activity. The body needs to be geared down through relaxation, just as does a car when the brakes fail. We do not have such equipment as brakes to immediately stop, unless by way of a heart attack or stroke, or the like. These serious conditions can never happen to people who obtain adequate, restful sleep. So insomnia, like indigestion, is one of nature's ways of telling us to correct our habits. Some helpful supplements for sufferers of insomnia include valerian and hops teas, tryptophan in megadoses and, sometimes, white willow bark tablets. But these will not correct the problem, so should not become habitual themselves — they will not induce possibly harmful side-effects, as can drugs, but they can induce a false sense of well-being and mask the original problem.

Kidney Problems These include a long list of pathological conditions, ranging from nephritis in its many forms, to the more critical problem of stones. The kidneys are so directly responsive to the diet, it is astounding that medical treatment for kidney disease does not include vital dietary guidance; but instead, resorts to surgery and dialysis with rapidly increasing frequency. Kidney breakdown would be regarded more seriously if man had only one unit in his body, but we need two kidneys because we sometimes need to take in large quantities of protein-rich foods, especially when undertaking hard and prolonged physical work.

The kidneys are vital to protein metabolism and elimination (of residues), so when kidney problems occur, we must undertake maximum rest — making fasting so ideal. If on a low-protein diet to minimise kidney activity, one's own activity must also be minimised. The diet should be primarily fresh fruit and vegetables — easiest to digest if taken in juice form. A fresh juice diet during alternating weeks can be a reasonable alternative to a total fast, but the rate of recovery will not be as rapid. Paw paws, mangos, bananas and watermelons are the most suitable fruits; celery, cucumber and zucchini the best vegetables. Smoking, alcohol and cola beverages must be discontinued, and especially tea and coffee, chocolate and cocoa. Oxalic acid is an ugly antagonist of the kidneys, for it combines with calcium and magnesium to form sharp crystals, gravel and, ultimately, stones. Certain herb teas can be extremely helpful in breaking down these stones, equisetum being the best of them; parsley, dandelion and rosehips teas are valuable kidney tonics; juniper and flax teas soothe when inflammation is present. Rosehips tea has been most beneficial to some people in helping break their coffee addiction. One of the most important vitamins for the kidneys is vitamin A — Dr Airola recommends up to 75,000 i.u. (22.5 mg) daily for the first three months, then 10,000 i.u. (3 mg) daily.

Lethargy Much said under the heading of Hypoglycaemia (see p. 247) pertains to lethargy. The dietary aspects of this condition of low energy are significantly related to toxicity and enervation, nutritional insufficiency and poor assimilation. It is always interesting to note the low energy level of people who have eaten a large meal of many courses and unthinkable combinations, compared to the energy evidenced by vegetarians after their usual main daily meal of protein-rich foods — it is exemplified by the tests at Yale University where a group of trained athletes (on the conventional diet) were pitted against a group of untrained (but normally fit) vegetarians in a long-distance race. The vegetarians far outdistanced their competitors. Meat-eating is one of the major causes of diet-induced lethargy, for meat demands such a high amount of energy in the body's efforts at metabolising it — an engine with such a poor performance would be scrapped as "unecological" and too expensive to run. For those who have sought to change and improve their health and energy, the Ideal Diet (Stage 10) offers vital guidance. To assist the body improve its performance and overcome casual lethargy, the best herb teas are ginseng, rosehips and cloves. Ginseng has long been regarded as a stimulant for the pituitary gland, thereby toning the body's performance level. Phenylalanine (see p. 94) has more recently been found to assist in this regard, being an essential amino acid and natural to the body's needs. A significant contributor to lethargy in children has been traced to lead poisoning, as found in the air of city streets. As lead is heavier than air, it tends to float lower, hence its increase in concentration nearer the ground where children breathe it in. Non-dietary reasons for lethargy have been discussed with hypoglycaemia and should not be ignored if a total recovery of energy is sought.

Leukemia This is a general name for a variety of pathologies whereby neoplastic (tumorous, wild) cells are formed by blood-forming tissues and bone marrow. These conditions are generally fatal unless urgent corrective steps are taken, for they are cancerous conditions which will be spread throughout the body by the blood. Medical forms of treatment rarely give any more than a short extension of life, but there is always the danger that the condition (or another cancerous propensity) will recur. And indeed it will, unless the corrective measures, as outlined for cancer (see p. 231) are immediately undertaken. As leukemia usually affects children, its occurrence is all the more saddening — and the responsibility of the parents all the more critical.

Liver Problems We have already considered hepatitis in depth and will now look into other liver problems, embracing cirrhosis, fibrosis, congestion, enlargement and fatty degeneration, many of which are interrelated. As the liver is the major detoxifying organ of the body, a diet to correct its problems will be of general benefit to the body's health. This diet is based on non-animal protein foods and all the other ingredients recommended throughout this book. Factors which overload the liver are saturated fats, cholesterol, refined sugar, alcohol and most of the chemicals used in food technology when they combine within the digestive system of the human body. Environmental chemicals are also highly damaging to the liver, and agricultural chemicals are critically dangerous. With this in mind, it defies logic why some health practitioners recommend animal liver for human digestion and therapeutic benefit — it might give a sudden boost to human B-vitamin needs, but its long-term penalty by way of added toxicity rules strongly against it. There are abundant natural sources of B-complex vitamins, as have been previously delineated. The speediest means of rejuvenating the liver is the total fast under supervision. Juice dieting is more slowly beneficial and a detoxifying diet of fresh fruits and vegetables (without concentrated foods) a little slower still. But they all help the liver to cleanse itself, thereby to better perform its role in properly cleansing the body. Special foods from which the liver will benefit include beetroot, paw paw, parsley and other green vegetables. Beetroot juice is also highly beneficial. Herb teas are dandelion and parsley. When the liver has recovered and a full diet is resumed, ensure that the primary protein foods are almonds, sesame and pumpkin seeds, ricotta cheese and dietary yeasts. Other nuts and seeds can be eaten with benefit, but go easy on macadamias and pecans, for they are exceptionally high in fats, with insufficient protein to justify the energy investment.

Lupus This is the "common" name for two severe skin conditions — lupus vulgaris and lupus erythematosus. The former is rarely encountered today, but the latter is becoming more extensive as human diet becomes more toxic. Apparent features of the syndrome are severe rashes of red patches on the cheeks, extending over much of the body, especially the exposed areas. As the scaly patches heal from the centre, scar tissue forms and this can tighten the skin to look rather contorted in places. The syndrome affects women far more than men for reasons unknown, but possibly related to hormonal imbalance. Sometimes fever, arthritis, pleurisy, anaemia and pneumonia accompany the chronic rash. The condition can become fatal unless rectified. Cortisone and other medical treatments only exacerbate the body's toxicity — medically, the condition is of "unknown cause".

The ideal treatment is to allow the body to thoroughly cleanse itself — by a long, supervised fast, or a series of shorter fasts. Once back on food, the Ideal Diet must be followed for total and permanent recovery and optimum health. The alternative to fasting, for those who do not have the unlimited time, is megadose vitamin therapy, but this should be undertaken under the supervision of a competent orthomolecular practitioner. Massive doses of B_3 should be supported by B_6 and C, with occasional use of E. But these are less effective if not accompanied by a detoxifying diet of fresh fruits and vegetables, with the occasional week on juices only. A very valuable food supplement for the skin is rice bran syrup, for it is the richest known source of silicon. Equisetum tea is also a worthwhile source and the best herb tea for this condition.

Ménière's Syndrome A series of uncomfortable and disquieting symptoms affecting older people was initially recognised by French physician, Prosper Ménière, in 1861. It is characterised by dizziness (vertigo), ringing in the ears (tinnitus) and nausea, often leading to vomiting; but the symptoms often only prevail for some hours, up to a day or so. The cause is medically unknown, and its treatment consequently haphazard. Naturopathically, the treatment is to immediately go to bed, taking a megadose of vitamin B_3 with as much niacin as the body can handle (up to 100 mg; the balance as niacinamide), with plenty of water. Maintain a high intake of B_3 thereafter, together with pantothenic acid (B_5) and vitamin C, being certain to drink at least ten glasses of water each day. The diet should be changed to the Ideal Diet described in Stage 10, for Ménière's is a warning that accumulated toxicity is affecting the body's nervous system, the gastrointestinal tract and the cerebral cortex. And unheeded warnings evoke a far more severe second attack. It is acknowledged that older people find greater difficulty in changing their dietary habits, but every support and encouragement should be given them by their families, who should, themselves, undertake necessary dietary changes in advance of severe warnings from the body.

Menopausal Problems Emotional and nutritional factors both contribute to make this period in a woman's life either easy or the most difficult imaginable. And if it is the latter, everyone in her circle (especially her husband) should realise that help is needed. The symptoms are extensive and unpredictable, but they can be lessened, even negated, by adopting the recommendations outlined in this book. If these are followed before the onset of menopause, it can be naturally delayed and eventually arrive without any physical or emotional stress. Menopause is as natural for women as is childbirth, but modern living habits have so upset the workings of the human body that few normal changes within now take their natural course — they struggle to develop through the toxic maze. Special assistance for women is achieved by undertaking a balanced exercise programme (featuring abdominal exercises, for these also offset the risk of uterus prolapse) to accompany their improved diet plan. Yoga and relaxation are also important, as well as maintaining an active interest in creative and/or communal affairs. Herb teas of particular benefit to women of the menopausal age are sarsaparilla, licorice and raspberry leaf. Special food supplements are dietary yeasts, kelp and lecithin — try to get at least 100 mg of B-vitamins B_3, B_5, B_6 and PABA each day, with good back-up of other B-complex vitamins; up to 1500 mg of vitamin E should be taken daily — as much as possible through food, the balance supplemented. Emotional counselling can also be highly beneficial. Tendencies towards emotionalism can be recognised for each person from the guidelines given in my book, *Secrets of the Inner Self* (Angus & Robertson Publishers, 1980).

Menstrual Problems To believe that the Creator ordained a monthly misery for mature women is to be ignorant of His wisdom and goodness. But when creatures live in conflict with nature's laws, prompt "karma" sends signals which need heeding. Failure to live in harmony with nature will always induce pain — it is a warning that a problem needs to be rectified. In those wilder regions of the world where Western civilisation remains foreign, female monthly cycles come and go without an ordeal, usually without notice, in fact, because their diets and lifestyles are primitive and natural. Sophisticated women of today in the West do not seek to return to the primitive (nor do the men), but we should certainly return to the natural means of keeping our body healthy and fit — properly nourished and exercised. Common symptoms of menstrual problems include depression, water retention, backache, cramps (usually abdominal), tender breasts and emotional indifference. Even with a prompt rectification of dietary patterns to the more natural, it will require some time for the body to accumulate an acceptable level of many nutrients. This implies the need for urgent supplementation, particularly of B-complex vitamins (B_3, B_6 and B_{12} primarily), iron and vitamin C taken together, iodine and calcium. Important health foods for inclusion in the diet are kelp, dietary yeast, lecithin, plus herb teas chamomile, hibiscus, raspberry, rosehips and especially pennyroyal.

Morning Sickness Nausea or vomiting occurring during the early months of pregnancy rarely implies anything more than dietary upset. It is a problem of the stomach and can be readily overcome by more careful selection of food. Avoid fatty foods, alcohol, tobacco, highly sweetened and spiced foods. Stay with natural, fresh foods and take heed of proper food combining rules to ensure best digestion and nausea-free mornings. If breakfast is not anticipated with an appetite, avoid it and wait until the body says it is ready for more food. The first meal of the day should be a fresh fruit salad, or a little whole grain cereal with apple juice or soya milk. At mid-morning, an ideal beverage is a warm cup of raspberry leaf tea — some expectant mothers prefer this also soon after rising. It will certainly be found beneficial for its immediate stabilising of the gastric juices and for the traces of nutrients it contains. Moderate activity during the day is well advised, such as yoga, light swimming, walking briskly and all the housework necessary. The diet should not deviate from the Ideal Diet (Stage 10), other than for the slight increase of foods rich in calcium (nuts, seeds, etc.), magnesium (same, plus wheat germ) and iron (dietary yeast, pepitas, wheat germ), plus a vegetable juice each day, plenty of parsley and fresh sprouts. Avoid all stimulants and, emphatically, smoking.

Multiple Sclerosis This is another of those modern illnesses for which medical science gives the origin as "unknown". Issue is taken with those who do not investigate beyond the confines of their bacteriological studies, for they mislead a public which has come to rely on them for guidance in matters of health. The cause of M.S. is no secret — it is a syndrome (one of the many facets) of malnutrition, deriving from an innutritive diet; not a lack of quantity, but of quality. Its symptoms manifest as initial weakness and clumsiness of the extremities, with possible visual disturbances. General physical and emotional weakness develops, sometimes with mental weakness evidenced as uncharacteristic apathy. Progressive deterioration of the central nervous system follows slowly upon the breakdown of the myelin sheath (nerve protective covering), resulting in unpredictable regions of the body becoming inoperative. The ultimate result is a crippled body which looks little different from the victim of a major polio attack.

Whereas poliomyelitis victims were once young and acutely afflicted, M.S. victims are older and gradually afflicted. But note please: the result is almost the same; the age difference almost reflecting the period during which massive immunisations for polio have been effected with trivalent vaccine. Could this have postponed the original acute manifestation, to insidiously and progressively erupt in the same result a few years later? Polio is described as an acute viral infection which travels along neural pathways throughout the body occasioning paralysis to muscle groups, usually in the lower body, but often in the arms as well. For some, polio was fatal; for others, paralysis was permanent; for most, partial recovery was accomplished (due to the acute nature of the illness). For M.S. victims, the vast majority have little hope of medically recovering from their immobility, so entrenched is the deterioration. But naturopathically, definite hope and a considerable degree of success are possible. In spite of the increasing incidence of M.S., increasing natural rectification is gaining general recognition, so that sufferers can now replace recovery for resignation in their minds.

It is incontestable that faulty diet is the primary cause of human disease, giving rise as it does to toxicity in which bacteria (the secondary factors) rapidly breed within the body. But the aspects of faulty diet which make the most significant contributions towards nerve and muscle breakdown are related to refined and processed cereals (acutely deficient in B-vitamins), refined sugar (robs the body of alkalising minerals), saturated fats (from animal foods, impairing blood circulation) and unnatural chemicals added to foods. Due to the long years of addiction to refined cereals, M.S. sufferers have actually built up an allergy to gluten (similar to coeliac sufferers), so all wheat and rye products must be removed from the diet, as well as all foregoing items. In fact, the only regimen by which the M.S. sufferer can hope to recover is to urgently embrace the totally vegetarian, raw food diet natural to man. Foods should be organically grown where possible, dairy products avoided and abundant amounts of sprouts eaten. The food intake should be highly alkaline and supplemented with certain health foods and vitamins. Before the diet change, a total fast would be ideal.

This will allow a vital resting period for the body, especially the gastrointestinal tract, preparing it for the complete change about to benefit it. After the fast, recovery for the gastrointestinal tract will be enhanced by the use of fresh fruit and vegetable juices, using only those from organic sources. With these can be introduced megadoses of vitamin B_1 (increasing to 2000 mg when solid food is being consumed), a well-balanced B-complex megavitamin, and up to 1500 mg vitamin E. Protein needs will be higher than usual, so abundant raw nuts and seeds must be included, almonds and pepitas being especially recommended. As the body gradually becomes more controlled, physiotherapeutic assistance will help reactivate unused muscles, but each active period needs to be punctuated with a period of rest to allow recuperation of energy. Another important facet of treatment for M.S. (and other muscular syndromes) is chiropractic. This course of manipulative corrections should be undertaken as soon as possible after the fast. It will include vital cranial adjustments and realignments of the spinal column and central nervous system to facilitate an unimpeded transmission of neural nourishment to the most needed regions. With total dedication to the corrective measures and natural living, the M.S. sufferer's condition may improve.

Other muscular and nerve syndromes may also respond to such a programme. This includes such illnesses as muscular dystrophy and atrophy, myasthenia gravis, Parkinson's and Huntington's diseases, meningitis, encephalitis, neuralgia, neuritis and all known and unknown syndromes associated with the central nervous system and spinal cord. Neurologic disorders are similar in essence to all other disorders of the body, being traceable to poor living habits. And unless these are corrected in the community at large, more and more disease syndromes will emerge, attracting some exotic names, but related to the same hapless source of ill-health — ignorance and wilful misrepresentation.

Nausea Pain is the body's fuse circuitry from which messages are transmitted to the brain (the body's switchboard) that something is wrong. If these messages come from the area of the stomach, the feeling conveyed is called nausea. It will generally indicate that the stomach has been overloaded, usually with combinations of foods which are too difficult to digest (see Stage 9). For its self-protection, the stomach might then regurgitate the food back through the oesophagus and out of the mouth, leaving a bitter and highly unpleasant taste. This is a warning that the stomach was mildly poisoned, a condition which could have been intensified had the contents been forced into lower regions of the gastrointestinal tract. Nausea can be caused by overeating, even on nutritious, natural foods (just as a car can be stopped from a flooded carburettor), but chances are that the overload came from less nutritive sources — people partaking of natural foods are usually highly responsible with regard to quantity as well as quality. Fatty foods, especially those emanating from "fast food outlets", are notoriously guilty. For prompt relief from nausea, drink a very warm cup of pennyroyal herb tea (if fatty foods have caused the problem) or alfalfa-peppermint tea (if large amounts of animal foods are at fault). Refrain from eating for at least 24 hours, drinking only pure water or suitable herb teas, preferably warm. If constipation is an accompanying problem, take a cup or two of licorice tea. If diarrhoea is the problem, let it flow, for that is the body's way of rapidly pushing it out of the system, when the disturbance has gone too far along the gastrointestinal tract to be vomited. Rest and complete relaxation are vital for a speedy recovery. Recovery will be permanent when your dietary habits evidence greater wisdom and knowledge.

Obesity Most people could live comfortably on half the amount of food they eat; the other half feeds their health practitioner! Obesity implies a heavy body — one which has accumulated fatty tissue in excess of its needs. It is most frequently induced by excessive food consumption, usually accompanied by insufficient exercise and activity. It is rarely a "gland problem", other than the salivary glands being over exercised. Modern advertising has been perniciously successful in seducing people to eat when they have no genuine appetite, thereby establishing a habit which becomes more difficult to break the longer it prevails. Many people overeat because they are emotionally upset, relating food to security and love, as they did when they were breast-fed or bottle-fed babies and cried when the tummy became empty. There is no harm in using food as a temporary palliative to the emotions, so long as the items selected are nutritious. But, instead of eating an apple or chewing a carrot, most people have a cup of coffee and a doughnut, or a hamburger — the sort of junk which induces emotional agitation and further eating. Simple ways to counter obesity include more exercise, eating natural foods, better food combining, avoiding stimulating spices, seasonings, salt and herb preparations. Avoidance of all refined and processed foods will increase the quantity of nutrients in relation to the number of kilojoules ingested, simultaneously minimising the build-up of toxicity. Regular days on total fasting or a juice diet will be the most positive way of helping the stomach to shrink to its normal size, and will help to revitalise the body. A vitamin-mineral preparation now available has proved to be of great benefit in normalising body weight — it contains kelp, lecithin and vitamin B_6 in a base of apple cider vinegar (often known by the initials: KLB6). These tablets, taken in pairs thrice daily, will allow the body to be fed less without a nutritional sacrifice, as well as working on breaking down fatty tissue. An excellent weight-loss diet is as follows:

Breakfast — A glass of fresh fruit juice, preferably grapefruit,
2 KLB6 tablets.
Lunch — A fresh fruit salad with options of
1) a small quantity of skim-milk yogurt,
2) addition of wheat germ and a little yeast.
Dinner — A fresh vegetable salad with sprouts,
up to 75 g raw unsalted nuts or 50 g raw seeds.

Lunch and dinner can be interchanged to suit personal needs, and with each, a pair of KLB6 tablets should be taken. Between meals, eat nothing (except an apple or pear if desperate), but drink plenty of pure water and take the occasional cup of herb tea (choose from the list in Stage 12 to suit your needs). Please note that this is primarily a maintenance diet, to be increased slightly in quantity when the desired body weight is reached. Special weight-loss diets can do harm to the health and are rarely successful in the long term, for they are generally not designed to improve the body's physical and emotional health — concentrating almost exclusively as they do on weight reduction. General guidelines constituting the essence of this book prove these points.

Osteoporosis This is a chronic syndrome of mineral deficiency, usually not becoming evident until later in life. The bones have been robbed of reserves of calcium, magnesium and phosphorus for most of the person's life, with gradual deterioration and porosity until a major fracture occurs and the condition becomes recognised. But by then, it is often too late for much more than token recovery, although further deterioration can be arrested. How often we hear of an elderly person falling and breaking their hip, when, in reality, they have broken their hip, thereby causing the fall. The hip breaks easily when bones are porous, due to the strong upward pressure normally exerted on the pelvis-femur joint by the weight of the body on the legs. Such a fracture sometimes never heals, requiring complicated and expensive surgery. Factors creating the general syndrome known as osteoporosis include prolonged drug-taking (especially cortisone), hormone imbalance (sometimes occurring after menopause), drinking tea, coffee, cocoa and eating chocolate — these are high in oxalic acid, thereby leaching available calcium and magnesium from the body's stores. Meat also does this, for it contains oxalic acid, although not as much as the other four. Meat also contains considerably more phosphorus than calcium, further contributing to a calcium deficiency. Milk-drinking also leads to calcium deficiency when people depend on milk for this mineral. Calcium in milk is barely assimilated by the human body once weaned — many youngsters have evidenced chalky teeth and bones in proof of this. Bone and teeth (see under Dental) problems will be averted if the body is properly fed from pre-natal times. To correct omissions now can only be achieved by prompt change to the Ideal Diet, with special emphasis on those supplements known to supply increased quantities of essential minerals and to aid in their assimilation. These include the foods already listed under Dental Caries (see p. 236), together with rice bran syrup and equisetum tea, both being rich sources of silicon, needed by the body in its assimilation of calcium. Adequate sunshine and vitamin D are also necessary for this assimilation — liquid chlorophyll and abundant alfalfa sprouts further assist, as do alfalfa tablets.

Pneumonia We read of many historical examples of the fatality of this syndrome, but not so frequently today. Not that it is less widespread, but that medical treatment can rapidly suppress the condition so that the body has more time to heal itself. But this becomes difficult when the lifestyle which induced the original condition is found to persist without change. And so we frequently discover the recurrence of pneumonia within a year or so of the original outbreak.

Pneumonia, itself, is a symptom in a long chain of suppressed illnesses affecting the respiratory system — see Bronchitis and Colds, pp. 231 and 234. It now involves the lung(s) and can include haemorrhaging, biliousness, fever, rapid pulse, severe headache, etc. Natural care has sometimes to be supplemented by medical if the call comes too late for the body to have enough energy left to throw off the many symptoms. Total rest in a well-ventilated, cool room is vital, with absolutely no food, but with small sips of water. Fasting is essential, for the body becomes so debilitated that there is no energy to metabolise food, the pulse rate is too high for proper digestion to take place and the little muscular energy the body has is vital merely for its survival. When the crisis has passed, continue the fast (of course, it must be under professional supervision) for as long as it takes the body to rid itself of the superficial toxicity. If the person is thin, fasting might need to be terminated and a juice diet continued for some days before further fasting. The rebuilding diet will be similar to the Ideal Diet, supplemented with high-nutrient health foods, such as dietary yeasts, lecithin, kelp, liquid chlorophyll and alfalfa tablets. A full range of vitamin supplementation should be used to assist the body to recover as soon as naturally possible. Vitamins C and E will be especially needed, as will B-complex, A and D, but to lesser degrees. So many cases of respiratory malfunctions are caused by smoking, one wonders how long it will be before this fatal habit is outlawed and tobacco production lands turned into the production of important food crops to improve human life, rather than to weaken it.

Prostatitis Inflammation of the prostate gland is a rather common problem with men in the latter stage of their life. If follows enlargement which affects 75 per cent of all men over 60 years, but the incidence of acute discomfort is less than 25 per cent. The syndrome can be actuated by cancer, kidney stones, a benign tumour or abscess formation, resulting in difficulty of urination, chills, acute fever, low back pain or, most seriously, total cessation of urination, by which time surgery is demanded.

Prostatitis is another manifestation of toxaemia and will beneficially respond to improved dietary habits, together with avoidance of tea, coffee, alcohol and heavy food seasonings, all of which are known antagonists to the prostate gland. Another antagonist is unnatural sex — intercourse without orgasm. In older men, this can be damaging to the prostate gland, as can sexual abstinence for a long period if frustration is experienced. Special foods to be included in the natural diet are pepitas (J. I. Rodale wrote an entire book on how these benefited the prostate), polyunsaturated cold-pressed oils (safflower, sunflower, wheat germ and sesame), pollen granules or tablets, lecithin and kelp. Prostatitis indicates a deficiency of zinc, more than any other mineral. This should be taken in chelated form to 25 mg daily initially, then rely on foods rich in zinc — pepitas, nuts, egg yolk, wheat germ and whole rye. Also beneficial will be foods rich in magnesium, in vitamins B_6 and A (see Stage 8), as well as a balanced exercise and activity programme, with special emphasis on walking and running.

Psoriasis Often called "crocodile skin", this is the common chronic syndrome of modern living which shows itself to the outside world as demanding correction. Yet conventional treatment does not succeed in anything but partially disguising it. Some people take years before they attend a naturopath for proper corrective guidance — others never make it, contending with the increasing irritation and unsightliness of scaly, scabby skin all their lives. As the skin covers such a large area, it is easily subject to a wide variety of toxic evidence and becomes a ready indicator of toxic levels in the body. This is the reason for so much acne and so many allergies. And psoriasis is part of that group, but more chronic than the usual acne.

Total fasting is the speediest way to overcome psoriasis and detoxify, when generally the skin will completely recover within one month. Juice dieting and alkalising foods will also do the job, but will require more like three months for the same degree of success, which is quite satisfactory for those people who cannot (or will not) take time away from their regular schedules to fast. A totally alkaline diet implies totally vegetarian, with only whole foods — nothing refined or processed, packaged or canned. No cereals (even though they be whole grain) are to be eaten with the exception of wheat germ and rice bran. Best protein-rich foods are almonds, cashews, sunflower and pepita seeds. Plenty of fresh green vegetables, including sprouts, should be eaten each day. One fresh fruit meal for breakfast and another occasionally for lunch (alternating with a green salad) is ideal. When eating fruit for lunch, dried figs can be included, for these are rich sources of calcium sulphate, helpful for the skin's healing. Avoid citrus fruits during the early stages of recovery; then minimise them. Wash the skin only when necessary, for the drier it is, the faster it will heal. When washing, use only pure coconut soap (the only addition recommended is wheat germ oil). Do not rub dry — pat with a soft towel until the skin has healed. Take plenty of opportunity to swim in sea water, but be sure it is well clear of areas near sewerage outlets. A little daily sun is good, increasing in time as the skin heals. Keep the skin as open to the air as possible, always avoiding polluted air. Vitamin supplements most desirable are A and E, with equisetum tea a very beneficial beverage to drink 2-3 times daily between meals. Rice bran syrup is amazingly beneficial, together with chelated zinc tablets.

Schizophrenia The name is a term for a group of mental and emotional disorders which have in common two aspects — they indicate malnutrition and emotional imbalance. Included are the many forms of psychoses, paranoia and autism found in increasing numbers as life becomes more complicated and diets less nutritive. Entire books have been written on the subject — and many more will be written in the future — so we shall not endeavour to describe its vast range of manifestations, other than in general. Sufferers are usually anti-social, becoming either aggressive or, more often, aloof. They manifest any number of suppressed emotional characteristics, including guilt, anxiety, confusion, frustration, hurt, hatred, envy, and so on. Then they can turn into angry, disturbed people who could undertake quite destructive acts. They certainly need wise and patient counselling, but this is only of lasting effectiveness when accompanied by a significant dietary improvement. There must be a removal from all artificially stimulating "foods", as discussed throughout this book. The Ideal Diet should be embraced, with special inclusion of those foods with known richness in vitamin B-complex (especially B_3), zinc and manganese. This includes dietary yeasts, wheat germ, seeds, nuts, mushrooms and plenty of alfalfa and salad greens. Fasting is particularly beneficial to these patients, the minimum period for benefit being four days. Juice dieting is also helpful after the initial total fast. Vitamin supplements recommended by Dr Abram Hoffer, leading authority on schizophrenia, focus on niacin in massive doses under close supervision. This is supported by vitamins C, B_1 and B_6, minerals manganese (best source is from alfalfa tablets) and chelated zinc, as recommended by leading authority on trace minerals in health, Dr Carl Pfeiffer, in his mammoth guidebook, *Mental and Elemental Nutrients*, published by Keats, Connecticut, 1975.

Senility Contrary to many opinions, senility is not a fact of life, but a syndrome of pandemic proportions which, in some ways, is related to schizophrenia. Senility usually affects older people, although it has been in evidence in recent years in people in their forties who have lived on junk foods and have allowed inordinate degrees of stress and mental strain into their lives. It is a form of enervation seen as gradual loss of memory, disinterest in life, loss of appetite and of thirst and loss of friends and family. Improvement can come about in two ways — by teaching the person to discover their purpose in life (see Stage 2) and by correcting the dietary deficiencies so that brain, nerves and bloodstream improve their performances. Senile people are found to have shrunk in stature. This gives the clue to their primary nutritional problem — they have dehydrated. This has also caused their brain to shrink, creating air spaces in the skull where none should be. Their bloodstream has thickened and nerve impulses dulled. Not a pretty picture, but one which can easily respond to corrective measures so long as the person seeks to co-operate. They must have a need to recover, which is where the emotional and mental counselling work must concentrate. Tests have shown that up to 15 glasses of water daily, when given to senile people together with vitamin supplementation (especially B_1, B_3, B_6, C and E), have helped these people to recover so that within six months they are thinking, feeling and looking considerably better. X-rays reveal that their brains have increased in size and even their bodies stand straighter and look more alert. Then, to encourage them onto the Ideal Diet is to see them live happily and healthily for a few more decades.

Stress In spite of the many books already in print and currently being written about the number one inhibitor to healthy heart functioning, stress remains a simple symptom of modern living. It is by no means a necessary component of modern commercial, industrial or social life, but one to have been wilfully engaged in by all who seek to manipulate. The seemingly relentless striving for power, recognition and security by many has unleashed within them an unnatural greed and competitiveness of obsessive proportions. This demands a constant tension and alertness of the person's nervous system to take a controlling position in any situation to arise, whether it be a major negotiation, a minor personal conflict or an occasional family disagreement. This fear of missing an opportunity produces constant demands on all the body's systems. The body needs time to relax to allow its best performance when it springs into action — just as a cat always lies relaxed, yet is confident in its ability to spring into action should the need arise. No physical body can remain constantly tense and perform at its best (neither can a machine!) There must be ample time to relax between performances, otherwise the nerves, bloodstream, lymphatic, digestive and all other systems will never be able to perform at their optimum when any sudden and urgent load is to be handled. Hence so many businesspeople who maintain constant tension "crack" and lose performance when a really urgent demand is placed upon them. This is a penalty of stressfulness. In any such person can be detected health problems, including allergies, indigestion, hypertension, muscular spasm, headaches and the like — ultimately leading to respiratory ailments and heart dysfunction or stroke (see below).

Stress is an insidious syndrome, most sufferers being unaware of its presence until its pattern has been deeply established. Treatment, then, must commence with an awareness and total recognition of its presence and various manifestations. This is followed by counselling the sufferer to establish his self-confidence, real purpose in life, pathway to achieving that purpose with best results and then to help him balance action and reaction for the most positive results. Accompanying emotional self-control must be dietary balancing. All stress-inducing food items must be deleted from the diet. These include tea, coffee, cola and alcoholic beverages, sugar and refined flour products, preserved meats, heavy spices and seasonings. Their diet should include as many natural foods as possible, especially those rich in B-complex vitamins for nerve nourishment. Excellent food supplements are dietary yeasts, lecithin and rice bran syrup; best herb teas are chamomile, hops and valerian. Another excellent relaxant is tryptophan (see p. 94).

Stroke (Apoplexy) One of the most crippling of degenerative syndromes, the stroke, as it is commonly called, is becoming progressively more common as people subject themselves to more stress and include in their diets ingredients which bring destruction to their bloodstream. A stroke will usually occur when the brain becomes starved of blood and oxygen by a clot, or becomes flooded with blood by a haemorrhage. The "sudden" occurrence of a stroke can delude many people, but this condition requires many years of healthless neglect to precipitate — the body will usually reveal such accompanying syndromes as chronic kidney dysfunction, hypertension and arteriosclerosis. From this weakened state, a heavy strain on the body can be "the last straw" — it might come from lifting, from a sudden emotional outburst, a drinking bout, a fall, excessive coughing or an overly large meal. A sudden total or partial unconsciousness, extremely flushed face and very heavy breathing will indicate the onset of the stroke. There will be paralysis down one side of the body — sometimes not immediately apparent, but it will develop over the following week, the degree depending on many factors, not the least of which is care. Once the stroke has occurred, the person must be given total rest. This means fasting. No other form of care is as effective, nor as easy to administer, because this patient cannot eat without difficulty, has lost his appetite and is extremely apprehensive, so must be kept very calm. Food will only stimulate the body and deviate its energy away from the gigantic healing process on hand.

The stroke victim must be kept warm, yet in a well-ventilated room. Suitable soothing music will be highly advantageous, as will relaxing colours in the room and in the view from the room (should such be available). Ensure the room does not overlook scenery which might remind the patient of the problems faced prior to the stroke (such as busy traffic, if he were a businessman). The duration of the fast and the type of recovery diet will, of course, depend on the supervising practitioner. Total recovery might not be possible, but the maximum amount of recovery will be facilitated by the new maintenance diet conforming with the Ideal Diet (Stage 10), supplemented by those foods and nutrients most beneficial for rebuilding the blood and its pathways, as well as the nerves. These special nutrients are iron, calcium, magnesium, vitamins B-complex and C.

Sunburn There appears to be a growing fetish in most Western countries that the browner one's skin becomes from sunburning, the healthier one is. While it is most important to obtain a certain amount of sunlight direct to the skin, excessive exposure can reverse the health-giving properties of the sun to danger-producing. The discipline of moderation must apply in all things suitable, for, in particular, too much exposure to solar rays in summer can so deeply burn the skin as to darken and harden it against healthy penetration by those rays which would otherwise be so valuable in vitamin D absorption. Those extremely dark suntans not only last longer, but kill so much of the skin as to cause it to crack, lose its elasticity, wrinkle and block the vital elimination work of millions of pores. Many of the burned skin cells become toxic and infected — some even become carcinogenic, eventually producing skin cancers varying from superficial to deep-rooted malignancies.

Before sunbathing, ensure your skin has been nourished with a suitable lotion or cream designed to allow moderate tanning with protection against damage. Essential ingredients in such a preparation should include aloe vera, PABA, and preferably lanolin and cocoa butter. Following exposure, a nourishing lotion or cream should also be applied and should include wheat germ oil and/or sesame oil, to prevent undue dryness. If, inadvertently, long exposure does occur and the skin becomes uncomfortably burned, soak in a bath of cool water to which a large pot of cool chamomile tea has been added. Afterwards rub in plenty of vitamin E lotion and take a short course of vitamins A, C and E in megadoses. Get plenty of rest and eat only raw fruits and vegetables for at least three days — a juice diet would be even better. This programme will allow the skin maximum healing opportunity.

Thrombosis The formation of a blood clot within the blood vessels must be avoided, for invariably, it will grow and move to block a major artery or a valve of the heart. Its travel to the brain and a resultant stroke (see p. 258) has become a major penalty of civilisation. Formation of clots in the arteries or veins is evidence of an unhealthy bloodstream and a poorly nourished body. They often develop in older people when they decide to take long periods of rest after a highly active life; too much inactivity then being a dangerous reversal. These people must not only exercise more, but must pay immediate attention to dietary rectification, for they will have undoubtedly consumed far too many saturated fats, cholesterol foods, common salt and heavy beverages, with insufficient natural moisture in their diets, deriving from fresh fruits and vegetables, supplemented by pure water. The development of any of the thrombotic conditions can be dangerously compounded when arteriosclerotic conditions (see p. 228) are also present in the body, as is often inevitable. For these people, the Ideal Diet has to be modified to exclude cooked foods. They should consume an exclusively raw food diet with emphasis on sprouts, especially alfalfa.

They should sprinkle a little cold-pressed safflower oil over their salads and supplement the diet with alfalfa tablets, lecithin and liquid chlorophyll. Most suitable vitamin supplements are E, C and P, but it must be emphasised that professional guidance is vital for ensuring against complications with this potentially unstable lump of accumulated blood. Regular dry skin brushing and exercise are also important.

Tinea Known in various parts of the world under different names (ringworm, athlete's foot, etc.), tinea is a fungal condition of the skin which occurs more in summer than in winter. Heat and humidity help it to grow from its initial appearance of a small, dark spot, increasing over the surface of the skin in a circular motion. It rarely causes disability, although it can produce soreness if left unattended with a level of bodily toxicity which feeds the fungus so that it deepens and cuts into the skin, especially near a joint. The condition can become inflamed, irritable and scabby if left unattended. It can create a social problem because it is contagious and can be transmitted in places where body toxicity provides breeding grounds, such as schools, swimming pools, gymnasiums etc. Usual parts of the body to be affected are scalp, groin, fingers and toes, especially between the toes. Its presence indicates that the body's innate toxicity is too high and must be reduced by an elimination diet of a few days on raw fruit and vegetable juices, or a short fast. Then be sure to eliminate from the diet those substances which are known to induce the development of toxicity (see Stage 10). Immediate relief from tinea can be obtained by the use of an ointment based on the herbs hypericum, calendula and comfrey, with tea tree oil, applied twice daily. Where possible, maintain a dressing of this ointment on the affected area, being careful to extend the dressing to cover a small distance beyond that appearing to be affected, knowing how this fungus can spread over the skin. If the condition is on the scalp, make a strong solution of sassafras tea and rub in twice daily, or use sassafras oil on the scalp after cleansing with pure coconut soap.

Tonsillitis When the tonsils become inflamed and infected, the body is conveying the message that its toxicity level is at crisis point. This is a first-level warning which, if ignored, will develop into a cold (see p. 234) to throw off unwanted toxicity. Tonsils are thus an important "fuse" in the body's self-protection mechanism whereby the first warning signs are indicated in the most natural way — the tonsils swell, the throat hurts and the person does not eat. That naturally induced short fast (including total rest) is the ideal natural way to reduce toxicity. If such heed is not taken, the body will develop a fever, the stomach will reject the food by vomiting it out and the head will ache to indicate the need for rest. This is not a viral condition, but a normal toxic reaction. It also indicates that the diet needs modification to remove those items guilty of contributing to the toxicity. If surgery has been unwisely undertaken, future minor toxicity crises will force greater discomfort upon the body, first by inflammation in the throat region, then by the various symptoms described as a cold, or for those who seek the more exotic name, influenza. The sore throats developed by the inflammations of tonsillitis, pharyngitis, laryngitis, etc., are best relieved by licorice tea or a compound of licorice, horehound, honey and aniseed. But this must be done in conjunction with at least a twenty-four-hour fast and total rest. It is very important to rest the throat and avoid talking — a withdrawal many people find difficult. This will allow nature to do its vital cleansing job unimpaired.

Toxaemia It is amusing (and rather sad) to read the limited definition of this condition in standard medical and health reference books. It is far more than the "absorption of bacterial toxins formed at a local source of infection". Toxaemia is a toxic bloodstream primarily produced from unhealthy habits in diet and hygiene (internal hygiene is more of a problem, since external hygiene is an accepted modern habit in the West). In such toxicity, bacteria breed and further add to the load, often inducing a localised eruption or a crisis point. Every disease syndrome discussed in this book has related and underlying toxaemia. Only by cleansing the bloodstream can toxaemia be permanently eradicated. This is most thoroughly and naturally achieved by fasting, juice diets or a simple fresh fruit and vegetable diet — each method being progressively slower than its former in achieving results. Each method should be undertaken for a limited period, based on the needs of the body, the obligations of the person and his or her environmental involvements. Professional guidance should be sought to ensure maximum benefits are achieved — most naturopaths and some medical practitioners now have experience with fasting and elimination diets. Once the body cleansing programme has been completed, adoption of a natural foods diet (referred to herein as the Ideal Diet) will do most to guarantee permanent freedom from toxaemia and its limitless manifestations.

Tuberculosis This is another deficiency disease, resulting from the breakdown of tissues and their wasting away by formation into a thickish pus and calcifying. This is either ultimately surrounded by healing, fibrous tissue, thereby creating the lesions characterising the healed condition, or if the body's general level of health is too low, calcification does not take place and the tissues continue to waste, ultimately inducing death. This latter possibility is removed these days, but did prevail as a constant problem to the health of our forefathers when their diets were so deficient in alkalising minerals. The tubercular condition can affect the body in various areas — in the skin (lupus — see p. 250), in the region of the brain (tuberculous meningitis), in the gastrointestinal tract, bones, joints and lymph glands, as well as in the most common region, the lungs. It is the pulmonary condition we have come to recognise as "T.B.", the old name for which is "consumption", meaning the wasting away, about which many stories have been written — Mimi in *La Bohème* is probably the most famous victim, with her choking cough and progressive debilitation. The incidence of T.B. is comparatively rare today, due to massive X-ray campaigns to detect it in early stages and suppress it with drug therapy. This leads to two dangers: 1) the suppression (supposedly, "countering" and "curing") does nothing to remedy the cause of the condition; 2) application of X-rays to the human body will often induce radiation syndromes upon toxic and sensitive tissues even when medically applied — one reason they cannot be used in pregnancy (for additional reading: *X-rays: More Harm Than Good*, Priscilla Laws, Rodale Press, Pennsylvania, USA, 1978).

Suppressing the development of T.B. should accompany a general body detoxification, for serious enervation and toxaemia will otherwise manifest in continually more serious forms. Many respiratory syndromes would have been suppressed in earlier life before T.B. developed in the undernourished body. In poorer countries, T.B. is still present, but with the higher intake of protein in the West, its incidence is rarer. Most countries have passed laws that T.B., as with cancer, V.D. and epilepsy, are "specified diseases" and can only legally be treated medically. So ensure you seek a doctor who has knowledge of fasting and natural nutrition to be guided onto the correct path for handling these syndromes.

As the tubercular body is so debilitated, it does not need feeding, but needs to direct all its energy towards the healing processes. Fasting and total rest are, therefore, mandatory, so long as the body has the reserves to handle the condition. Recovery on juices, then the Ideal Diet (Stage 10), should be speedier than is usual when drugs are administered (for the body would have to contend with these). For the ex-T.B. sufferer, additional proteins, vitamins and minerals are required through the foods, especially dietary yeasts, nuts and seeds; vitamins C and E will need to be taken as supplements as well as a B-complex. Comfrey tea will be found most beneficial between meals during recovery and thereafter as desired.

Ulcers These can develop outside or inside the body, depending on where the skin or mucus membrane weakness exists. It is a breakdown of the area's integrity by gradual disintegration and necrosis of the tissues. External ulcers can vary from minor occurrences in the mouth (canker sores, see p. 232), to ugly and huge inflamed bulbs on the legs. Outer skin ulcers are initiated by a wide variety of factors, all of which can only develop into ulcers when skin integrity is lost due to toxaemia. Abrasion, pre-existing skin problems (such as scleroderma), openings which have accepted bacterial or fungus invasion, can all develop into the more chronic ulcer, revealing the desperate need for a detoxification and then a lacto-vegetarian diet with more than the usual amount of protein. Nuts, seeds, cheeses and eggs will be needed to compensate for the protein deficiency which would have precipitated the ulcerous condition (generally accompanied by too many carbohydrates).

Internal ulcers are invariably found in the gastrointestinal tract. They are a development of excessive animal foods in the diet creating a flow of excessive hydrochloric acid into and from the stomach, compounded by a stress-induced weakened mucosa. Most effective remedial treatment for ulcers of the gastrointestinal tract is fasting under supervision, but this can be initially painful for sufferers from peptic or duodenal ulcers (gastric ulcer sufferers can usually handle it better); for them, a frequent intake of vegetable juices and the occasional salad with a few nuts blended into it is the best remedy, fasting when it can be done without too much discomfort.

Comfrey tea is beneficial for sufferers of internal ulcers; comfrey ointment and poultices for skin ulcers will speed healing so long as no infection is present — if it is, sterilise with calendula extract first. Licorice tea can also benefit sufferers of peptic and duodenal ulcers.

As ulcers often indicate deficiencies in assimilated protein and vitamins, it is wise to supplement the diet, once returning to food, with dietary yeast, lecithin, a well-balanced multi-vitamin-mineral formulation and added vitamins C and E. A delicious liquid meal, rich in B-vitamins and protein and most suitable as a whole meal for ulcer recoverers, is the Soyvita Shake. Its recipe is as follows:

  1 cup pure water
  3 heaped dessertspoons Soyvita instant soymilk powder
  1 level dessertspoon dietary yeast
  1 level dessertspoon lecithin powder or granules
  2 dessertspoons pure maple syrup (or equivalent honey)
  1 raw egg yolk (no white)
  blend or whisk until mixed

It is important for ulcer sufferers to take smaller meals more frequently than the conventional large meal thrice daily. They should avoid citrus and other acid foods until the ulcers are healed and they should avoid over-exertion. Plenty of rest must be taken until the body has totally healed itself; then include adequate exercise in the build-up programme, especially when stress has played a role in developing internal ulcers. All highly seasoned and spiced foods should be avoided indefinitely, for strong curries, peppers and spices are known to be responsible for inducing damage to the sensitive linings of the gastrointestinal tract.

Underweight The human body has individual specific minimum requirements for fatty tissue and muscle bulk. They each must supply the body's needs from adequate reserves stored around the human skeletal frame, the sum total of which is registered as a body weight reading. In orthodox health circles, those people registering less than average weight for their height and frame structure are considered "underweight". And here lies the essence of the misunderstanding. Average weights should not be confused with *normal* weights (and this refers only to our Western civilisation). The average citizen is overweight, the result of eating too much and doing too little. For the past few hundred years, average weights have been increasing when compared to normal — what a person should weigh for their height and frame type. So we now find that many people with *normal* weight-for-height are considered slightly underweight. And those now classified as "quite underweight" are only slightly under normal; but these are not the people with problems. Most "underweight" people therefore pose a psychological threat to those heavier than themselves, for their presence implies the overweight of the others; it also reveals how much fitter and healthier being underweight can be. The people who are really underweight are those whose body weight registers around 25 per cent or more below the average for their frame and height. This does not take into account weight differences for age increase — nor should it, because a person should not increase in weight with age, in fact, they should decrease slightly, for as they get older, their body needs less musculature and uses less energy. And there is no need for the ageing heart to lift more weight around than it needs. (People put on weight as they age because they continue to eat more than they need, being addicted to quantities set when younger, more active and using more calories.)

But all statistics aside, a person is actually underweight when their body looks uncomfortably thin, when they tire quickly or have insufficient strength for the needs of their lifestyle. For these people, dietary and emotional changes are probably equally needed. They are probably nervous, with sharp, rapid movements and over-alert as though in constant danger. They talk very quickly, eat just as quickly, and often eat quite hearty meals, snacking frequently between meals. To these people, meditation and relaxation are words without meaning. They are stressed people (but will rarely admit it), anxious, ambitious, often frustrated and easily irritated. Wise emotional counselling is their first need, for this will effectively slow them down to a normal pace, conserve their nervous energy, they will chew their food better and improve their metabolism. Their food needs to be more wisely selected. It should be based on the Ideal Diet (Stage 10), with special emphasis on those foods rich in B-vitamins as listed for stress (see p. 257). They would do better to eat smaller meals more often than the two or three large meals in which heavier people have the habit of indulging. They should always allow a short time to relax after a meal and ensure they are relaxed when eating the meal. A cup of warm chamomile tea will help in this regard, if sipped 20–30 minutes ahead of the meal. A soyvita shake, as recommended for ulcer sufferers (see p. 262) is an excellent meal occasionally, but it must be drunk slowly, "chewing" each mouthful. Underweight people can increase their weight, if they wish, by limiting their intake of fruits and increasing their intake of complex carbohydrates and protein foods. They must also allow themselves at least one day each week for relaxation and recreation of a casual nature — no body was meant to be kept at its most active for seven days every week.

Varicose Veins When veins in the legs swell with stagnant blood, the condition becomes varicosed and visible through the skin. This occurs with leg veins more than elsewhere because these are farthest from the heart and the anti-gravitational pull to draw the blood into the heart for purification is sometimes too great for the enervated condition of the veins. As the veins and their one-way valves lose their elasticity, the varicose condition develops. It occurs in women twice as frequently as in men, being often induced at or soon after pregnancy — more than 50 per cent of all women over 36 have varicose veins. Other significant factors relating to their development are obesity, common salt, saturated fats, cholesterol from animal foods, lack of exercise, too much standing (particularly in the one spot), insufficient fluid intake (contributing to a thickening of the blood), weakened heart, unsuitable diet and/or constipation. All these problems are considered throughout this book in detail and the sufferer of varicose veins would do well to digest them thoroughly, for this condition can be overcome — the degree of success will depend on how long and how entrenched is the condition. Vitamin supplements B-complex, C and E will be of added benefit — the massaging of witch hazel ointment over the vein area will also assist in diminishing the varicosity. Resting with the feet higher than the head for many periods during the day will provide further aid — a slant board is ideal, for it can also be used to perform invaluable abdominal exercises regularly. Sleeping with the bed slightly elevated at the foot end has helped many people.

Venereal Disease This is both a social and a dietary syndrome with just as much prevalence now as a century ago; in fact, more cases are being reported now than ever before — not to say that more exist, but that their seriousness is now recognised more extensively with less social stigma than previously. V.D. includes two major syndromes — syphilis and gonorrhoea. The former is the more critical, being easily spread beyond and around the body, inducing death if unchecked; the latter is more often localised. Both are easily detected on the man by the hard sore on his penis from syphilis or by the exuding of pus from his urethra when gonorrhoea is present. Women are not so aware of being infected carriers, so they should undertake frequent clinical checks if they share intercourse with various partners. It is primarily through sexual intercourse that gonorrhoea is spread — syphilis can be contracted much more superficially due to its more ubiquitous nature. But these syndromes, as with any other "contagious disease", will rarely be of consequence to the non-toxic person (who is relatively rare, too!) When toxaemia is present in the bloodstream, even though its level might be well below crisis point, the presence of infectious invaders will have a suitable medium for spreading and growth into infection. Therefore, abundant health should always be sought, and this is achieved through the practice of guidance contained in this book. If toxicity is present, the most effective manner of eliminating it is by fasting, for indeed, this discipline is particularly effective where V.D. is present. A greater personal awareness of morality and the real understanding of love are other vital factors in controlling V.D..

Vitiligo When white spots appear on the skin and grow in size or number; when rather premature greying appears in the hair and tends to spread, the possibility appears that a skin deficiency syndrome called vitiligo is present. Most people are concerned with the cosmetic consequence of this deficiency, but more care should be evidenced towards its inference of dietary deficiency, generally of the B vitamins, in particular choline, PABA and pantothenic acid (B_5). Dietary guidance to correct this problem involves the inclusion of whole grain cereals, especially high-protein wheat, rye, triticale, buckwheat and millet, wheat germ, dietary yeasts, lecithin and the supplementary vitamins as researched by Dr Carlton Fredericks and his group and found highly successful: choline 2000 mg, PABA 60 mg and pantothenic acid 30 mg daily. It is important to realise that the condition took many years to manifest, so do not expect an immediate reversal — it can take many months and will be the more effective when processed items and animal meats are eliminated from the diet, for they include chemicals known to interfere with the skin pigmentation of some people. (Pork has been known to induce premature baldness on rare occasions, with the hair regrowing after a total fast and abstention from pig meats thereafter.)

Water Retention This syndrome is present in some of the foregoing conditions, especially in gout and arthritis, kidney problems and where common salt is taken in large quantities. Sodium chloride is hygroscopic, attracting to it moisture wherever it might be in the body. When this is added to food, the body separates it and shunts it out of the way, generally around the joints, the favourite being the ankles, with the help of gravity. Excess water in the body finds gravity the same help and is soon attracted by those thirsty salt crystals. Water retention is responsible for adding excess body weight, inducing lethargy and aching legs, limiting joint flexibility and creating discomforting and ugly oedema. It is not caused by too much drinking, but by too much unsuitable fluid intake. Were the intake only water, the problem would possibly not occur, but it is caused by too much common salt intake, as well as the consumption of carbonated beverages and the like, beer and cola drinks being two of the worst offenders. Many people disclaim adding salt to their food, yet suffer water retention problems. An investigation into their diet will often reveal hidden sources of salt, such as in bread, bacon, ham, sausages, margarine and butter, packaged breakfast cereals, canned seafoods, cheeses, crustaceans, buns and biscuits, salted nuts and crackers — the list is almost endless. When a person suffering from water retention is put on a fast, their initial weight loss is astounding — up to 2 kg daily over the initial few days is not unknown. This proves how much excess weight the body carries, overloading the heart and all other organs, impairing their normal work and the person's health. A salt-free diet of vegetarian foods is imperative for these people, and for immediate relief (if unable to fast), a daily intake of 50 mg vitamin B_6, plus homoeopathic sodium sulphate cell salt tablets or drops are effective water dispellers.

Worms Intestinal worms, the most common of which is the tapeworm, have been found living within the human body since man began eating animal flesh and sea foods. They can be taken into the gastrointestinal tract quite unknowingly and hatched in the warmth of the human body without the person suspecting. Worms very rarely inhabit vegetarians, but are frequent in people who eat pork — hence the age-old Chinese preoccupation with the problem. Two herbal remedies have been proved effective over the years — garlic and paw paw seeds or tea. Garlic can be eaten fresh or taken in capsule form; paw paw seeds should be chewed before a meal and swallowed when the stomach is empty, to be washed down by dried paw paw leaves when infused into a tea. Future freedom from intestinal worms will only be guaranteed by a total vegetarian diet, another advantage of supplying the body's natural food needs.

Psycho-sclerosis

Intentionally out of alphabetical order, this syndrome has not yet appeared in medical or health texts, yet it is found to prevail in so many people. It is "hardening of the attitude". Among other things, it is the syndrome of those who fear change, who seek to persist with established habit even when their intelligence or their intuition tells them it is unsuitable and unwise. In our consideration of the foregoing common illnesses and health inhibitors, we find that diet always exerts a major influence. But before a person will effectively change diets and revert to the natural foods approach, a change in attitude must occur. They must realise that everything they swallow has an influence on their health, just as every thought they entertain has an influence on their attitude and emotional harmony. It all works together.

STAGE FOURTEEN

The Organic Revolution

> *Revolutions are not made, they come. A revolution is as natural a growth as an oak. It comes out of the past. Its foundations are laid well back.*
>
> Wendell Phillips (1811-1884),
> American orator and reformer

Good health is impossible without good food. Good food is impossible without healthy soil. Healthy soil can only be achieved in conformity with nature's laws.

We know good health to be dependent upon more than food alone; we also recognise that food which contains optimum nutrients will sustain a higher standard of health, all other factors being equal.

Nutrients in foods must offer properties beyond those quantitatively measured by chemical analysis. They must possess as well the qualitative property of life force, detectable by the senses, especially by taste and psychometry.

To provide nutrient-rich food for human consumption is a noble undertaking when performed in conjunction with environmental harmony. It offers satisfaction to the consumer as well as the producer. But this satisfaction can only be obtained by the use of organic methods, age-old systems which are again achieving renewed popularity by being entitled "the organic revolution".

Such a description implies that agriculture is revolving back to nature, and none too soon. It indicates dissatisfaction and disillusionment with the chemical system of farming which pays virtually no attention to ecology as it takes everything from the soil, and returns sterilising, poisonous chemicals. It encourages farmers to denude the land of trees, farm every square metre on their property and use liberal doses of a wide range of chemical poisons and hormonal preparations to stimulate a high crop yield.

For years, the decline of ethical agriculture continued largely unnoticed, save for the perceptions of a few observant "radicals", such as Rachel Carson, J. I. Rodale and the pioneering ecologists before them.

Today, we witness the success of those early, untiring efforts. In spite of frequent newspaper criticism of the organic revolution (sometimes accusing the organic movement of the very fraud it works to expose), the widespread following it now commands is impossible to halt. The truth it brings is being heard by responsible citizens who are recognising the need to alter chemistry's collision course with nature.

Nutritional Advantages

With people expressing their right to obtain poison-free, properly ripened, correct-tasting foods, to breath poison-free air and enjoy unpolluted lands and waterways, the organic revolution is gaining more attention than ever before in the world's history.

Even when a person antagonistic to the organic concept is conducted on a tour of an organic farm and feels the almost inexpressible harmony it possesses; when he tastes the delicious flavours of organically grown food and experiences the pleasure of it satisfying both appetite and thirst — then there is no more argument. This conversion we witnessed so often on our own organic farms that it became one of our most pleasant occupations. When newspaper reporters, professional and academic horticulturalists and farmers could be converted against their previous training and belief then we must have had something very special to offer.

In fact, every organic farm has something special and unique to offer and every organic farmer should be prepared to share it with anyone who is interested enough to investigate.

One of the most interesting conversions I witnessed was that of the head of the government agricultural advisory service for that part of Australia where our organic farms are located. At first very sceptical, his interest developed when we showed him the huge paw paws, some weighing up to 4 kg, just harvested after a period of partial drought. Then, when he tasted one and discovered how smooth a texture and sweet a flavour it had, he was incredulous. A few weeks later, he devised a test which substantially proved our point.

The branch of the Department of Primary Industry at Nambour, Queensland, prepared a taste test on paw paws grown in the region. Taste, as you know, is a very reliable guide to a food's qualities. They invited each of the twelve farmers who produced paw paws in the region to submit one of their fruit for the test.

Each paw paw was numbered so that its identity was unknown to the people who were invited to sample and report their preferences. Staff of the department were included; so were local businessmen, farmers and people walking by the office.

You have guessed the result. Our paw paw was chosen *unanimously* as the best of the twelve — a surprise to everyone but the organic farmers. This test was carried out early in 1970, just two years after we had bought the farm.

Tests carried out by the Soils Department of the University of Missouri have been quoted in the writings and lectures of world-renowned British agricultural expert, Dr W. E. Shewell-Cooper. "Drs Wittwer and Schroder discovered that the amount of carotene (from which vitamin A comes) varies from as low as 0.50, in the case of carrots grown in chemically fertilised soils, to as high as 31.0 milligrams per 100 grams weight of carrot grown in compost-rich soils."

A brochure handed out to visitors to the Rodale Experimental Farm at Emmaus, Pennsylvania, tells of tests that have been made at the farm on the nutritional values of chemically vs. organically grown wheat and oats. Using a set of circular plots and a system named after its inventor, Sir Albert Howard, two sets of crops were produced, one organically, the other by chemical fertilisation. Howard had used this system in India with the British government, proving how much more nutritional food could be produced from a given area of land if organic techniques were employed.

To obtain precise test figures of the nutritional differences between the two systems of crop production, J. I. Rodale sought the services of a Philadelphia biochemist, Dr Howard E. Worke.

Using precision equipment, Dr Worke undertook to analyse samples selected at random from both crops of wheat and oats. He used the chemically fertilised group as the control so that any change in the nutrient value of the organically fertilised group would be registered as a percentage increase or decrease. The results were summarised as follows:

Nutrient		Wheat		Oats
Protein	increase of	16%	increase of	28%
Vitamin B$_1$	"	108%	"	92%
Vitamin B$_2$	"	131%	"	171%
Niacin (B$_3$)	"	63%	"	100%
Calcium	"	29%	"	25%
Phosphorus	"	1%	"	3%

Averaging the results over all samples, every nutrient tested showed an increased concentration in the organically fertilised crops when compared to those chemically fertilised. Proponents of the organic system have always attested to dramatic increases in vitamin content of foods thus cultivated. Now these test figures actually prove beyond doubt the extent to which chemical fertilisation decreases the optimum nutritional qualities of food. This is especially evident with the B-complex group of vitamins.

With each of the three principal vitamins within the B-complex range, the test figures reveal that chemical fertilisation produces an average of only half the plant's optimum capability. Could this explain a phenomenon which for years this writer and many other independent nutritional scientists have been endeavouring to bring to the attention of Westerners? Man's health is not only decreasing because modern processing of foodstuffs reduces their nutritional properties, but also because the foods themselves, even before processing, are nutritionally deficient. Such test results as those above prove the seriousness of the charge.

When the very agricultural methods employed by man actually halve the potential B-complex vitamin content of his food, what damage must he be sustaining, not only to his crops, but also to his soils and his health?

Every practitioner connected with human health today is concerned about the incipient decline being registered by the progressive increase in symptoms of sickness. There is unanimity of opinion that man is becoming physically weaker, more nervous, less patient, more intolerant, more constipated, more depressed and less energetic. All these symptoms can be directly related to an inadequate intake of nutritious foods, especially those rich in the B-complex vitamins. Not only is man consuming more processed and less whole foods, but the very method of producing his crops gives him a serious nutritional handicap.

Further testimony is apparent by the increasing occurrence of anaemia in Western societies. The remedy is not to supplement the diet with isolated concentrations of vitamin B$_{12}$, but rather to ensure that this newly discovered vital trace vitamin is not depleted by a departure from nature's own system of producing food, the organic system.

Undernourished Plants

Of special interest in the comparison of nutritional properties of foods produced by different agricultural methods is the content of protein. When a method of fertilisation actually restricts the development of nearly a quarter of the crop's potential protein availability, it is depriving man of his most vital nutrient.

When plants are subjected to enforced growth, rather than fed to promote natural development; when they are chemically stimulated and deprived of natural, organic nutrients upon which to feed, such plants react by a wild development of cellular structure which is deficient in trace elements and amino acids. Put simply, both the plant and its produce develop an overabundance of carbohydrates (in the form of starches and cellulose) at the expense of protein. Such poorly constituted crops cannot avoid, and must inevitably attract, any prevalent form of disease.

That the nutrient imbalance in plants created by chemical fertilisation predisposes towards disease development can be nowhere more conclusively proven than when nearby organically fertilised plants, of the same variety, remain virtually unaffected by the same disease. Many an organic farmer and gardener has demonstrated this.

At our own organic farms, not one paw paw tree was lost during the severe disease epidemic of 1973 which followed eastern Australia's 1972 partial drought. Every newspaper reported the severe plant losses of up to 90 per cent of plantations from "three strains of virus ... The exact cause of the virus and their treatment has not been positively identified by the Department of Primary Industry's researchers. However, there is strong evidence to suggest that the paw paws are suffering from a calcium deficiency."*

It was no strange or mystical phenomenon that our farm, with its organically mulched plants, registered not even a decline in crop production while other farmers in the district were bemoaning their huge losses. Yet few even learned by the experience. Some farmers sold out; others replanted but continued to rely on chemicals for fertilisation, scavenger poisoning, etc. The consequence is that the price of paw paws on the Australian open market hit an all-time high in 1973-74, but that was no benefit to those with no paw paws to sell.

The Meaning of "Organic"

It is erroneous to regard organic cultivation as the "alternative" to chemical. Organic is by far the older, having been practised since man first learned how to grow his own food. It is the chemical method which is the alternative; it has been tried, found initially promising in terms of crop yields, but has since become wanting.

With considerable research and huge financial investment in the chemical method, its promoters obviously felt challenged by the long-proven organic method. Why else should they resort to an intimidation campaign which, among other methods, attempts to constrict the use of the word "organic" to a branch of chemistry, implying that the ecologically minded farmer is intruding upon their territory with its use?

In actual fact, the use of "organic" far antecedes modern chemical practice. It is Greek in origin. It referred to that unique aspect of plants and animals — their organised physical structure. It was thus used to describe regulated life, from which the term "organised" arose. In its broader sense, it came to be respresentative of life, of organised growth.

In the fourteenth century, as the infant study of anatomy developed, "organic" attracted further use in being applied to the description of functions of "organs". But a new use for the word arose 150 years ago with the development of a branch of science devoted to the study of chemicals containing, or derived from, hydrocarbon radicals. Hence, "organic chemistry" became known as the study of compounds deriving from once-living plant or animal substances. It has since expanded to embrace any chemical related to life.

---

* Extracts from front page of *The Australian Financial Review* of September 18, 1973.

The chemist has obviously taken a liking to the use of this word "organic", and now regards himself as its exclusive custodian. But as far as the original and unconfined use of the word is concerned, organic chemistry is no more organic than the chemicals applied to cultivation. "Carbon chemistry" would be a more explicit, less confusing description. Thus, when organic farmers make correct use of the term, so necessary to distinguish between their methods and those using synthesised chemicals, they are accused of "plagiarism" by the very people who are themselves the pirates.

Although many organic chemicals might be structurally duplicated by the chemist, his efforts are incomplete. To believe that the synthetic is identical with the natural is to overlook one vital factor — the life force. A synthetic chemical can appear to represent a natural one only to the extent that a waxen image is a dummy of its living model.

As "organic" implies "organised", it necessarily also implies balance and harmony. This describes an environment which is ecologically in tune; where all components peacefully and synergistically co-exist by enacting natural adjustments to any slight imbalance occasioned by lack or excess of individual components — rain, wind, sun, soil, etc.

Chemicals Against Nature

Ecological balance is maintained by the operation of that inviolable law of cause and effect. This law of compensation, of "karma" (if you know it better under that name), ensures that an equal and appropriate reaction balances every action. However, when actions involve flagrant applications of sterilising chemicals to the soil, to plants or the atmosphere, nature reacts by attempting to negate such counter-ecological conditions in quite unexpected ways. These induce further, more toxic efforts on the part of the chemists. And so the decline magnifies into accelerating misery for all concerned.

Exemplifying this unhappy karmic cycle is the farm of John Barnett in Florida, USA. For years, he had been producing the sweetest, reddest tomatoes ever to stimulate your gastric juice. In 1968, a well-trained chemical salesman convinced him that if only John would use his company's new fertiliser prior to planting, then dust with its specially prepared hormone as the crop commenced to mature, the next crop would be at least half as big again. Somewhat reluctant to alter his proven pattern, John was convinced when the salesman reminded him how much more quickly he would be able to pay off his new tractor with the added income — and with no more work, he was promised.

As the salesman promised, the next crop of tomatoes was actually nearly 60 per cent heavier than the previous one. What excitement, and the only extra cost was a hundred dollars' worth of chemicals.

John and his wife and children had always enjoyed eating their tomatoes. And that year, they had them a whole month earlier to enjoy. But their enjoyment was somewhat diminished because the crop was not as sweet as in past years, nor did they seem to keep as well when picked. It must have been because of the earlier maturing, the salesman convinced them; hormones and sulphate of ammonia couldn't possibly do that!

Anxious to see even bigger crops, John bought more chemicals and increased their application by 25 per cent. Unfortunately, the crop did not respond. In fact, it was a little less than that previous bumper harvest. Then, a strange thing happened. As John commenced harvesting, he noticed some yellowing of the leaves. That hadn't happened before.

But a worse occurrence was yet to come. When he was only two-thirds of the way through harvest, John noticed that some tomatoes had small holes from which fluid was weeping. Surely not the fruit fly! Why, he had been farming for years and had never been inflicted by this scourge, although he knew of many who had.

The friendly chemical salesman was on vacation at the time, but as soon as he returned John told him of the loss of nearly one-quarter of his crop due to fly damage. Yes, the salesman had the perfect answer — oh, he had plenty of experience with this sort of thing. His company had just released a new anti-fly spray which should be applied to the plants when in flower. It was highly toxic, but its effect would wear off before the fruit was ready to harvest, John was assured; it would last just long enough to spell death to only the fruit fly, nothing else. The new chemical was called malathion.

John did as he was told. The night after he sprayed the new-flowering tomato plants, John was forced to retire early to bed. He had a most unusual, splitting headache. He was never one to suffer from this sort of thing. To make matters worse, he had to run into the bathroom twice during the night to vomit. He had not done that ever before in his memory. John's wife was worried.

Next morning they sat down to breakfast together and talked long and hard about last night's nightmare experiences. John was still far from well. His mouth felt the way the bottom of the parrot's cage looked. Even his hands were not steady. At thirty-five, he was too young to be getting old.

Obviously, that poisonous spray was a deadly weapon. If he had inhaled some of it, as he must have done, what would it do to everything in the atmosphere? He only wanted to kill the fruit fly, not every living organism, bird and animal on his farm. They loved their animals and the birds. This could not go on. John would not run the risk of another night like the one he had just gone through.

What a gamble for that extra income, they thought. How could they have conceived that it involved such a risk?

No longer would they use chemicals; they intended to revert to the old system of compost, mulch and loving care. But this revised resolve had yet to meet the acid test. When harvest time came around, John noticed with unbelievable horror that the fruit fly had laid its eggs in most of his crop and he remembered the salesman's warning: "You must spray this malathion at least twice, John." He refused; he also had his income cut very severely that year.

Next year, John and his family decided not to plant tomatoes. They would spend the whole year trying to rebuild the soil and remove those obnoxious chemicals. They wisely grew a crop of string beans, harvesting only the first maturing beans and ploughing the rest into the soil.

The following year, it was almost back to square one. The tomato crop was not as big as the last time he had produced it organically, but the old, delicious flavour was almost as good. And then the following year, there was a complete return to the good crop and the full, sweet flavour. Nature, it seemed, had forgiven him.

And you know, the whole family felt strangely very happy again, almost as though they had insulted God, but then asked His forgiveness. They obviously received it. They learned that it is better to trust Him and nature all the way, than give lip service to God's commandments on one day and contravene nature's laws on the other six days.

Man is a very delicately balanced living organism. Everything he does should honour that situation, for he can use such balance with infinite power, wisdom and benefit, but not by poisoning himself and his environment.

Before the recorded history of man, people lived naturally, worked adequately, ate suitably and populated at fancy. They were the natural things to do. Ethics were propounded, morals predicated and practised, pyramids and chariots, boats and palaces built — all based on natural principles observed in action. Agricultural and pastoral communities provided food and raw materials for shelter and clothing. The human race seemed to effectively evolve into this present era, this unique period in the history of our planet which supports the greatest numbers ever.

People had to be temperate in their demands upon resources, so all this was achieved with reasonable satisfaction. And without the aid of man-made chemicals? How was it possible?

Primitive man learned to fear nature, but in that fear, he developed great respect for its power and developed methods of co-operating with it. He had neither the technology, nor the desire to fight nature; instead, he learned to thoroughly understand it in its expression. Most importantly, man learned to use nature, rather than abuse it.

As man's intelligence developed, he learned how to live in harmony with nature. He was ignorant of the chemical composition of water, but realised that compost and mulch, similar to those on the forest floor, were necessary to preserve the moisture (and the fertility) of his soil. He did not know the reason for the moon's orbiting around his own planet, or whether earth actually revolved around the moon, but he did observe how the phases of the moon affected the growth of his plants. So he cultivated accordingly. He had not the technology to construct huge dams to control floods, but he observed the regularity of floods and avoided huge losses by them, learning to gather and prize the silt they left as an extra fertilising of his soil. He had not discovered how to construct a deep-freeze unit, yet was able to preserve foods for considerable periods of time with the aid of natural phenomena for the arresting of decay.

In forest areas, a high level of natural fertility is maintained by the constant mulch cover provided by droppings from birds, trees, etc. In the presence of adequate moisture, such as is always attracted by abundant tree growth, mulch decomposes into compost right there where it is most suited. The natural soil cover attracts plenty of soil animals, especially those valuable earthworms whose food chain is so vital to soil fertility. Thus we have an adequate supply of mulch material, the means of its breakdown with the release of essential nitrogen in the process, and its reuse by plant communities to maintain their own growth and to propagate.

Sound agricultural practice is to emulate nature in the forest. It implies a deliberate effort on the part of the farmer or gardener to ensure that his soil is supplied with adequate organic material for its constant feeding. By suitable mulching, compost is obtained where it is needed; by adequate watering, organic matter is decomposed and the minute animal kingdoms are encouraged. To maintain this practice requires just a little time, but far less cost than to omit it and have it replaced by expensive chemicals.

But post-war man was generally too impatient to take the time to garden organically. Besides, he had also been conditioned to the mechanisation and chemicalisation which characterised recent warfare. How could he resist the promises of the redirected war machine as its production turned from homicide to insecticide? The rot had set in.

Chemical fertilisation temporarily overcame the small yields and small individual sizes of produce resulting from infertile soils. By stimulated growth, plants erupted into production; but their enforced products reflected the nutritional imbalance we now know to be characteristic of artificial fertilisation.

A further consequence of chemical fertilisation became progressively apparent. Such potent chemicals were found to effectively sterilise their host soils, diminishing the colonies of minute soil animals and vital earthworms until, with repeated usage, the chemicals finally depleted soil life altogether. Soils became dry and powdery, as is to be expected when deprived of moist organic matter. Layers of topsoil yielded easily to even moderate breezes and were lifted miles away, creating dust storms, to be finally dumped into waterways and washed out to sea.

In the balance of nature, it is the function of scavenger insects to feed upon unhealthy organisms. Their prolific breeding then renders the host somewhat unfit for human use. If the environment is in balance, predators will maintain a check on scavenger proliferation; but when unhealthy substances abound, excessive numbers of scavengers are attracted.

So it was with the action of insects on unhealthy, chemically fertilised crops and the comparative ineffectiveness of predator colonies to contain them. Man induced the imbalance by his chemicals, so more chemicals were developed in an effort at containment. This only produced temporary respite, and gave more permanent exacerbation to the imbalance. Lower forms of life mutate easily. Predator birds and large insects were decimated by the new poisons, but the scavenger colonies merely adapted after their initial shocks. And so the rot accelerated.

Soils are poorer, lighter and actually diminishing in quantity as well; plants are weaker and their products nutritionally depleted. Crops produced chemically contain fewer vitamins and minerals than similar crops produced organically. Their protein content is lower, and carbohydrate content higher; but this is not even a balanced carbohydrate — it is composed of more starch than sugar, reflected in the diminished sweetness of chemically produced foods.

At last the unified voice of ecology-conscious man is being heard. At first it was regarded as no more than a crank rumble in the distance. But now it is becoming fashionable to join such protests. Even politicians now find this to be a vote-getter! May such protests achieve a curbing of *all* unnatural, counter-ecological acts, not only the abandoning of nuclear activity, limitation to city sprawls and cessation of dumping untreated sewage, but also the veritable mining of soils which is known as chemical agriculture, with its attendant poisoning of the atmosphere and man's most vital food, fresh fruits and vegetables.

Returning to Nature

When Eve gave Adam that "apple", he didn't even wash it. If it happened in most of the world's apple orchards today, we would not have the population explosion. Adam would have probably been poisoned and unable to reproduce as prolifically as he must have for the present population of our planet to reach its unprecedented numbers. But even with such a population, the amount of arable land now available is adequate, if only sensible use would be made of it.

There is no disputing that with the passing of each year, the amount of arable land is decreasing. Man's activities are solely to blame. If he devoted the time and money demanded by chemical research into organic reconstitution of the soil's fertility, we would see deserts diminish instead of increase. Then, if he would produce crops for his direct consumption instead of feeding the huge herds of animals he has so thoughtlessly bred, and instead of producing all those non-food crops — the world would not know of a food shortage. It is a strange paradox that many of the countries which cry for food are vigorously producing non-food crops such as tea, coffee, cocoa, plant drugs, spices, sugar, etc.

When all complexities fail, man learns that by returning to nature his problems are solved. This is no more cogently apparent than in the agricultural sphere, so let us now turn back to the simple facts of farming and restore this earth to its Edenic state.

The means whereby we may return to Eden will depend on the degree of deterioration created by chemical applications. To provide specific remedies in one book for each and every possible set of circumstances is totally impossible, just as it is to offer accurate diagnoses and treatments for every type of disease symptom within the human body. But just as it is possible to define the ideal diet and the ingredients for human health, so it is possible to offer a basic, proven guide for the correct method of ensuring the health of the soil and its inhabitants.

Variations of the basic organic method are legion. A huge variety of factors will indicate the wisdom of suitable modifications, but all these are easily recognised and employable when one learns to observe Nature at work, to be guided by his own inherent intuition and to maintain a firm adherence to altruistic principles.

Some of the influencing factors are: climate, including rainfall, prevailing winds, etc.; topography and altitude; existing vegetation; previous use of land; use of surrounding land; availability of organic matter; suitability to specific crops.

Crop Selection

It is always easier to swim with the current. Likewise, it is much easier to grow plants which have natural tendencies to a region, than to introduce foreign plants and work hard at adapting them to the climate or the climate to their needs. For example, the ingenuity of man does not fall short of building a tropical climate within a glass house in a sub-temperate part of the world. But no matter how perfectly man thinks he has simulated the natural, the resultant fruit will never be quite as flavoursome as its naturally produced counterpart.

The first step in any sensible agricultural method is thus to select crops which are naturally suited to the region. Alternatively, select the region for the crops one wishes to produce. Priorities must be given due prominence — if it is more important to grow paw paws and bananas than to live in Melbourne, then move to northern New South Wales or to Queensland.

Other vital factors of influence in crop selection include the availability of adequate water (either as rainfall or for irrigation), as well as its seasonal distribution. For instance, it is impossible to produce a fine crop of almonds in an area which has a record of heavy summer rains. The importance of a permanent stream for supplemental irrigation cannot be too highly stressed. But rainfall will always constitute the primary source of water for plants, as it also brings freshly ionised trace elements from the atmosphere, especially if created by storms.

Prevailing winds present a factor in farming about which little can be done. Wind breaks can be erected at some expense, or can be grown by planting a stretch of suitable trees. But even if they are fast-growing trees, they require some years before becoming effective. Therefore, if seasonal winds are strong and/or induce any temperature extremes, such factors must be considered in the selection of suitable crops. For instance, it would be economical suicide to try to grow fruiting trees in an area which experiences strong winds during their flowering season — early loss of flowers would prevent cross-pollination and subsequent fruit setting.

While soil types do not imply as much influence in the selection of crops or location of the farm, recognition of their influence can certainly be beneficial. Whereas chemical agriculture does nothing to improve soil fertility (rather it causes depletion), the organic method not only greatly succeeds in the enrichment of soil, but very often effectively alters the nature of the soil in so doing. It is only a matter of a few seasons before loose, light soils are converted to rich fertility, or heavy, clayey soils are converted to dark, friable loams.

It is obviously more efficient to select the crop for greatest suitability to the basic nature of your soil type. Otherwise, the period required for soil conversion will be one of lowered income return. We know that carrots grow best in light, friable (even sandy) soils, so to convert heavy clays to this type of soil suggests a couple of years before carrots can be successfully produced. By reverse, tall, shallow-rooted plants such as paw paws will not do well in light, sandy soils; they require a heavy, rich soil to provide both adequate nourishment and root stability.

We should be mindful that plants are very sensitive to their environment. Over a limited range, they do possess some power of adaptability, both physically and metaphysically. Their searching for suitable nourishment by the extension of their root network is widely recognised. So, too, is their ability to absorb atmospheric nutrients through their leaves — indeed, this means of feeding can be more important to a plant than the generally accepted root feeding, assumed by most people to be the only way by which a plant can take up nourishment.

The "biodynamic method" of Dr Rudolf Steiner is designed to utilise a plant's ability of leaf feeding, its application in agriculture always bringing successful results, as we shall discuss farther on.

A plant's root system is vital for the absorption of moisture and for the physical security of the plant. The ability of roots to find assimilable nutrients is also part of their searching function, often inducing them to seek the upper surface of the topsoil if too much disturbance of the subsoil has resulted in its loss of trace minerals. Such near-exposure of sensitive root ends makes them susceptible to atmospheric conditions, to climatic extremes to which they cannot adapt.

We are aware of most of the physical atmospheric influences on plants, but currently more and more people are becoming aware of the metaphysical forces which produce significant reactions in living plants. Bookstores everywhere now sell popular paperbacks attesting to the various ways in which plants react to psychic influences, most of which are human in origin. Man's thoughts seem to have effects on the growth patterns and production of plants. Farmers, therefore, should be especially aware of their mental influences, learning to cultivate a loving attitude towards each plant in their field or orchard. Response from the plants will be doubly beneficial — it will return to the farmer an appreciation by way of harmonising "vibrations", and simultaneously reflect that harmony in a more abundant output of fruit, both in terms of quality and quantity.

Not only is the relationship of farmer to plant of importance — the relationships between plants themselves must be considered. This will be taken up in conjunction with a further aspect, crop rotation. Meanwhile, we should be mindful of the implications of companion planting, for its proven effects are most important in contributing to successful agricultural practice, especially regarding crop selection.

Abandoning Monoculture

In every field of commercial enterprise, the emphasis is directed towards the highest financial return for the least outlay. The economics associated with the result always wield far greater influence in industrial undertakings than satisfaction derived from the method. Such is man's short-sightedness; the basis of so much of his frustration.

As farming becomes progressively more influenced by industry and as it becomes regarded more as a competitor with industry in terms of financial return on investment, farmers are persuaded to employ the products of industrial output to regulate their farming habits in a manner hitherto unknown in agricultural history. Agriculture is becoming so mechanised that the pristine peace of the countryside is being converted into an extension of the industrialised city, bringing with it the pollution, tension and noise with which industry regrettably has become identified.

In revolting against the industrial revolution's stranglehold on farming, man has seen the need to revert to the organic method of crop production in every way. This implies not only mulching and composting the soil, but other important phases which are often overlooked such as proper ripening, crop rotation, fallowing and crop selection. And a vital consideration of crop selection is the choice of a range of suitable plants to provide a balanced farming enterprise, devoid of the pressures to cultivate vast areas of one type of plant, such as we see in modern agriculture's mono-methods.

By specialising in one type of crop, the modern farmer can apply his chemicals on a broad scale, sowing his crop with complex machinery which is also adapted to extensively disturb his soil with its plowing attachments. His reapers and harvesters can then take over to capture the crop in a fraction the time otherwise required. But this is not the way to produce nutritious food for man.

With its compatible selection of crops, the ideal organic farm comprises a range of output which contrasts most acutely with the monocultural ideas of chemical farmers. In not having to use chemical fertilisers or deterrents, the organic farmer derives no benefit from vast acreages of the same crop to facilitate mechanised chemical application. In not using chemical hormones to induce early and uniform ripening, the organic farmer has no need for further expensive harvesting equipment or mechanised packing to handle the flood of his crop all being picked at one time, after which the equipment lies idle for weeks and months on end.

Employing the organic method, the farmer will choose a variety of crops such as are suitable to his climate and geography. They will be compatible with each other and will provide a variety of produce which can be picked over an extended period to give a constant, regular income as well as satisfy the food needs of his own family.

Monoculture is never found in nature. Natural forests typify successful agriculture — they comprise differing types of trees, shrubs and vines, all at different stages of growth, all in harmony and all well-nourished. We learn by observing nature, then in adapting our methods to her proven laws; thus we too can benefit from a wise selection of crops. Such practice will significantly contribute towards the total health of all plants on the farm, guaranteeing their disease-resistant ability and the optimum nutritional value of their crops.

Ground Preparation

Clearance of the ground for cultivation should always be done with a minimum of disturbance to the soil and its life. Heavy ploughing is unwise for many reasons:

1. Interfering with the subsoil will disrupt the water table, interfering with the natural drainage pattern of the farm.

2. Turning the soil has the effect of bringing heavier minerals from the subsoil to the surface and of turning in the lighter topsoil minerals, in a reversal of the soil's natural mineral structure. This creates havoc with plant root systems which have developed to feed on those minerals most suited to the plant's needs, as well as to anchor the plant at the most suitable subterranean level. Plant roots which would normally extend into the subsoil for nourishment are induced to the surface when subsoil minerals are ploughed up, thereby failing to adequately anchor the plant and rendering it subject to collapse in

times of strong prevailing winds — taproot depth being very important for tall plants.

3. Such extensive aeration of soil levels induces stimulated germination of millions of weed seeds lying dormant below the soil's surface.

If the ground has been cared for, its soil will not require breaking up or disturbing in any way. If it has been neglected, preparation for its suitability to agriculture is best achieved in the manner most closely related to the natural.

A thorough and profitable way to break up hard ground is to plant a crop of potatoes or sweet potatoes. Their burrowing is most effective in loosening compacted soil. After the crop has been dug, turn in the plants with a light chisel ploughing so that they are merely just below the soil surface. Give a dusting with dolomite, and water this into the soil to facilitate the decomposing of residue potato plants. Allow a period of one or two months, during which a suitable mulch cover can be applied to the topsoil. Then your farm is ready for planting. Of course, if prepared compost is already available, it can be applied to the soil with suitable regard for the nature of the crop to follow.

An alternative method of ground preparation is to employ a light chisel ploughing, penetrating no more than 15 centimetres. Then sow a crop of nitrogenous plants, such as peas, beans, lupins, etc. These legumes are hardy growers and should be allowed to develop until their flowers begin to die and the pods form. They should then be cut and slashed into a mulch cover. After a few days of weathering, they can be sprinkled with dolomite and lightly turned into the soil; then they should be allowed to decompose for a month or so. Again, the application of prepared compost will facilitate a rapid increase in the soil's fertility and hasten its suitability for optimum crop production.

One of the most important aspects of farming is usually ignored in modern practice when the land is totally cleared of all tree growth and natural wooded cover. With the high cost of good farming land, it is understandable that the farmer seeks to achieve the maximum possible production from his holding. But unless he is conscious of the need to maintain a balance between productive and unproductive areas, he will seriously upset a natural ecological pattern, with high penalties being inflicted on him by nature.

As a general rule, one-quarter to one-third of a land holding should be retained in its state of natural growth. It should comprise tall trees and shrubs in just the same manner as in any natural wooded area; for then it will be found to house the predator birds and insects vital to the natural containment of any crop scavengers which might otherwise be attracted to the farm by the odd unhealthy plant. The exclusion of this natural wooded area from ground preparation is an investment in biological insect control and an insurance in a balanced ecological harmony which can never be compensated by any artificial means.

Whether the natural wooded area should be in one place only or whether it should comprise two or more selected locations around the farm will depend on the size of the land holding, its topography, the proximity of surrounding forested areas and other pertinent considerations. Careful study and wise choice at the beginning will provide the best return of any investment possible. This is another of those important occasions when a thorough study of nature is urged, whereby man recognises his intimate dependence on and co-operation with those forces of which he is, both directly and indirectly, a vital part.

Organic Fertilisers

Organic fertilisers for the farm or garden must only comprise living matter in which the life force is still present. This embraces any botanical material which can decompose to release its inherent nutrients. These are more intended for enriching soils than feeding plants directly — it is the soil animals which ensure the latter activity, feeding as they do on the organic matter contained in the home soil to which they are attracted.

Organic fertilisers ensure an abundance of moisture-inducing matter in the soil which can never be simulated by technological alternatives. Such fertilisation is derived from compost, supplemented by a suitable mulch application to the topsoil. The ways in which this may be achieved probably constitute the most divergent aspect of organic agriculture. It is influenced by such a variety of factors as: local availability of compostable or mulchable material; types of crops intended for cultivation; personal preferences for different systems; availability of labour to prepare material, etc.

Some farmers make use of animal manures; others prefer to avoid them. Some prepare a compost heap; others prefer to use only the compost which develops from mulch covering. Of those who make compost heaps, wide variation in composition and style is found, depending on the factors listed above.

There are many arguments for and against the use of animal manures. It is this writer's experienced opinion that, so long as adequate botanical matter (plant life) is available, or can be grown for use, animal manures should be avoided. Some of the reasons are:

1. Most commercial animals harbour some intestinal diseases, which are frequently passed through the intestines and into the soil.
2. Animal manures are highly acidic, requiring heavier applications of dolomite or lime to retain a reasonable acid-alkali balance (there is already plenty of natural manure in those soils which have abundant earthworm and minute animal life).
3. Animal manures are highly odorous, unpleasant and unhygienic, and their gathering a labour-intensive expense.
4. With so many antibiotics fed to animals in commercial herds, the risk of their passing into the soil and their decimation of its minute animal life poses a very real problem.
5. We should do everything possible to discourage the intensive commercial farming of animals, especially in regard to their unhealthy living conditions, the effluent of which could hardly be considered suitable to fertilise crops for human consumption.

Compost and mulch made of vegetable refuse is a natural way to ecologically recycle otherwise unusable material. Such material can comprise any refuse from food processing and milling, any kitchen vegetable throw-outs, grass cuttings, leaves, sawdust or any crops especially grown for the purpose. Some of these materials can only be used in limited quantities, due to their particular natures, as shall be detailed as we look into the most suitable methods of producing the compost pile or applying the mulch cover.

The basic difference between compost and mulch is the mode of application. Both become humus as they decompose into the soil, compost being more readily assimilable due to its already-decayed state.

Compost is the adequately decayed refuse which has been prepared in a specially constructed heap; when applied to the soil it is allowed either to seep in from the top, or it is lightly dug into the topsoil. By contrast, mulch is applied directly to the soil and is, in effect, compost in situ. In the former method, the material decomposes in the heap after which it is applied to the soil; in the latter, it decomposes directly onto the soil. Let us look at each individually.

Compost Formation

The best method of building the compost heap is to arrange the layers of material so that speediest decaying is facilitated uniformly throughout the heap. The layer method is the most commonly used by people who recognise the need for uniformity and speed. When built in the following manner, the heap will be ready for use in about half the time taken by the toss-it-all-in-anywhere system.

Layer compost heaps were developed into quite a sophisticated technique by Dr Rudolf Steiner in conjunction with his biodynamic method of agriculture, about which we shall give more detail later. The method employed by this writer on his organic farms has been based on that taught by Dr Steiner and should be developed in the following steps:

1. Prepare an area of ground in the proportions of 4 × 3 — it can be four feet by three feet or four metres by three metres or two yards by 1½ yards, so long as the proportions are maintained roughly thus.

2. On this area is laid the first course, a 5 cm thick bed of coarse material such as tall grasses, hay or similar substances (near our farm was a factory which produced wood scrapings from pine logs for packing fruit being sent to market — we obtained the continuous supply of all their refuse).

3. The second layer constitutes another 5 cm but consists of finer material which is laid immediately on top of the first — it can be lawn clippings, chopped leaves or similar material.

4. Third layer is one of vegetable refuse spread to 5-10 cm thickness, depending on the amount of refuse available.

5. These layers should be covered by a generous sprinkling of dolomite — the more vegetable refuse used, the heavier the sprinkling.

6. Cover the dolomite and the heap so far built with a layer of friable soil to a depth of about 3 cm over the top and sides. As each layer is added its sides should be tapered, enabling the heap to become self-supporting in a truncated pyramid fashion, as shown:

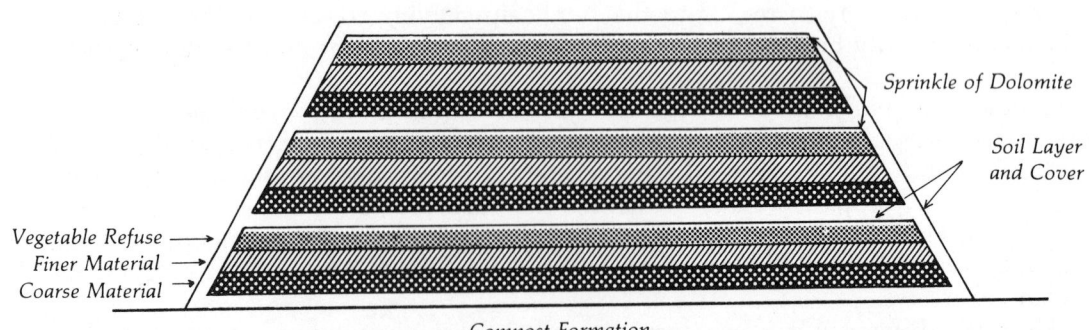

Compost Formation

At no time should a compost pile be allowed to dry out, nor should it become too moist. Thus, the best area in which to construct it is one which is not exposed to heavy rain — if the pile does become too wet, some of its essential nourishment will be leached away and it might collapse. If a sheltered area cannot be chosen, then be prepared to cover the heap in times of heavy rain.

To guard against drying out, a reasonable sprinkling of water should be applied to each layer of soil as the heap is being built. When the final layer of soil is applied, a more thorough watering can be given the heap. During very hot or drying periods of weather, it is wise to cover the final heap with a layer of leaves or light straw as a form of mulch, to ensure that it retains a reasonable level of moisture.

The basic concept of composting is to provide moisture and warmth to facilitate speedy decomposition of the chosen material into readily applicable humus. This is most efficiently achieved by the layer system as described, using three or four sets of layers to construct the compost pile.

Special care should be taken when fine lawn clippings or sawdust are used. Although suitable as part of the second layer, if used without any other material they should not be applied to any greater thickness than 3 cm. Fine clippings of grass, like sawdust, have the natural habit of "matting" into a tight layer which can act to exclude air and moisture, greatly inhibiting decomposition. When using grass clippings or sawdust, mix them with chopped leaves or similar, less dense materials.

All material used in our compost pile is of vegetable origin, except dolomite. Although regarded as organic and prized for its value in organic agriculture, dolomite is actually crushed rock of a special type. It is a double compound of magnesium carbonate and calcium carbonate ($CaCO_3 \cdot MgCO_3$), occurring naturally as rock; but it is of greater value than mere limestone ($CaCO_3$), to which it is closely related.

Composting vegetable matter is generally highly acidic. Both dolomite and lime are alkaline and act to maintain a more suitable neutrality by balancing the acid-alkali relationship. They also act as catalysts in accelerating the decomposing process. However, when dolomite is used, it releases magnesium, a vital trace element deficient in most of the world's soils. For this reason, it is a very valuable addition to the compost heap and, fortunately, is relatively inexpensive. If not available, lime can be used until dolomite is found.

During the process of decomposing, many heaps are found to give off unpleasant odours. This will be avoided if animal manures are not used and when dolomite is used in adequate proportions. Animal manures greatly increase the acidity of compost. If used through lack of other suitable material, they should be heavily covered by dolomite to neutralise some of their acids, especially uric acid. This, added to the naturally forming carbonic acid, can be a serious scorcher of plants if applied in the raw state to soils.

Carbonic acid is formed as a normal aspect of decomposing vegetation. It derives from the combination of carbon dioxide and water ($CO_2 + H_2O = H_2CO_3$), carbon dioxide being the natural effluent of decaying organic matter. The production of carbonic acid is an important function of compost; it is nature's instrument for etching minerals from large rock particles, rendering them into colloidal form for plant nutrition.

Compost piles are generally more suited to small intensive gardens, such as at home, than to larger commercial farms. Although this layer system of compost preparation eliminates the onerous task of "turning the pile", which people who use the haphazard mode of pile-building find necessary, it is nevertheless more demanding of time than the system of layer or sheet mulching.

Mulching is a vital aspect of organic farming even when compost is used. Forest soils always support some measure of mulch cover, teaching us how wise it is to learn by the best teacher of them all. Thus, when compost is applied to the soil, it should be covered by a light layer of suitable mulch material such as lawn clippings or hay. A light sprinkling of dolomite on top of the mulch, followed by a reasonable watering, and the mulch cover will be induced to gradually decompose. It will thereby provide follow-up compost a month or two after the original compost has been applied.

Many people ask how long it takes for a compost heap to become ready for application to the soil. This is impossible to categorically define, for there are so many variables. Decomposition will be quicker in summer than winter, in humid rather than drier weather; it will vary with the nature of the material used to construct the heap, the amount of moisture applied, etc. Assuming the area to be free of freezing temperatures, one can safely give the range of time as being one to three months. The biodynamic preparations with their catalytic action are so effective that normal time will be halved, as will be described farther on.

A word of warning. Do not apply compost too heavily. Plants, like humans, have definite requirements as to their total nutrient need. If tempted by too much food, the tendency is to over-eat, especially when it is "delicious" organic food. Humans will, in turn, put on too much weight; so will plants. If the ratio of humus to soil is too high, plants will certainly grow rapidly; but most of their efforts will be in structural and leaf growth, with less devoted to fruiting.

Many gardeners have proved this by the plants which grow out of their haphazard compost heaps. Invariably they manifest abundant, luxuriant growth, but very little fruit in comparison. Thus, when compost is applied to the soil, its concentration should be regulated to the soil's needs. The amount will vary with the prior condition of the soil's fertility, from a heavy sprinkle to perhaps as much as 5 cm for barren ground.

Layer Mulching

Fertilising the soil in a graduated manner is by far the best method once a basic fertility has been developed. To achieve this by regular applications of compost, protected by a light cover of mulch, is far too time-absorbing and in no way an economical proposition for the farmer. Compare the manifold advantages of a layer mulch technique:

1. Mulch provides continual compost exactly where and when it is needed.
2. It encourages a concentration of healthy, active life in the soil under its protection.
3. This protection is especially successful against erosion by wind and rain, thereby not only guarding against the loss of topsoil, but actually increasing its depth as the lowest layer of mulch composts into the soil.
4. It inhibits weed growth, yet protects surface-feeding plant roots.
5. It facilitates moisture retention and reduces the soil's temperature variations, thereby avoiding any disturbance in the vital work of minute soil animals.

Equally effective and reliable in home gardens or on the commercial farm, layer mulching is nature's way of regular organic fertilisation of the soil in an undisturbed manner, simulating the activity of the forest floor. And who would not want their soils to be as lush as those found in the depths of the forest?

During visits to hundreds of organic farms and gardens throughout the world, I have rarely seen the practice of layer mulching developed to provide soils with those very desirable advantages just listed, but in Australia, we developed a layer-mulch technique that had proved so very successful on our own organic farms in the subtropics of Queensland. It has been successful everywhere else it has been practised, with modifications to suit climatic conditions.

Layer mulching is extremely versatile. It can be adapted to suit any climate, any crop and any variety of mulchable material. Its general mode of application follows these steps:

Layer 1 — A light scattering of well-decayed humus directly upon the soil. This is most desirably from a compost pile. Alternatively, the soil can be sprayed with a molasses solution, comprising about one part of raw molasses to five of water. Lacking either of these, a solution of manure can be used, comprising one part of weathered manure to about three of water.

Layer 2 — This will be readily compostable and comprise such material as vegetable refuse and/or leaf compost, finely chopped clippings, peat moss, etc. Application should be to a depth of 4-8 cm over the full area, depending on the type of crop, season and rainfall. (We used a mixture of sawdust and leaf compost.)

Layer 3 — A liberal sprinkling of dolomite is now applied — somewhat heavier if Layer 2 comprises the maximum 8 cm of compost. This we broadcast by hand.

Layer 4 — This is a medium-heavy layer of grass clippings, wood scrapings, coarser vegetable refuse or similar material. (We found it advantageous to plant a small crop of beans the previous season to have them slashed and ready for applying as Layer 4 to our mulching. Any leguminous crop is suitable.) A layer of 6 cm should do.

Layer 5 — The heaviest material is used to comprise the top layer: longer grasses, hay, megass (refuse after the extraction of juice from sugar cane). It should be applied to a thickness of 8-15 cm, again depending on the crop, season and rainfall. Should no rain fall within a week of the mulch being laid, a good watering is advisable — it will probably be the final one you will need apply, unless a drought period occurs.

It will be recognised that the method of applying mulch layers is the reverse of that used in building the compost pile, when the heaviest material was on the bottom. Now we need to have the lightest material available for speediest breakdown. This is facilitated by the attraction to the soil's surface of a concentration of minute animals, earthworms and bacteria, encouraged by the nature of our first layer. These important little creatures will act like a vast line-up of contestants in an eating competition, rapidly activating their minute mouths to ingest the material in our second layer of mulch soon after it is applied.

Of course, the easiest way to apply mulch is upon unplanted soil. However, if an orchard or plantation is to be converted to enjoy the numerous advantages of this system, mulching must be undertaken around existing plants. When doing this, be especially careful to maintain a clearance distance of about 10 cm from tree trunks to facilitate their continued breathing. At least 3 cm clearance should be allowed for the small plants.

Layer mulching should never be done in the cold weather. This will only trap the coldness in the soil. If performed correctly, mulching will be most successful in maintaining a reasonable residue of summer warmth in the soil throughout winter.

Likewise, it should not be applied when the soil is saturated with moisture, such as occurs during periods of heavy rains. Allow a reasonable amount of evaporation to occur before applying your mulch cover. The best time to apply it, therefore, is several days after good, soaking rains, when the soil is warm, and before planting.

Crop planting is then made through the mulch by parting the covering to soil level to provide only sufficient space for the actual seed or seedling. This will happen year after year, because your soil will never again become exposed to the light, except, after very heavy rains, allowing the soil to partially dry out. A well-designed mulch will last for an entire year in temperate climates; just prior to next planting season, it will only require topping with a sprinkling of dolomite, then a renewal of Layers 4 and 5.

In tropical climates, it will be found that mulch is more rapidly decomposed into the soil. Wise modification to the system in the tropics includes the application of mulch after the rainy season; thus by the arrival of the next year's rains, little or no mulch will remain, allowing the soil to dry somewhat before the next mulching is undertaken.

Critics of the layer-mulch method generally centre their comments around the costs of collecting and applying the various layers. It does not require the expertise of a cost accountant to realise that this is no more than a one-time labour charge, conducted only for a short number of days or weeks, depending on the area to be mulched. When we realise that this method virtually eliminates irrigation needs, weeding, chemical fertilisation, plowing, etc., plus high equipment costs, we will soon see who is financially ahead. And let us not overlook the fact that mulched crops are more healthy and free from disease, avoiding the chemical farmer's high expenses of poisonous spraying and his need to pick crops early to avoid their inability to hold and mature naturally.

It is a fact of farming that organically grown foods are more wholesome than their chemically produced imitations. Not only do they retain their flavour longer, but they have the vital advantage of travelling better when sent to market, and of always enjoying top market prices for their superior quality.

Fallowing

Just as an overworked human body demands regular rest and the occasional fast, so too will the soil be found to benefit from its own form of fasting — the age-old concept of fallowing. As far back as man's prehistory, fallowing was found to benefit the quality of the following crop.

Many farmers and gardeners have practised fallowing to the present day, although their number has diminished considerably with the promotion of chemical fertilisers to induce "eternal miracles of continual productivity from the soil". But after decades of raping natural nourishment from the soil and replacing it with sterilising chemicals, farmers are beginning to realise that their crop yields are diminishing, and that perhaps a season of fallow would help. This is at least a step in the right direction.

It is especially important to allow a full season of fallow if the area is to be reverted to organic farming. This will allow some reduction in the toxicity of previous chemical applications by weathering. The following season should be devoted solely to building up the soil's natural fertility by applying a mulch cover comprising the layers previously enumerated. No planting in this soil should take place until the third season, when legumes or other nitrogenous crops can be suitably planted. These will further improve soil fertility if they are turned in for mulch once their crop is picked.

Depending on the season, crop types, topography, etc., a system of fallowing should be applied by rotation of the entire farmed area. Where climate allows continual growing seasons, one in seven should be allocated to fallow, crop type permitting. In cold northern climates, every winter is a period of natural fallow, precluding the need for any other.

Where permanent tree crops are planted, it is obviously impossible to engage in periodic fallowing. However, adequate mulching will be compensatory. When, finally, the tree crops are to be replaced, a whole year of fallow should be employed before the new planting.

It is very important to remember that during periods of fallow, the soil should not be left bare. Its covering protection of layers of mulch will allow the soil to rapidly return to optimum fertility, as well as protect it from any form of erosion.

Crop Rotation and Compatibility

The logic behind the idea of crop rotation is that different plants extract different nutrient combinations from the soil. Therefore, by rotating the types of plants, the soil is allowed to rebuild while still producing.

The concept of rotation applies to annuals as well as permanent tree crops. Of course, we would not consider transplanting permanent trees each year. But we do suggest that when their cycle of production has expired, they be replaced with a different type of tree, or with a few seasons of annuals.

No hard and fast rules can be offered for the rotation of crops. So much depends on the suitability of particular crops to the area — this will obviously limit the selection. However, it is wise to take note of the fact that there are five different groups of annual vegetable plants and that these should be rotated and/or intercropped. They are differentiated according to their native characteristics, as determined by the physical form of their development and the vibrational influence each exudes and attracts. The five groups are:

Tuberous — potatoes, carrots, turnips, beetroot, jerusalem artichokes, sweet potatoes, etc.;
Surface — lettuce, cabbages, cauliflower, spinach, celery, Brussels sprouts, etc.;
Shrubs — tomatoes, capsicums, beans, peas, eggplant, okra, etc.;
Grains — corn, millet, rye, wheat, oats, barley, buckwheat, etc.;
Vines — cucumbers, zucchini, squash, pumpkin, melons, climbing beans, etc.

For the farmer who wishes to cultivate single crops in each bed, it is suggested that he begin with potatoes or sweet potatoes — their powerful burrowing will ensure that the soil is adequately broken up. Carrots, in contrast, will not burrow if the soil is too heavy. Instead, they produce stubby tubers which are generally coarse and deformed. The selection of crops for successive planting can follow the sequence of groupings listed. For example, celery could follow potatoes, then capsicums, then sweet corn, then cucumbers; then fallow.

But single cropping is not the most scientific, nor the most suitable for best output. A study of plant companionship reveals that if specific varieties are intercropped — two or three in alternating rows in the same plot of soil — they will encourage each other to better production. In contrast, haphazard selections of plants to share the same plot could result in depleted production if such plants are not naturally compatible.

Very little experimental data is as yet available, for science appears to regard this branch of study as of somewhat dubious value. Many scientists and horticulturalists are even prepared to completely ridicule the concept of companion planting, yet anyone who has undertaken his own experiments will soon acquire proof of its validity.

A new scientific name is "allelopathy" — so new that it had not appeared in the 1972 edition of the Oxford English Dictionary. Allelopathy may be defined as the science of the study of the effects of plants upon each other. It is indeed an ever-developing science in which we can expect to see gigantic progress over the next few years, now that people are generally becoming aware of the vibratory properties of plants.

One very interesting and successful suggestion by Helen Philbrick and Richard Gregg (*Companion Plants and How to Use Them*, Devin-Adair) is the intercropping of sweet corn, climbing beans and cucumbers. This proved very successful on our own farms, where we planted the beans two weeks after the sweet corn broke through the soil. This allowed the corn plants enough start to be always ahead of the beans, which we found happy to climb up their neighbouring corn. A month later, we planted a row of germinated cucumber seeds on the shade side of the corn-bean combination, row for row. The cucumbers loved the shade and all three seemed to prove they were not "a crowd".

Harvesting

An essential aspect of organic agriculture is that the crop be allowed to mature on the plant. In chemical farming practice, so long as the crop has commenced its maturity, it is often picked for ripening by further chemical means. Chemical dyes and gases are in frequent use for tomatoes, bananas, oranges, etc. While this somewhat appears to ripen the fruit or vegetable, its texture and flavour reveal otherwise.

Only four kilometres from our farms in Queensland was a conglomerate of citrus orchards owned and developed along modern chemical lines. At the time (1970), that part of Australia had no facilities to artificially "ripen" oranges (they now have them in the capital cities, as they have had for years in Florida and California). These orchards, therefore, had to pick the fruit as close to ripeness as possible. But they found that if they did not rush the fruit immediately to market and sell it within a day, it would begin to break down rapidly. The fruit acquired the nickname among local farmers as "the 24-hour oranges".

Organically grown fruits and vegetables are so much more balanced in their texture and nutritional properties that they will generally outlast any two consecutive chemically produced counterparts. Their balanced constitution enables organically produced foods to be picked when more than merely mature — when actually tree-ripened. They do not bruise as readily nor lose their flavour so quickly after picking, ensuring better condition during transportation and higher market acceptability.

By being allowed to tree ripen as much as is practically possible, foods develop a higher level of sweetness as their starches convert to fructose. Properly constituted crops acquire this delicious advantage because they can remain on the plant without falling off prematurely, as often occurs with malnourished crops produced by chemical enforcement.

The Biodynamic System

When asked by many of his pupils to direct his genius to the problems of trying to farm depleted soils as then existed in Central Europe, Dr Rudolf Steiner said that he was sure that the same principles he was inculcating in his philosophy could be applied with equal success on the land.

His unique combination of physical, moral and metaphysical studies endowed Rudolf Steiner with a rare ability to investigate an apparent mystery in life and unravel its secrets. His development of the biodynamic system of agriculture was no exception.

When asked to define Steiner's biodynamic system, we can best describe it by the statement: "It is a sophisticated method of organic cultivation." The biodynamic method employs certain special organic preparations for specific purposes. Some are used to accelerate the development of humus in the compost heap, others to attract more etheric nutrients from the atmosphere onto the plants' leaves. It is an important aspect of Dr Steiner's teaching that a vital part of the nourishment for living entities emanates from the ether. Plant life is no exception to this rule, for plants take in so much food through the leaves.

That this system was an unqualified success is now history. From Central Europe, in less than a century, the biodynamic (meaning "life force") system has spread throughout the civilised world. Associated with it are thinking people who are constantly developing its potential for improving our world by improving our food and environment.

Wherever man interferes with and alters the pattern of nature, a serious imbalance arises which always reflects upon the instigator. Suffering inflicted on nature's gifts is always amplified in its rebounding upon man, who is encouraged in his pursuit by the promise of greater financial profit. But the donkey will never catch this carrot. Too many losses are created by the practice — ecological studies are revealing this. Studies in human health are gradually, ever so reluctantly, recognising this, too.

Greed will always seduce man away from wisdom. If he can be induced to employ less effort with the promise of more profit, his common sense abdicates.

Initially, organic farming will involve a higher outlay in terms of manpower and the gathering of compostable materials. But what you invest in nourishing the soil today will repay handsomely in following years. The food you produce will taste better, provide optimum nourishment and, most importantly, you will feel a deep sense of satisfaction such as can only develop where total harmony prevails, where all vibrations are in phase, from soil to psyche.

Into the New Age of Awareness

I will follow that system of regimen which, according to my ability and judgment, I consider for the benefit of my patients, and abstain from whatever is deleterious and mischievous. I will give no deadly medicine to anyone if asked ...

From The Oath of Hippocrates

Abstaining from everything deleterious and mischievous might have seemed to us, at an earlier age, not only impossible, but undesirable. Who would not have asked: "How can we enjoy life without a bit of fun?"

Fun? What did we mean by fun? To many people who act on impulse, fun is anything which is "illegal, immoral or fattening".

But how much wiser we have become. With one's initiation into that small group of people who have learned the purpose of life there comes a responsibility by which our own individual purpose will be achieved. But this does not stop us from enjoying life. In fact, it enables a very full enjoyment to be obtained, one based on the most satisfying, the most rewarding act a man can perform — that of service to one's fellow man.

We have already recognised that to be of service, we must know a person's needs, rather than his wants. To be so informed, we must first recognise the distinction between the two. This we have done. In so doing, we have successfully discriminated between wants and needs in our own life, bringing us now to this further point in time where we must look ahead to the rapidly approaching New Age of Awareness.

As the world's population continues to rise at an increasing rate, as our knowledge of the world and of life grows from constant experience, so we begin to perceive a factor which we would not have hitherto recognised, least of all admitted, even to ourselves. Each and every one of us being so prepared through awareness has a vital role to play in the exciting emergence of this New Age.

The world is evolving towards a unique part of its development and we each have a small, but vitally important part to play in that evolution. We shall witness, and be instrumental in developing, man's compassion for man and for all life; and also man's ability to conquer time and space, and again become a spiritual being, capable of perfect health and total understanding; in tune with nature and his Creator.

Of course, this will not take place without some considerable measure of adjustment. We see that already transpiring. But it is in this critical period of adjustment that the greatest challenge, our most valuable help, is demanded.

Many of man's established material conventions will collapse. They must, to allow the more spiritual to develop. Non-thinking people will grow uneasy at the changes, feeling a loss of identity. This is where we will be the greatest help. We know why the changes are taking place and will lead others to that awareness. No good fruit ever came from a tree which had not been heavily pruned in preparation.

True, monarchies will fall. Some already have. Still others will. People will want less of external rule. Individuality is asserting itself. This is already becoming apparent in national struggles for freedom. Nations are craving for autonomous responsibility.

Just as nations demand freedom, so does individual man. Ever so much more important than most people are prepared to recognise is human individual freedom, but not freedom from everything. Man needs freedom from fear, freedom from the physical confines and conventions which inhibit the development of his individuality. Man needs freedom to follow his individual guidance. This is his great need — this is the promise of the New Age of Awareness.

May peace and love be with all beings.

Bibliography

Many of the subjects covered throughout this work are dealt with in greater depth by allied books of which further details are listed below, with page references indicating where they apply to *New Dimensions in Health*. However, it should be recognised that a great number of these books are written by specialist scientists, many of whom base their investigations on orthomolecular concepts, but a few are still somewhat restricted by their original medical training. This is not to detract from their work, but rather to suggest that the overall natural health viewpoint is far more wholistic, as revealed in this text. ("Various" indicates many mentions.)

AFTERDEATH JOURNAL OF AN AMERICAN PHILOSOPHER by Jane Roberts; Prentice-Hall, New Jersey, 1978; p 42

APPLE CIDER VINEGAR by Paul Bragg; Health Science, California; p 175

AUSTRALIAN HEALTH FOOD RECIPE BOOK by Dr David Phillips; Angus & Robertson Publishers, Sydney, 1983; various

BEE POLLEN AND YOUR HEALTH by Carlson Wade; Keats Publishing, Connecticut, 1978; p 192

BREAKTHROUGH TO CREATIVITY by Dr Shafica Karagulla; DeVorss & Co., California, 1967; p 45

COLOR THERAPY by Linda Clark; The Devin-Adair Co., Connecticut, 1974; p 60

COMPANION PLANTS by Philbrick & Gregg; The Devin-Adair Co., Conn., 1975; p 285

CONSUMER BEWARE by Beatrice Trum Hunter; Simon & Schuster, New York, 1971; various

DICTIONARY OF MAN'S FOOD by Dr William Esser; Natural Hygiene Press, Chicago, 1972; various

DIET, CRIME AND DELINQUINCY by Alexander Schauss; Parker House, California, 1980; various

EVERY SECOND CHILD by Dr Archie Kalokerinos; Keats Publishing, Connecticut, 1981; pp 129, 235

FLUORIDATION, THE GREAT DILEMMA by Dr George Waldbott; Coronado Press, Kansas, 1978; various

GRAPE CURE, THE, by Johanna Brandt; various publishers; pp 232

GUIDEBOOK TO NUTRITIONAL FACTORS IN FOODS by Dr David Phillips; The Pythagorean Press, Sydney, 1977; Woodbridge Press, California, 1979; various

HANDBOOK TO HIGHER CONSCIOUSNESS by Ken Keyes, Jr; Living Love Publications, Kentucky, 1972; p 243

HERB BOOK, THE, by John Lust; Bantam Books, New York, 1975; p 211

HERB TEA BOOK by Dorothy Hall; Keats Publishing, Connecticut, 1981; p 208

IMPROVING YOUR CHILD'S BEHAVIOR CHEMISTRY by Dr Lendon Smith; Pocket Books, New York; various

ION EFFECT, THE, by Fred Soyka; Bantam Books, New York, 1980; various

JOURNEYS OUT OF THE BODY by Robert Monroe; Anchor Press/Doubleday, New York, 1977; p 42

LIFE AFTER LIFE by Dr Raymond Moody; Stackpole Books, Pennsylvania, 1975; p 42

MENTAL AND ELEMENTAL NUTRIENTS by Dr Carl Pfeiffer; Keats Publishing, Connecticut, 1975; p 257

MERCK INDEX, THE, Ninth Edition; Merck & Co. Inc., New Jersey, 1976; various

MIRACLE OF GARLIC, THE, by Dr Paavo Airola; Health Plus Publishers, Arizona; p 179

NUTRIENTS TO AGE WITHOUT SENILITY by Dr Abram Hoffer; Keats Publishing, Connecticut, 1980; pp 116, 123

NUTRITION AND PHYSICAL DEGENERATION by Dr Weston Price; The Price-Pottenger Foundation, California, 1977; p 236

ORTHOMOLECULAR NUTRITION by Dr Abram Hoffer; Keats Publishing, Connecticut, 1980; p 116

PREVENTION OF ALCOHOLISM THROUGH NUTRITION by Dr Roger Williams; Bantam Books, New York, 1981; various

PROBLEMS WITH MEAT by Dr John Scharffenberg; Woodbridge Press, California, 1979; p 93

PURE, WHITE AND DEADLY by Prof. John Yudkin; Davis-Poynter, London, 1972; p 158

REFLECTIONS ON LIFE AFTER LIFE by Dr Raymond Moody; Stackpole Books, Pennsylvania, 1977; p 42

SACCHARINE DISEASE, THE, by Dr T. L. Cleave; Keats Publishing, Connecticut, 1975; p 172

SAVE YOUR LIFE DIET, THE, by Dr David Reuben; Ballantine Books, New York; various

SCIENCE AND FINE ART OF FASTING, THE, by Dr Herbert Shelton; Natural Hygiene Press, Chicago, 1978; p 224

SECRETS OF THE INNER SELF by Dr David Phillips; Angus & Robertson Publishers, Sydney, 1980; various

SELENIUM AS FOOD AND MEDICINE by Dr Richard Passwater; Keats Publishing, Connecticut, 1980; p 109

SILENT SPRING by Rachel Carson; Penguin Books, London, 1965; p 127

SUGAR BLUES by William Dufty; Warner Books, New York, 1975; various

SUPERIOR NUTRITION by Dr Herbert Shelton; self published, 1967; p 153

TRACE MINERALS AND MAN, THE, by Dr Henry Schroeder, The Devin-Adair Co., Connecticut, 1973; p 106

TRIUMPH OVER DISEASE by Dr Jack Goldstein; Arco Publishing, New York, 1977; p 235

VITAMIN BIBLE by Earl Mindell; Warner Books, New York, 1979; various

WHY SUFFER by Dr Ann Wigmore; Hippocrates Health Institute, Boston, 1964; p 232

WHY YOUR CHILD IS HYPERACTIVE by Dr Ben Feingold; Random House, New York, 1974; various

WORLD WITHOUT CANCER by G. Edward Griffin; American Media, California, 1974; p 123

X-RAYS: MORE HARM THAN GOOD by Priscilla Laws; Rodale Press, Pennsylvania, 1978; p 261

Index

Abdominal distension 241
  muscles 38-39, 211
Aboriginal children 235
abstinence (see temperance)
acid-forming foods 150-152, 181-182
acid-forming minerals 104-109
acne 226
activity (see exercise)
adaptability 1, 7, 24, 33, 34
addictions 9, 80
adhesions 206
adipose tissue 101
adrenal glands 95
adrenalin 81, 94, 119, 157
advertising claims 4, 34, 55, 75-78, 152
aggression 65, 157
ageing 2, 21-22, 62, 116
Airola, Dr Paavo 179
alanine 95
alcohol 11, 79, 113, 115, 117, 118, 120, 122, 126, 138, 219, 226-227
Alexander The Great 66
alfalfa 86, 134, 172
  tea 203-204, 205
alkaline-forming foods 150-152
alkaline-forming minerals 104-109
allantoin 205
allelopathy 285
allergies 227
allicin 179
almonds 77, 95, 190
alpha tocopherol (see vitamin E)
aluminium cookware 167
Alzheimer's disease 125
amino acids 75-76, 93-95, 124, 139
amygdaline (see vitamin B_{17})
amylase 138-139
anabolism 30, 91, 137
anaemia 107, 118, 119, 120, 121, 126, 186, 209, 227-228, 269
animal feed 6-7, 21, 158
animals 6, 157-158
aniseed tea 203-204
anorexia 124, 175, 205, 228
antibodies 79
antiseptic, herbal 205
apoplexy 258-259
appendix 139-140
appetite 90, 152-153, 156-157, 163-164, 188, 228

arable land 73-74
architecture 32-33
arginine 94
Arguello, Dr Carlos 220-221
arteries 101, 228-229
arteriosclerosis 125, 228-229, 259
arthritis 43, 92, 117, 229
ascorbic acid (see vitamin C)
aspartic acid 95
aspirin 16, 126, 200
asthma 79-80, 229-230
atheism 31
atherosclerosis 122, 228-229
athlete's foot 260
atmosphere 18, 23-26
attitudes 41, 56
autism 118, 257
automobiles 25, 34, 91
avidin 124
avocados 100, 142
awareness 12-14, 18-19, 44-46, 52-54, 58, 80

baby foods 78-79, 118, 150, 254
Babylon 48-49
backache 230, 251
Bailey, L.O. 70-71
balanced diet 163
baldness 127, 128, 211, 230, 265
bananas 60, 97-98
Barnes, Dr Joseph 157
beans 149, 151
bee pollen (see pollen)
beef 76-77
Beethoven, Ludwig van 58
belching 159, 241
Besant, Dr Annie 69
Bible 2-3, 64, 68, 174, 181
bile salts 101, 108, 138-139, 213
biliousness 241
biochemistry 104
biodynamic agriculture 286-287
bioflavonoids (see vitamin P)
biological insect control 278
biotin 124
Bircher-Benner Clinic 70, 173
birth defects 117
bladder 94
bleeding gums 135
blenders 183
blood circulation 62, 76, 117, 122, 134, 235

293

stream 91, 95, 101, 133, 157, 185, 211, 258, 259, 260-261
body fat 38, 101-102
  odours 230-231
  warmth 76
bones 95, 105
boredom 247
bowels (see colon)
Bragg, Paul 175
brain 53-55, 78-79, 118, 124-125, 215
bran 96-97, 172-173, 199
Brazil nuts 75, 92, 94
bread 83-84, 173
breakfast 11, 163-164, 169-170
  cereals 148, 159, 170, 173-174, 232-233
breast feeding 78-80
breathing 24-25, 38, 53-54
brewer's yeast (see yeast, dietary)
broken bones (see fractures)
bronchitis 206, 231
bruising 135
buckwheat 99, 181
Buddha 57
bulghur wheat 174
Burkitt, Dr Denis 172
burns 133
Burton, Dr Alec 219, 220
butter 188-189

caffeine 113, 117, 209, 244
calciferol (see vitamin D)
calcium 32, 77, 78, 88, 105, 121, 178, 195
calendula 205
calisthenics (see exercise)
calorie content of meat and nuts 76-77
calories (see kilojoules)
cancer 17, 43-44, 123, 129, 140, 146, 216, 231-232, 249, 259
canker sores 232
carbohydrates 72, 88, 96-99, 139, 145, 178, 190
carbon 105
  dioxide 38, 96, 105, 197
carbonated beverages 161-162
carbonic acid 281
carcinogens (see cancer)
cardiac failure (see heart disease)
cardio-vascular disease 105, 109, 122
Carey, Dr George W. 104
Carlyle, Thomas 12
carnivores 71-73
carob 174-175
carotene (see vitamin A)
Carson, Rachel 127
caseinogen 79, 137
cashew nuts 92, 190
catabolism 30, 91, 137
cataracts 109, 240
cattle 73
cause-and-effect (see karma)
cell salts 104
cellulose (see fibre)

chamomile tea 204
cheese 77-80, 105, 142
chemical fruit ripening 97-98, 286
chemicals in agriculture 161, 249, 269-274, 277, 286
  in foods 30, 140, 156-159, 177-178, 231, 286
chewing 71-72, 137
chickenpox 233, 245
chickens 158
chicory tea 204
childhood illnesses 7, 233-234
chiropractic 17, 230, 242, 253
chlorine 106, 132
chlorophyll 106, 134, 172, 175
chocolate 159, 174-175
cholesterol 76-77, 79, 100-101, 112, 116, 125, 127, 185, 243, 264
cholic acid 101
choline 124-125
Christ, Jesus 15, 50, 56-57, 66-68, 83
Christianity 2-3
Christmas 68, 189
church 68
Churchill, Sir Winston 13-14
Cicero 90
cider vinegar 175
cinnamon tea 204
circulatory disorders 234
cirrhosis 122, 125, 249-250
cities 1-2, 85, 102
Cleave, Dr T. L. 172
Clement of Alexandria 68
clothing 31-32
cloves tea 204
cobalt 109, 119-121
Cockburn, Mrs F. M. 71
cocoa (see chocolate)
coconut 100, 142, 196
cod liver oil 131
co-education 48
coeliac disease 95, 134, 137, 232-233
co-enzyme A (see vitamin B_5)
  R (see biotin)
coffee 16, 127, 211
cola beverages 161-162
cold-pressed oils 102-103
colds 31, 44, 129, 221, 234, 260
colitis 134, 234-235
colon 72, 76, 139-140, 216, 234-235
colonic problems 134, 201, 206, 234-235, 253
colour 43, 59
  therapy 60
comfrey 175-176
  tea 205
Commandments, The 67-68
companion planting 285-286
compassion 22, 56-57, 60
compost 278-284
concentration 51-53
confinement 83-84
conformity 75

conjunctivitis 239-240
conservation (see ecology)
constipation 76, 140, 159, 172, 206, 234-235
contraception 113, 117, 118, 120, 126, 132
convenience foods 84, 156, 159, 178
convulsions 118-119
Cook, Captain James 129
cooking 103, 113, 126, 153, 166-168
Copernicus 42
copper 108
corn 99, 100, 115, 116, 178, 179
cortisone 115-116, 250
cot deaths 129, 235
cramps 235, 251
creativity 41
Creator (see God)
crime 8, 152
crop compatibility 285
    rotation 285
    selection 275-277
Crotona 42, 47, 49
CSIRO 76
currants 177
cyanide (see vitamin B_{17})
cyanocobalamin (see vitamin B_{12})
cycling 37
cysteine 95
cystine 95
cystitis 208, 235-236

dandelion tea 205
dandruff 127
Daniel 15, 49
da Vinci, Leonardo 69
dates 176
deamination 92
death 2, 12, 101
Delphi 49
dental caries 79, 159, 236-237, 255
Department of Primary Industries 268, 270
depression 33, 115, 118, 129, 191, 237, 251
dermatitis 117
deserts 65
detoxification (see fasting)
diabetes 237
diarrhoea 27, 210, 234-235
dietary oils 99-103, 195-196
dietetics, science of 60-61
digestion 29
dill seed tea 205-206
dinner 165-166, 168-169
diphtheria 233
disciplines 49-63
discrimination 62
disharmony 5, 18, 30, 33, 44, 51, 54, 59-60, 225-226
diuretics 210, 212-213
diverticulitis 234-235
dolomite 176, 280-281
dong quai 248
dreams 29, 214

dried fruits 98, 143, 176-178
drinking 26-28, 162-163, 216, 257
dropsy (see kidney problems)
drugs 44, 110-134, 140, 160-162
duodenum 101, 138-139
dust storms 25,65

earthworms (see soil animals)
ecology 23-24, 196, 249, 267, 271-274, 278
eczema 124, 128, 226
EDTA 193
education 5-9, 20-21, 40, 47-50, 58
efficiency 62-63
eggs 77-78, 124, 141
Egypt 48
electricity 33, 43-44
elimination diets 217-218, 239
embarrassment 55-56
Emerson, Ralph Waldo 10, 69
emotional illnesses 237-238
emotions 44-46, 79, 152, 228, 229, 240, 251, 256-257
emphysema 238-239
encephalitis 253
endosperm 84
endurance 65-66, 71
energy 101, 116-117, 163, 179, 215-216
    vibration scale 43
enervation 30, 239, 261
Enoch 57
enteritis 234-235
environment (see ecology)
enzymes (see gastrointestinal tract)
epilepsy 239
equisetum tea 206
essential fatty acids (see polyunsaturated fatty acids)
eucalyptus tea 206
exercise 36-39, 61-62, 228
exhaustion 124
eye problems 114, 239-240

faeces 72-73, 139-140
faith 31
fallowing 284
fashions in clothing 32
fasting 9-10, 26, 35-36, 60-61, 214-224, 227, 235, 240, 256, 257, 259, 262, 265
    animals 6-7
    for 105 days 216
    practitioners 219-220
fats 76-77, 99-103, 116, 125, 138, 145-146, 149, 178, 190, 195-196
fear 50
    of fasting 218
fenugreek tea 206-207
fever 240
fibre 72, 76-78, 96-97, 140, 172-173, 179, 190, 235
fibroids 206
fibrosis 249-250

fidgeting 51
Fielding, Henry 136
figs 176
fish liver oils 102
flatulence (see indigestion)
flavonoids 134-135
flax tea 206
flour 178-179, 184, 199
fluoride 27, 244
fluorine 107
folic acid 125-126
Food and Drug Administration 103, 123
food classifications 141-144, 149
    combining 136-154
    processing 84, 113, 115, 117, 140, 156, 225, 252
    shortage 74, 152
fortitude 54-55
fractured bones 255-256
Franklin, Benjamin 69
Fredericks, Dr Carlton 264
free car 74-75
freedom 12-14, 289
freezing foods 85, 132
friendship 56-57, 166
frigidity 240-241
fructose 96-98, 127, 148, 159-160, 179, 237
fruit fly 272
fruitarians 95
fruits 85, 143-144, 147-149, 162
frying foods 153, 167
Funk, Casimir 111

Galilei, Galileo 42
gallbladder functions 94, 211, 213
    problems 241
garlic 150, 179
gastric juice 91, 137-139, 145-146
    lipase 138
    ulcers 55, 147
gastrointestinal-tract 137-140, 262
German measles 233
germ theory 17
Gilbert, W. S. 34
ginseng 180
    tea 207
glacé fruits 180
gland problems 254
glass 32-33, 103
glaucoma 240
glutamic acid 95
gluten 232-233
glycine 95, 101, 119
glycogen 94, 95, 139
goat's milk 78
God 18, 44, 56-57, 64, 223, 272
goitre 108, 183, 242
Golden Age of Greece, The 48, 66
gonorrhoea 264
gout 92, 229
Graham, Rev. Sylvester 1, 69

grains 98-99, 151, 180-181
Greece 7
grey hair 108, 117, 125, 128, 264
grinding mills 184
Guthrie, Thomas 214

haemoglobin 94, 107, 108, 227-228
haemophilia 134
haemorrhoids 244
hair 37, 114, 124, 127, 204, 206, 212, 230
halitosis 175, 231
hamburgers 82
Hamey, Ian 59-60
happiness x, 14, 21, 34, 61
harvesting methods 286
Hauser, Gayelord 80
hawthorn tea 207
Hay, Dr W. H. 153
hay fever 191-192
headaches 16, 17, 242-243
health food stores 171
hearing 41-43
heartburn 200, 210
heart disease 17, 27, 101, 207, 243-244
    stimulation (see Vitamin E)
hepatitis 205, 244-245
herb teas 202-213
herpes 245
hesperidin (see vitamin P)
hexane in oils 103
hiatus hernia 245-246
hibiscus tea 204, 207
Hindus 223
Hippocrates 206
Hippocratic Oath 288
histamine 115, 119
histidine 94
Hoffer, Dr Abram 28, 43, 115-116, 247, 257
Holt, Harold 16
honey 181-182
Hopewood Health Centre 219-220
hops tea 207-208
horehound tea 207
hormone stimulant 212
hospitals 8, 59, 83
Howard, Sir Albert 268
humus (see compost)
hunger 163
hunting 65-66
Huntington's disease 253
hydrochloric acid 72, 76, 91, 118, 137-138, 146-147, 150, 203, 208, 262
hydrogen 105
hydrogenation 188
hydroxyglutamic acid 95
hydroxyproline 95
hygiene 5, 21, 233, 261
hyperacidity 227, 232, 246
hyperactivity 30, 204, 213, 238
hypertension 228, 243, 246-247, 258
hyperthyroidism 242

hypochondriacs 3-4
hypoglycaemia 239, 247
hypovitaminosis D (see rickets)

iatrogenic disease 5, 221
Ibsen, Henrik 75
ice cream 99
ichthus 68
ideal diet 34-35, 162-170
ignorance 54
ileocaecal valve 139
impotence 240-241
inactivity (see lethargy)
indigestion 59, 136, 144-145, 247
individuality 11, 16, 288-289
indulgence (see overeating)
industry 23-25, 32-33, 60, 75
infant feeding 78-80, 94, 118, 150, 160
infants 30, 137, 150
infertility 218-219, 247-248
inflammation 206, 260
influenza (see colds)
innervation 248
inositol 126-127
insecticides 27, 127
insomnia 29-31, 207, 248
insulin 108, 115, 139, 172, 237
intelligence 16, 52, 54-55, 82
intestinal bacteria 140
intrinsic factor 120
intuition 45-46
iodine 95, 108-109
iodogorgoic acid 95
iron 77, 88, 107, 178, 195, 227-228
irritability 33, 51, 81, 118
Islets of Langerhans 107, 139
isoleucine 94
isometrics 37-38

jasmine tea 208
Jennings, Dr Isaac 69
Jensen, Dr Bernard 194
Judaism 48-49, 223
juicers 183-184
juniper tea 208

Kalokerinos, Dr Archie 129, 235
Karagulla, Dr Shafica 45
karma 15-16, 251, 271
kefir 182-183
Kellogg, John Harvey 70
kelp 95, 109, 183
kidney disease 16, 92, 118, 161, 248-249, 258
    stones 118-119, 203, 206, 248-249
kidneys 26, 72, 92, 94, 208, 248
kilojoules (4.186 = 1 kilocalorie: "calorie") 76-77, 88, 178
kirlian photography 45
kitchen appliances 183-185
kitchen gardening 85-86
Krebs, Dr Ernst 122, 123

lactose 79
laetrile (see vitamin B_{17})
large intestine (see colon)
law of compensation (see karma)
laxatives 209
learning 78-79
lecithin 78, 124-125, 126-127, 141, 185
legumes 185-186
lemon balm tea 208-209
    grass tea 209
lethargy 37, 59, 94, 191, 207, 249
leucine 94
leukemia 249
licorice 186
    tea 209
life expectancy 1-3, 5, 21-22
    force 81, 135, 270-271
light 32-33, 43
lindane 127
linden tea 209
linoleic acid 100, 196, 206
linseed 196
lipase 138
lipids 99-103, 138
liver 91, 94, 95, 112, 122, 129, 139, 186-187, 244-245, 249-250
Loma Linda University 157
longevity 2-3, 21-22
love 19, 55-57, 79, 235
Lowenthal, Sir John 17
lumisterol (see vitamin D)
lunch 165, 168-169
lungs 24-25, 38, 261-262
lupus 250
lymph 94, 139
lysine 94

macadamia nuts 99-100, 142
MacFadden, Bernard 70
macrobiotic foods 183, 187
macro-nutrients 105-107
magnesium 77, 106, 121
malathion 271-272
mammals 78
mammary glands 95
manganese 108, 172
manure 279
maple syrup 187-188
margarine 188-189
marriage 54
maté tea 209
mathematics defined 49
Mayans 194
meat costs 73-75
    eating 71-76, 101, 112, 146-147, 157-158
medical practitioners 45-46
    profession 4, 46, 110, 261, 288
meditation 50-52, 223-224
melanin 94
Melchizedek 57
melons 143, 148

memory 29, 52-54, 214
Ménière's Syndrome 250
meningitis 253
menopausal problems 133, 135, 251
menstrual problems 134, 251
metabolic rate 165
metaphysics 40, 44-46
methionine 75, 94, 95, 125
Methodism 68-69
Middle Ages 42
migraine 17, 242-243
millet 181
milk 78-80, 137-138, 146, 150, 174, 192, 199, 201-202, 229-230, 236, 255
milk powders 189
mind control 52-54, 214
minerals 104-109
miscarriage 126, 133
misfortune 56
mitosis 126
moderation (see temperance)
monoculture 276-277
monosodium glutamate 167-168
monotrophism 153, 217
mono-unsaturated fatty acids 100
morning sickness 118, 211, 251-252
mother's milk 78-80, 212
mouth 137
   ulcers (see canker sores)
mucus 137, 146
muesli 170, 173-174
mulch 273-274, 281-284
multiple sclerosis 43-44, 121, 252-253
mumps 233
mung beans 88
muscle tone (see exercise)
muscles 37-39, 53, 62, 94, 95, 101, 105, 107, 117, 192, 215
muscular atrophy 253
   dystrophy 253
   spasms 213
music 49, 58-60
Muslims 182, 223
mustard oil 150
myasthenia gravis 253

Nader, Ralph 82
names — importance 52
Natural Health Society of Australia 71, 220
natural hygiene 69, 153, 225
nausea 27, 112, 118, 119, 241, 251, 253
needs 90
nephritis 248-249
nerves 105, 252-253, 258
nervousness 125
nettle tea 209-210
neuralgia 253
neuritis 253
New Age 41-42, 49-50, 288-289
Newton's Law of Motion 15
niacin (see vitamin B_3)

night-blindness 239-240
nitrogen 92, 94, 105
norleucine 95
nucleic acids 125
numbers as symbols 35, 49
nut butters 190-191
nuts 75-78, 92, 99-100, 141, 142, 151, 189-191

oats 268-269
obesity 79, 98, 101-102, 119, 152-153, 157, 159, 160, 221-222, 253-254, 264
oesophagus 137
oestrogen 113, 115, 117, 118, 126
Ohsawa, Georges 187
oils, edible (see dietary oils)
oils, mineral 99, 131, 132, 134
old age 1-3, 14
oleic acid 100
olives 100
onions 150
oral contraceptives (see contraception)
oranges 135
organ transplants 34
organic chemistry 104-105, 270
   fertilisers 278-284
   meaning of 270
organically-grown foods 267-287
orotic acid (see vitamin B_{13})
osteomalacia 131, 161
osteoporosis 131, 159, 254-255
osteosclerosis 27
ovaries 95
overeating 54, 98, 136, 152-154, 156-157, 160, 253-254
overfeeding plants 282
oxalic acid 119, 161, 203, 209, 248
oxidation 26, 164, 199, see vitamin loss factors 112-133
oxygen 24-25, 104, 105

PABA 127-128, 259
pain 9, 14, 15, 200
pancreas 94, 138-139
pangamic acid (see vitamin B_{15})
pantothenic acid (see vitamin B_5)
papaya tea 210
paralysis 252-253, 258
paranoia 257
Parkinson's disease 119, 253
parsley 105
   tea 210
Pauling, Dr Linus 43, 129
peanuts 141
pecan nuts 99-100, 142
pellagra 115
Penn, William 155
pennyroyal tea 253
pepitas 194-195, 256
peppermint tea 210
pepsin 137, 203
perfection 18-19

pernicious anaemia 120, 186-187, 228
Peru 80
Pfeiffer, Dr Carl 257
Pherecydes 48
phenylalanine 94, 191
philanthropy (see compassion)
Phillips, Wendell 267
philosophy 48-49
phospholipids 101, 103, 185
phosphorus 32, 77, 78, 88, 105, 119
Pitman, Sir Isaac 69
pituitary gland 94, 119, 180, 207
plant feelings 276
pneumonia 255
poisons 54
polio 252
pollen 191-192, 256
pollution 23-28
polypeptides 138
polyunsaturated fatty acids 100
population growth 73-74
pork 265
potassium 77, 88, 105
potassium sorbate 177
potatoes 98
prana 25
predator insects 274, 278
pregnancy 118, 119, 126
prejudices 45-46, 82
premenstrual tension 118
prevailing winds 275, 278
primates 65
primitive man 65-66
Pritikin Diet, The 244
proline 95
promotional frauds 75-81
prostatitis 255-256
protein 72-74, 77-80, 88, 90-95, 96, 141-142, 149, 178, 181, 189, 190, 195, 197
  digestion 72, 75-76, 91-92, 137-142, 145-147, 150-151
  supplements 192
proteins, complete 75-76, 93, 181, 197
prunes 177
psoriasis 256
psyche 29-30, 40-46, 50-52, 58-60
psychic development 42, 45-46
psychosclerosis 82, 265-266
psychosis 256-257
ptyalin 72, 97, 137-138, 147, 233
pulses (see beans)
pumpkin seeds (see pepitas)
pylorus 138
pyridoxine (see vitamin B_6)
Pythagoras ix, x, 1, 7, 12, 13, 15, 18, 42, 47-50

racehorse diet 21
radio transmission 43
raisins 177
Ramadan 223

rancidity 103, 112, 132, 190, 199
raspberry tea 210-211
reincarnation 42, 46
religion 2-3
relaxation 28-31, 162, 165, 206, 207, 213, 257-258
rennin 79-80, 137-138, 150
research 8, 17, 110-111
respiratory disease syndrome 185
  problems 27, 206, 231, 255, 261
  system 95
responsibility 16, 288-289
rest 16, 28-31, 215
retinol (see vitamin A)
retirement 8, 9
revolution 267
rheumatic fever 233
rheumatism 229
riboflavin (see vitamin B_2)
rice 99, 180-181
  bran 113
    syrup 192-193, 245
rickets 31-32, 131
ricotta cheese 142
ringworm 260
ripening of fruits 85, 97-98
Robbins, Harold 10
Rodale Experimental Farm 268
Rodale, J. I. 207, 268
rosehips tea 211
rosemary tea 211-212
rubella 233
rutin (see vitamin P)

sabbath 221
saccharine 159
safflower 100, 196
sage tea 212
salad dressings 193
salicylic acid 200
saliva 72, 137-138
salt, common 106, 109, 193-194, 264, 265
Samos 48, 49
sandwiches 165
sarsaparilla tea 212
sassafras 260
saturated fatty acids 76, 79, 100-101, 116, 252, 264
Savoy, Gene 80
sawdust fertiliser 281
scarlet fever 233
scavenger insects 273-274, 278
schizophrenia 43-44, 115-116, 129, 157, 238, 256-257
Schuessler, Dr W. 104
Schweitzer, Dr Albert 69
scleroderma 262
scurvy 129
seeds, edible 76-78, 99-100, 141, 194-196
selenium 109
self-control 80-81

senility 28, 54, 116, 257
sensitivity 80-81
serine 95
serotonin 94, 198
sesame seeds 195
Seventh Day Adventism 69, 232
sexuality 55, 66, 115, 214, 219, 236, 240-241, 242, 245, 255-256, 264
Shaw, George Bernard 69
sheep 73
Shelley, Percy Bysshe 68
shelter 31-33
Shelton, Dr Herbert 43, 70, 82, 153, 219, 224
Shewell-Cooper, Dr W. 268
shingles 245
Shute, Drs E. & W. 133
shyness 56
sickness 1
siesta 165
sigmoid colon 139
silence 50-52
silicon 106-107, 193, 206
singing 25
skin 31-32, 34, 76, 114, 118, 133, 206, 250, 256, 259, 260, 264-265
   brushing 37-38
   pigmentation 31-32, 108, 130-131, 259
sleep 28-31, 198, 206, 215, 248
slippery elm powder 196
small intestine 139-140, 151
smoking 8, 11, 79, 129, 133, 219, 238, 255
snacking 98, 160
soap 196-197
sodium 77, 88, 106
soil animals 273, 283
   erosion 25, 273-274
   fertility 273-284, 286-287
   ploughing 278
sorbitol 159
soyabeans 74
soya milk 170, 262
spearmint tea 212
specialisation 17, 104
spiritual development 223-224
spirulina 197
spleen 94
sports 36-37, 102
sprouts 86-89, 99
starches 137, 143, 147, 149
starvation 216
steaming foods 167
Steiner, Dr Rudolf 25, 70, 280, 286
sterility 117
sterols 101
stomach 72, 91, 137-138, 150-153, 253
strength 65-66, 76, 79
stress 51-52, 120, 129, 152, 207, 225, 257-258, 262, 263
stroke 9-10, 258-259
success x, 47
sugars 96-99, 147-148, 158-160, 174, 175, 181-182, 236, 237
suicide 1-2, 60
sulphur 94, 95, 105-106
   dioxide 177
   drugs 117, 126, 128
   drying 177
sultanas 177
sunbathing 31-32, 128
sunburn 31-32, 128, 259
sunflower seeds 77, 94, 195
sunshine 31-32, 130-131
superstition 76
surgery 44
Swedenborg, Emanuel 69
syphilis 264

tabouly 174
tahini 195
Taiwan 177
Tanzania's cashews 92
taste 137, 151, 268
   buds 157
taurine 101
teenage acne 226
teeth 27, 72, 79, 95, 105, 146, 163, 236, 255
temperance 54-55, 152-154
tension 28-30, 51-52, 59, 152, 187, 204, 218, 257-258
textured vegetable protein (see TVP)
Theosophy 69
thiamine (see vitamin B$_1$)
threonine 94
thrombosis 259-260
thyme tea 212
thymus 94
thyroid 94, 95, 120, 180, 242
thyroxine 94, 95, 108, 115, 242
Tilden, Dr John 70
tinea 260
tinnitus 250
tobacco 8, 129, 255
tocopherols (see vitamin E)
tolerance 7, 24-25, 54-55
Tolstoy, Leo 69
tomato production 271-272
tongue 217
tonsillitis 233, 260
tooth decay (see dental caries)
topsoil 273-274
torula yeast (see yeast, dietary)
toxaemia 4-5, 33, 69, 220-221, 256, 260-261, 264
trace elements 107-109
Trall, Dr Russell 69
transamination 93
transmutation 86
triangular relationship 57
triglycerides (see saturated fatty acids)
triticale 180-181
tropical fruits 66
   ulcers 95, 262